# Healing by Heart

# Healing by Heart

*Clinical and Ethical Case Stories
of Hmong Families and Western Providers*

Edited by

Kathleen A. Culhane-Pera,

Dorothy E. Vawter,

Phua Xiong,

Barbara Babbitt,

and Mary M. Solberg

Vanderbilt University Press

NASHVILLE

Published by Vanderbilt University Press
First Edition 2003

This book is printed on acid-free paper.
Manufactured in the United States of America
Design by Dariel Mayer

Library of Congress Cataloging-in-Publication Data

Healing by heart : clinical and ethical case stories of Hmong families and Western
providers / edited by Kathleen A. Culhane-Pera ... [et al.].— 1st ed.
p.    ; cm.
    Includes bibliographical references and index.
    ISBN 0-8265-1430-8 (cloth : alk. paper)
    ISBN 0-8265-1431-6 (paper : alk. paper)
    1. Hmong Americans—Medical care—Case studies. [DNLM: 1. Asian
Americans—psychology—Asia, Southeastern—Case Report. 2. Asian Americans—psychology—United States—Case Report. 3. Delivery of Health Care—
methods—Asia, Southeastern—Case Report. 4. Delivery of Health Care—
methods—United States—Case Report. 5. Cultural Characteristics—Asia,
Southeastern—Case Report. 6. Cultural Characteristics—United States—Case
Report. 7. Professional-Patient Relations—Asia, Southeastern—Case Report. 8.
Professional-Patient Relations—United States—Case Report. W 84 AA1 H434
2003]    I. Culhane-Pera, Kathleen A.
RA448.5.A83H43 2003
362.1'089'95942073—dc21

                                                    20030 02518

# Contents

# Illustrations

# Preface and Acknowledgments

This is a book of stories—stories of Hmong people's anguish, suffering, desire, struggles, and successes as they have sought compassionate health care. Refugees from the Vietnam War in Laos, the Hmong came to the United States believing they would receive excellent health care from doctors and nurses. Sometimes they did. But often they encountered disagreement, conflict, and disrespect. These are the stories of their experiences and also the stories of their U.S. health care providers. This book is filled with insights into demonstrating respect and building trust across cultures—in short, about healing by heart.

In the mid 1990s health care professionals were expressing deep concern that they were failing in their relationships with Hmong patients and families. They wanted to better understand traditional Hmong health beliefs and practices and to learn how to develop more respectful, trusting, and satisfying relationships with Hmong patients and their families. Thus, the Minnesota Center for Health Care Ethics, inspired by its mission "to explore the perspectives that diverse faith and cultural traditions bring to health care decisionmaking" and its partner organizations' shared commitment to social justice, set about, under the leadership of Dorothy E. Vawter, to develop and sponsor several collaborative projects with the Hmong community.

The strategy, with foundation and private support, was to invite Hmong health care providers and leaders to meet regularly with the Minnesota Center to decide what information was most important to convey to U.S. health care professionals. Barbara Babbitt made the first overtures to English-speaking leaders in the Hmong community and invited them to consider whether a collaborative effort could improve health care for Hmong patients. She assembled a core group who graciously agreed to partner with the Minnesota Center—individuals with exceptional patience and generosity of spirit.

Over a four-year period of monthly meetings, the work group developed and presented three conferences for U.S. health care professionals—where the majority of speakers were Hmong—and organized several other educational activities, including the production of two videos of Hmong families' bewildering experiences with Western health care.

Early in the process, the work group planned a critical meeting with the Twin Cities' clan elders to seek their advice about the work group's proposed purpose and methods. Whether the efforts of the work group—consisting primarily of relatively young members of the Hmong community and U.S. health care ethicists—would be embraced by the Hmong community elders was on the line. Most of the three-hour meeting was conducted in Hmong, but even to those who did not understand Hmong, the suffering recounted by people in their interaction with U.S. health care professionals was unmistakable and the emotion in the room was palpable. The clan elders indeed embraced the work group's efforts and underscored the importance of helping health care professionals show respect and build trust with Hmong patients and families.

Poignant stories were the common currency of the work group meetings and conferences. The power of the stories led to the collection and development of more than forty for use in various venues. It soon was evident that the insight that these cases provided into Hmong health beliefs, practices, and values, the delivery of culturally responsive health care, and tools to assist with identifying and addressing ethical issues in cross-cultural health care were not readily available in the literature. To respond to this lacuna, the Minnesota Center resolved to develop this book, *Healing by Heart*.

As project director, Dorothy E. Vawter invited four colleagues to collaborate with her on this book. The editorial team represents the fields of family medicine, health care ethics, medical anthropology, nursing, theology, and social work and includes Kathleen A. Culhane-Pera, a family practice physician and medical anthropologist who has lived, worked, and conducted ethnographic research with the Hmong in Southeast Asia and the United States; Phua Xiong, one of the first three Hmong women to become a physician in the United States, who has researched, educated, and provided health care to the Hmong communities in St. Paul, Minnesota, and Philadelphia, Pennsylvania; Barbara Babbitt, who has training in health care ethics and many years of experience in psychiatric nursing, cross-cultural communication, and community efforts to improve health care delivery to immigrant and refugee populations; and Mary M. Solberg, a professor of religion and a former social worker with cross-cultural experience and editorial skills.

The heart of this book is the stories and wisdom shared over many years in informal conversations and interviews, in clinics and in hospitals. The editors and the Minnesota Center for Health Care Ethics owe an exceptional debt of gratitude to the patients, families, and providers who offered the gift of their stories. This book is dedicated to them.

In addition we thank the thirty-four other contributors to this volume. This book would not be as rich in cultural complexity without their contributions, which often included far more than their written offerings. We are similarly indebted to the Hmong people in Chang Khian Thailand and Minneapolis–St. Paul who graciously permitted photographs of themselves to enliven these pages.

We are grateful as well for the support and guidance we received from many other people, including Kathi Antolak, Mila Aroskar, Bee Vue Benson, Lisa Boult, Miriam Cameron, Mary C. Casey, Xong Moua Cheupao, Deborah Ciracy, Elizabeth Coville, Yang Dao, David Dudycha, Eric Egli, Roberta Goldman, Kaying Hang, Yee Leng Hang, Yer Hang, Karen Harrison, Neal Holton, Nancy Johnson, Pa Lee, Pao Lee, Prasit Leepreecha, Robert Like, Deacon Va Thai Lo, Foung Lo, Marion Louwagie, James McCord, Timothy McIndoo, David J. Mersy, See Moua, Mouala Mouacheupao,

Timothy Pera, Don Postema, Ellen Rau, Maria Rubin, Beth Spottiswoode, Chue Blong Thao, ChueHue Thao, Poj Sua Theresa Thao, Sheng Thao, Xoua Thao, Rev. Chue Ying Vang, Gao Ly Vang, Sy Vang, Blong Xiong, Lee Pao Xiong, Mao Vang Xiong, Tong Neng Xiong, Wang Xang Xiong, Qhua Neeb Yaj, Gaoly Yang, Maykia Nina Yang, Tseng Zong Yang, and William Yang.

High praise and heartfelt thanks go to Julie Robbins, for her exceptional skill and dedicated attention to shepherding the book to completion. Thanks also to Kevin Christopherson for his fine research assistance.

Generous financial support for the Minnesota Center for Health Care Ethics' work on cross-cultural health care ethics has been provided by the Medtronic Foundation, the Partners in Justice Fund of the Sisters of St. Joseph of Carondelet of the St. Paul Province, the estate of Lloyd Simms—a founding member of the Board of the Minnesota Center for Health Care Ethics—and the College of St. Catherine's Bush Foundation Grant, "Diversity and Democracy in Higher Education." In addition, Kathleen A. Culhane-Pera held a Bush Medical Fellowship from the Bush Foundation.

We thank the leaders and representatives of the partner organizations of the Minnesota Center for Health Care Ethics for their vision and support—David R. Page, Robert M. Meiches, and Charles P. Ceronsky of Fairview Health Services; Timothy Hanson, Joseph R. Clubb, and the Reverend Scott W. Hinrichs of HealthEast Care System; Sr. Andrea Lee, Sr. Amata Miller, Susan Cochrane, Nan Kari, Margaret McLaughlin, and Tone Blechert of the College of St. Catherine, and Sr. Margaret Belanger, Sr. Margaret Kvasnicka, Sr. Ann Walton, Sr. Delore Rochon, Sr. Christine Ludwig, Sr. Susan Oeffling, and Sr. Karen Hilgers of the Sisters of St. Joseph of Carondelet.

This book is born of an unusual confluence of good fortune, opportunity, and rich experience in an area of cross-cultural health care that remains underdeveloped. We are grateful to Michael Ames, director of Vanderbilt University Press, for embracing this project, and to the Editorial Committee of Vanderbilt University Press for granting *Healing by Heart* the Norman L. and Roselea J. Goldberg Prize for the best project in the area of medicine for 2002. We are humbled and honored.

Minnesota Center
for Health Care Ethics
*Karen G. Gervais*
*Dorothy E. Vawter*

Editors
*Kathleen A. Culhane-Pera*
*Dorothy E. Vawter*
*Phua Xiong*
*Barbara Babbitt*
*Mary M. Solberg*

*Hla dej yuav hle khau.*
*Tsiv teb tsaws chaw yuav hle hau*
—White Hmong Proverb

When crossing a river, remove your sandals.
When crossing a border, remove your crown.

# Introduction

Members of minority communities who have lived in the United States for generations—Asians, Africans, Latinos, and American Indians—have long complained about being treated as second-class citizens by a health care system that does not understand or meet their needs. The dramatic influx of recent immigrants and refugees, including, among others, Mexicans, Somalis, Ethiopians, Hmong, Cambodians, Bosnians, and Russians, is strengthening the pleas for change in the practice and delivery of health care services. Fleeing war, famine, poverty, and persecution in their homelands, immigrants and refugees continue to arrive in large numbers in search of something better. The 2000 census confirms that the number of foreign-born residents and children of immigrants and refugees as well as the percentage of non-European Americans are the highest they have been in the history of the United States. Demographic projections based on current trends indicate that "minorities" will be in the majority in 2060 (U.S. Census Bureau, 2000).

The scale and pace of these demographic changes are leading health care professionals, administrators, and policy makers to recognize with new urgency the inadequacy of rote applications of Western biomedicine to every person who enters a health care facility. Fueled further by recent studies describing racial and ethnic disparities in health status, the constellation of social and historical factors is at last compelling health care professionals, administrators, and policy makers to seek greater cultural awareness and competence (American Medical Association, 1999, 2001; Institute of Medicine, 2001; Smedley, Stith, & Nelson, 2002; U.S. Department of Health and Human Services, 2000, 2002).

Delivering culturally responsive health care* is both difficult and rewarding. It requires providers to be self-aware and culturally knowledgeable and to apply complex communication skills and demonstrate attitudes that help build trusting and respectful cross-cultural relationships. Providers want to provide care that is respectful of the patient, medically correct, nondiscriminatory, and consistent with professional integrity. Often providers can achieve these goals. Sometimes, however—espe-

---

*People are using a wide variety of terms, such as "culturally sensitive," "culturally competent," "culturally effective," "culturally appropriate," and "culturally congruent" to refer to the obligation health care providers and organizations have to respond to patients' cultural needs effectively. The phrase "culturally responsive" suggests that clinicians can respond to pertinent aspects of patients' cultural practices, beliefs, and values in clinical settings and stresses the application of knowledge, skills, and attitudes without requiring that clinicians be "competent" in other people's cultures (Goldman, Monroe, & Dube, 1996).

cially in cases involving cultural differences between providers and patients—questions arise about how to balance and prioritize these objectives. Providing health care to patients from diverse cultural backgrounds may generate confusion and conflict, requiring clinicians to make difficult decisions about which objectives to sacrifice when not all can be fully realized.

When U.S. providers do not understand the choices and actions of patients and families from diverse cultures, they may inadvertently use their status and power to impose their perspective on patients and families. Alternatively, they can choose to learn about the social issues, core beliefs, moral commitments, and emotions that underlie what seem to them strange choices and actions and remain open to negotiating options that are acceptable to all. Providers who learn more about the perspectives of their patients may also be better able to make creative changes in their practices and the institutions where they work. The results should lead to fewer misunderstandings and conflicts, more satisfied patients, families, and practitioners, and—ultimately—better health outcomes.

A comprehensive consideration of how to enhance the delivery of health care across cultures requires attention not only to health care professionals but also to the health care organizations in which they work. An organization's culture—its policies, practices, and attitudes—affects practitioner-patient relationships and shapes the space within which practitioners may be able to modify their own practices to improve their care of individual patients. State and federal health care policies, for their part, strongly influence the capacity of health care organizations to respond to the needs of all groups they serve. Finally, clinicians, health care organizations, and policy makers are all constrained by historical and current social and economic circumstances.

## Overview of the Book

Based on ethnographically informed reflection on the health-related cultural beliefs and values of the Hmong community, *Healing by Heart* explores clinical and ethical challenges in cross-cultural health care. It contrasts traditional Hmong health-related moral practices and commitments with those that are widely held by U.S. practitioners and offers a model of key learning areas for delivering culturally responsive health care. (See Figure 16.1: A Model for Culturally Responsive Health Care.)

The model identifies a set of key ethical issues arising from and within cross-cultural healing relationships that each provider must decide. How providers respond to these cross-cultural ethical issues will affect profoundly the decisions they make, the care they provide, the quality of their healing relationships, and the satisfaction of both providers and patients. The model also offers an approach to working through serious cross-cultural ethical conflicts.

This book emerges out of our years of ethnographic study, clinical experience with Hmong patients in the United States and Thailand, training of medical students and other health professionals in cross-cultural health, partnerships with leaders within the Hmong community in Minnesota, and commitment to improving relationships between U.S. health care professionals and Hmong families. It reflects our attempts to understand the role of culture in health, to deliver culturally responsive health care to Hmong patients, and to address the cross-cultural ethical issues and conflicts.

At the heart of the book are stories—our own and those of others—that puzzle, disturb, amaze, and move. The experiences the stories relate have taught and inspired us to replace some ingrained clinical habits, customs, and rules with other ways of knowing, relating, and serving. Culturally responsive health care does not happen in the abstract; it happens in the context of clinical interactions. Sharing stories of suffering, confusion, and success enlivens the model of culturally responsive health care and offers an effective and accessible method of learning about others and ourselves. *Healing by Heart* encourages emotional understanding of other people's suffering and enhances appreciation for how the body, mind, and spirit all contribute to health and illness.

Since the Hmong began arriving in the United States as refugees from Laos in 1975, serious misunderstandings and conflicts have arisen between Hmong families and U.S. health care professionals (Barrett et al., 1998; Bliatout, 1988; Cha, 2000; Culhane-Pera, 1989; Culhane-Pera & Vawter, 1998; Deinard & Dunnigan, 1987; Fadiman, 1997; Kirton, 1985; Minnesota Center for Health Care Ethics, 1995, 1997; Mouacheupao, 1999; Muecke, 1983; O'Connor, 1995; Osborn, 1992; True, 1997; Westermeyer & Thao, 1986). While change is occurring and conflicts may be less frequent, clinicians remain confused by Hmong families' reluctance to trust and accept their treatment recommendations, and Hmong families remain confused about U.S. health care professionals' interference with their decisions and decision-making practices.

Health care professionals have expressed to other providers their disappointment that Hmong families refuse the best care they have to offer, their anguish when families refuse life-saving interventions, their frustration with spending extended time with families without arriving at a satisfactory agreement, their anger at families who treat them in ways they consider disrespectful, and their ambivalent feelings of relief and sorrow about obtaining court orders to compel families to comply with their treatment recommendations.

Likewise, Hmong families have told their stories to other Hmong people about their frustration, mistrust, and anger. They are amazed by the disrespect with which they are treated and angry that providers do harmful things to them against their will. They rail that providers use them for educational or research purposes or as a source of body parts for Americans. They are bewildered and angry that providers can call the police and force their children to be treated—perhaps even tortured—without their families' permission.

Contrasting worldviews and ideas about health, illness, and healing can thwart goals that clinicians, patients, and families share: for patients and providers to feel respected and to be satisfied with both the healing methods used and the outcomes (Jecker, Carrese, & Pearlman, 1995). The range and depth of the differences in health-related beliefs and moral practices between Western-trained clinicians and traditional Hmong families make it an exemplary case to explore cross-cultural health care and health care ethics.

This book offers resources to clinicians and institutions committed to delivering culturally responsive care, paying special attention to building successful healing relationships with traditional Hmong patients and families. In the context of a model for delivering culturally responsive health care, it describes and interprets traditional Hmong health beliefs and practices, provides personal reflections by patients, families, and practitioners on their cross-cultural experiences, and offers recommendations to help reduce misunderstandings and address serious cross-cultural ethical conflicts. The wide range of case stories is accompanied by perspectives from thirty-seven case commentators.

Hmong terms and phrases are included throughout the text to make the meanings more precise for those who read Hmong and for other interested readers. Most of the words are in the White Hmong dialect; but Green Hmong is used in two commentaries. Because the words are not spelled in phonetic English, readers unfamiliar with the romanized script should consult a pronunciation guide (e.g., Heimbach, 1979; http://ww2.saturn.stpaul.k12.mn.us/hmong/pronunciation.html).

Chapter 1 describes aspects of Hmong culture pertinent to health status, beliefs, and practices as they existed in Southeast Asia and are changing in the United States. It recounts some of the historical, political, and economic events that brought about a war that disrupted the agricultural lifestyle of the Hmong in Southeast Asia and made them refugees, contributed to increases in the incidence of such diseases as hypertension, diabetes, depression, and posttraumatic stress disorder, and resulted in their needing to modify some of their cultural practices. Photographs illustrate several of the healing practices the Hmong use, both in Southeast Asia and in the United States.

As a summary of Hmong culture, the wide variations in cultural beliefs and practices transmitted through families for generations may seem to be lost in generalizations. We caution the reader not to take the generalizations as stereotypes but to use them as initial information upon which to build when interacting with individual patients and families.

Chapters 2–15 include sets of clinically realistic case stories of Hmong patients, their families, and U.S. health care providers, accompanied by discussion questions and followed by two or three commentaries. The cases are written from the biomedical perspective. Patients across the life span and in different states of health interact with clinicians in multiple disciplines (hospice, surgery, pediatrics, family practice, internal medicine, emergency medicine, obstetrics and gynecology, and psychiatry and psychology). The case stories illustrate intra- and intercultural differences as well as diverse perspectives on the successes and failures of particular health care relationships, interventions, and outcomes. They also exemplify important cross-cultural health-related moral practices and commitments, among them respectful treatment of the ill or dying; trust of health care professionals and traditional healers; roles, responsibilities, and prerogatives of the ill person, the family, practitioners, and institutions; disclosure practices; best-interest and risk/benefit assessments; and decision-making practices.

Eight of the fourteen case stories are based on real-life situations and the others are composites and constructions, inspired by multiple clinical situations. We gathered cases from community members, health care providers across the country, and our own experiences. Patients or family members of real-life situations graciously consented to share their difficult and painful experiences with the hope that others would learn from them and that health care for Hmong patients and others will improve. We are grateful to these families for allowing us to include: "Woman with Pregnancy Complications," "Children with High Fevers: Neng's Story," "Infant with Down Syndrome and a Heart Defect," "Man with Diabetes and Hypertension," "Young Woman with Kidney Failure and Transplant," "Hospice Patient with Gallbladder Cancer," "Pregnant Woman with a Brain Hemorrhage," and "A Widowed Mother's Search for a Good Place to Die." In "Young Woman with Kidney Failure and Transplant" the patient chose to use her real name. Other families preferred fictitious names and other changes in the facts and identifying characteristics to protect their privacy. In the remaining cases, the names, circumstances, and geographic information are fictitious; any similarities in name or location or to actual persons or events are coincidental and unintended.

These commentaries include suggestions to assist clinicians with providing culturally responsive health care. Chiefly, however, the commentaries in this book offer insight into the moral, spiritual, social, political, and emotional perspectives of Hmong patients and their families. They have suffered physically from old familiar diseases and new diseases since living in the United States; and they have suffered psychically because of rapid and profound changes within their sociocultural system, spiritually because they have been uprooted from a religious perspective that pervaded all aspects of life, and socially because of the discrimination they experience in a racist society.

Among the commentators are clinicians (nurses, physicians, psychologists, and social workers), medical anthropologists, health care ethicists, clergy, patients, family members, and a shaman. Most of the authors are Hmong. For the actual cases, the patient, a family member, or a traditional healer involved in the case wrote (or was interviewed by someone who wrote) a commentary from his or her intimate perspective. Hence, the book offers a mix of perspectives, including those of Hmong authors not previously published in English and scholars with years of professional experience working with the Hmong in Laos, Thailand, and the United States. As a collection, these commentaries illustrate the value of multiple perspectives.

Chapter 16 presents a model for delivering culturally responsive health care. It offers recommendations for developing each of nine learning areas and suggestions for applying the knowledge, skills, and attitudes to particular clinical encounters, with extended guidance on developing communication skills and working with Hmong families. The model identifies ethical values for practitioners and health care organizations to focus on as they seek to understand the health-related moral commitments and practices of the cultural groups they serve and raises key ethical questions individual providers confront when serving culturally diverse patients. Finally, it offers a guide for working through ethical conflicts in cross-cultural health care. While it focuses on providing concrete recommendations for clinicians who seek to enhance their understanding of the influence of culture on health, the quality of their cross-cultural healing relationships, and their knowledge and skills in cross-cultural health care ethics, it also offers recommendations for health care institutions and policy makers.

## How to Read This Book

Each chapter of *Healing by Heart* can stand on its own. Thus, readers who are most interested in culture and in Hmong culture in particular may prefer to start with Chapter 1 and then read the cases and commentaries in Chapters 2–15, or vice versa. Readers who are most interested in health care ethics or the model for culturally responsive health care might begin with Chapter 16.

## How to Teach with This Book

Teachers can work with the cases in this book in several different ways depending on their discipline, the level of their students, available time, and preferred educational methods. After reading Chapter 1, the students could discuss the cases together in class, guided by the questions at the end of the cases and the commentaries. Students could do role plays, guided by specific information about their character (patient, spouse, family member, doctor, nurse, social worker, ethicist, etc.); they could act out specific disagreements or conflicts in the cases. Alternatively, students could read specific cases and their commentaries before class and then discuss the major issues raised in those cases. Or students could act out parts of the cases, by choosing a specific orientation and then "defending" that stance in front of their fellow students, whether an audience of health care providers, anthropologists, ethicists, lawyers, or Hmong community members.

Once students have studied specific cases, they could then read Chapter 16 and reexamine those cases in the light of how individuals, institutions, and policy makers could improve delivery of health care and improve health care outcomes. They could also use the model in Chapter 16 to further explore the ethical issues involved in the cases, particularly where they have identified that health care providers have objections based on professional integrity to following patients and family's wishes. Alternatively, they could begin by reading Chapters 1 and 16 and then explore specific cases and the commentaries.

## References

American Medical Association. (1999). *Cultural competence compendium.* Chicago: Author. Retrieved January 30, 2003, from *www.ama-assn.org/ama/pub/category/4848.html*

American Medical Association. (2001). *Enhancing the cultural competence of physicians: Recommendation from the Council on Medical Education* [Report 5-A-98]. Retrieved December 27, 2002, from *www.ama-assn.org/meetings/public/annual98/reports/cme/cmerpt5.htm*

Barrett, B., Shadick, K., Schilling, R., Spencer, L., del Rosario, S., Moua, K., & Vang, M. (1998). Hmong/medicine interactions: Improving cross-cultural health care. *Family Medicine, 30*(3), 179–184.

Bliatout, B. T. (1988, March 5). *Hmong refugees: Some barriers to some western health care services.* Paper presented at conference on Southeast Asians in the United States, Arizona State University, Tempe, AZ.

Cha, D. (2000). *Hmong American concepts of health, healing, and illness, and their experience with conventional medicine.* Unpublished doctoral dissertation, University of Colorado, Denver.

Culhane-Pera, K. A. (1989). *Analysis of cultural beliefs and power dynamics in disagreements about health care of Hmong children.* Unpublished master's thesis, University of Minnesota, Minneapolis.

Culhane-Pera, K. A., & Vawter, D. E. (1998). A study of health care professionals' perspectives about a cross-cultural ethical conflict involving a Hmong patient and her family. *Journal of Clinical Ethics, 9*(2), 179–190.

Deinard, A. S., & Dunnigan, T. (1987). Hmong health care: Reflections on a six-year experience. *International Migration Review, 21,* 857–865.

Fadiman A. (1997). *The spirit catches you and you fall down: A Hmong child, her American doctors, and the collision of two cultures.* New York: Farrar, Straus and Giroux.

Goldman, R. E., Monroe, A. D., & Dube, C. E. (1996). Cultural self-awareness: A component of culturally responsive patient care. *Annals of Behavioral Science and Medical Education, 3,* 37–46.

Heimbach, E. E. (1979). *White Hmong-English dictionary.* Ithaca, NY: Southeast Asia Program Publications, Cornell University.

Institute of Medicine. (2001). *Crossing the quality chasm: A new health system for the 21st century.* Retrieved December 29, 2001, from *www.nap.edu/catalog/10027.html*

Jecker, N. S., Carrese, J. A., & Pearlman, R. A. (1995). Caring for patients in cross-cultural settings. *Hastings Center Report, 25,* 6–14.

Kirton, E. S. (1985). *The locked medicine cabinet: Hmong health care in America.* Unpublished doctoral dissertation, University of Santa Barbara, Santa Barbara, CA.

Minnesota Center for Health Care Ethics. (1995). *Western medicine through Hmong voices* [videotape, 11 minutes]. Minneapolis: Author. Available from Minnesota Center for Health Care Ethics, 601 25th Avenue S., Minneapolis, MN 55454; 651-690-7895.

Minnesota Center for Health Care Ethics. (1997). *Trading beliefs: Four Hmong families consider relinquishing their traditional health beliefs* [videotape, 20 minutes]. Minneapolis: Author. Available from Minnesota Center for Health Care Ethics, 601 25th Avenue S., Minneapolis, MN 55454; 651-690-7895.

Mouacheupao, S. (1999, April 17). *Attitudes of Hmong patients to surgery.* Paper presented at annual spring research forum of the Minnesota Academy of Family Physicians, Minneapolis.

Muecke, M. (1983). Caring for Southeast Asian refugee patients in the USA. *American Journal of Public Health, 73*(4), 431–438.

O'Connor, B. B. (1995). Hmong cultural values, biomedicine, and chronic liver disease. In B. B. O'Connor, *Healing traditions: Alternative medicine and the health professions.* Philadelphia: University of Pennsylvania Press.

Osborn, D. G. (1992). Conflict and collaboration in cross-cultural health care. *World Health Forum, 13,* 315–319.

Smedley, B. D., Stith, A. Y., & Nelson, A. R. (Eds.). (2002). *Unequal treatment: Confronting racial and ethnic disparities in health care.* Washington, DC: National Academies Press.

True, G. (1997). 'My souls will come back to trouble you:' Cultural and ethical issues in the coerced treatment of a Hmong adolescent. *Southern Folklore, 54*(20), 101–114.

U.S. Census Bureau. (2000). *Population projections program, population division.* Retrieved January 30, 2003, from *www.census.gov/population/www/projections/natproj.html*

U.S. Department of Health and Human Services. (2000, December 22). *National standards on culturally and linguistically appropriate services (CLAS) in health care.* Office of Minority Health, *Federal Register.* Retrieved March 2, 2001, from *www.omhrc.gov/clas*

U.S. Department of Health and Human Services. (2002). *Healthy people 2010* (2nd ed.). Retrieved May 31, 2002 from *www. health.gov/healthypeople*

Westermeyer, J., & Thao, X. (1986). Cultural beliefs and surgical procedures. *Journal of the American Medical Association, 255*(23), 3301–3302.

# PART I

# Health-Related Cultural Beliefs, Practices, and Values

# Hmong Culture:
# Tradition and Change

*Kathleen A. Culhane-Pera M.D., M.A.,*
*and Phua Xiong, M.D.*

This chapter provides an overview of the central elements of traditional Hmong culture in Southeast Asia and the changes that have occurred since large numbers of refugees resettled in the United States in the mid 1970s. It reviews the history of the relationship between Hmong and Americans and describes those aspects of Hmong traditional and changing culture that ground Hmong health-related beliefs, values, and practices. This historical and cultural information is crucial for U.S. health professionals and institutions committed to providing culturally responsive health care to Hmong patients and their families.

A note of caution: while general statements about culture are useful as starting points, they can become dangerous stereotypes if applied unconditionally. Also, general statements will not hold for all Hmong people because of significant variations in Hmong culture influenced by differences in Laos (such as animistic rituals, geographic locations, political affiliation, the war, and refugee experiences) and differences in the United States (such as formal education, employment, and religion). Health

Information for this chapter is based on texts cited, the authors' clinical experiences and interviews with Hmong patients in health care settings from 1983 through 2002, and the authors' research projects from 1986 through 2002. Kathleen A. Culhane-Pera has conducted qualitative research on Hmong people's reactions to operations, blood draws, and septic work-ups in St. Paul, Minnesota; on providers' responses to Hmong refusal of treatment in St. Paul; on Hmong concepts of health, causes of disease, traditional healing practices, preventive care, children's illnesses, and decision making for children's illnesses in Thailand; on the role of hemp fiber in life-cycle rituals; on the effect of changing village socioeconomic conditions and household decision making on children's health status in Thailand; on adult health status in Thailand; and traditional healing, concepts of childhood illnesses, childhood immunizations, childhood anemia, medical decision making for children's illnesses, and childhood home safety in St. Paul. She is currently researching the effects of group visits on Hmong patients with type 2 diabetes mellitus. Phua Xiong has conducted qualitative research on Hmong people's reactions to Western medicine and immunizations; traditional and changing shamanic healing practices and how these influence health care utilization and decision making; Hmong cultural and religious practices; traditional Hmong health concepts and beliefs; the construction and use of storycloths; the design, method, and meaning of White Hmong *paj ntaub* (embroidered cloth); Hmong cultural and social adjustment to American society; and trust and distrust of Western health care.

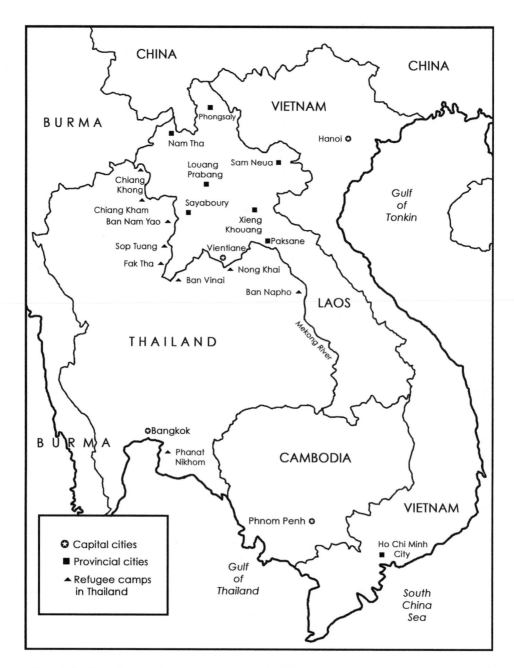

**Map 1.1. Southeast Asia in the Late 1970s**

care providers should consider this general information as a resource from which to learn more and to generate questions for individual patients and their families.

## Traditional Life in Southeast Asia

According to ancient Chinese texts, the Hmong lived in northern central Asia, approximately the area of present-day Mongolia, in 2300 B.C.E. (Ruey Yih-Fu, 1962; cited in Tapp, 1989). Over the centuries, people migrated south into Tibet and China and finally into Southeast Asia in the 1800s as a result of warfare with the Han Chinese and a decrease in fertility of mountaintop soil (Cooper, 1984; Savina, 1930; Tapp, 1989). Despite their conflicts, the Hmong and the Han Chinese have many cultural and linguistic similarities, including their social structures, their practices of geomancy, their beliefs in the importance of ancestors, and their metaphysical concepts of the yin/yang balance (see Schein, 2000). Many Hmong migrated to Laos, where for almost two hundred years they lived separate from the native Lao people geographically, socially, and culturally. After the 1975 communist takeover in Laos, Hmong soldiers and their families fled to Thailand. In the ensuing two decades, they were resettled from refugee camps in Thailand to countries around the world. The Hmong diaspora numbers about five million Hmong people in China and almost one million in other countries, including Argentina, Australia, Canada, France, French Guyana, Laos, New Zealand, Thailand, the United States, and Vietnam.

### Agriculture

On the shallow but fertile mountaintop soil in Southeast Asia, Hmong people practice subsistence, slash-and-burn agriculture (Cooper, 1984; Kunstadter, Chapman & Sabhasri, 1978; Lemoine, 1972b; Geddes, 1976; Tapp, 1989; Yang, 1975, 1993). Before clearing the land and after harvesting the crops, men perform rituals to honor, thank, and appease the land spirits. Life is physically demanding; with no machines or animals to help with the fieldwork, people perform the arduous tasks of cutting down trees, clearing shrubs, burning brush, planting seeds, hacking weeds, and harvesting crops. In some instances horses transport food home, but this work too is mostly a human activity. All family members, from young children to elders, work according to their capacity to benefit the household, for without everyone's hard work, people do not have enough to eat. They harvest what they plant—field rice, corn, beans, pumpkins, and various green leafy vegetables—and supplement their diet with food gathered from the forests, such as bamboo shoots and bananas. Many people also grow opium as a cash crop and hemp as a fiber for clothes. Although animals, especially chickens, pigs, goats, and cows, are raised for meat, meat is not consumed daily; herds are small and some animals have to be saved for rituals and breeding. When the land becomes infertile in eight to ten years, families move to a patch of virgin mountain land.

Time is measured by the yearly cycle of the seasons and related field activities: planting in the early rainy season, harvesting at the end of the rainy season, and collecting opium resin and weaving hemp cloth in the cold season. Days are counted according to the moon's cycle: one to fifteen days of waxing *(hli xiab)* and sixteen to twenty-nine or thirty days of waning *(hli nqeg)*, with twenty-nine days in the odd months *(hli tab)* and thirty in the even months *(hli txooj)*. In the Hmong zodiac system *(tsiaj nres xeem)*, which is similar to the Chinese system, months and years could be characterized by twelve animals (e.g., year of the horse 2002; year of the snake 2001) (Hmong Cultural Center, n.d.). As the Hmong did not count years systematically, they did not have birthdates until assigned by the French-based Laotian government or the Thai refugee camp administrators.

### Social and Family Structure

Hmong traditional society is patrilineal, patrilocal, and patriarchal (Cooper, 1984; Donnelly, 1994; Geddes, 1976; Leepreecha, 2001; Lemoine, 1972b; Tapp, 1989; Yang, 1975, 1993). The patrilineal system of tracing family lineage through the father has social as well as spiritual significance. All people with the same family clan name are related and people refer to each other using an elaborate system of kinship terms (G. Y. Lee, 1986b). Most frequently, eighteen clans are acknowledged (though scholars have disagreed, counting fifteen to twenty-two clans [Yang, in press]). (See Table 1.1.) The incest taboo applies to people with the same last name; marriages occur only between members of different clans. When social, political, financial, or health problems arise, men turn to their extended families for assistance, including the families of their brothers, uncles, and great-uncles. Husbands' family members *(kwv tij)* have more social obligations to each other than they have to their wives' family members *(neej tsa)* (Cooper, 1984). (See Chapter 3.) The household's ancestral spirits *(dab niam dab txiv)* have special relationships with the household members. People remember and revere their ancestral spirits, and the ancestral spirits protect the living. (See below, Changing Spiritual Concepts: Animism; and Traditional Beliefs about Illness Causation: Supernatural etiologies: Spirits; also Chapter 15.)

Animist rituals are passed from fathers to sons, so that close relatives share ritualistic details. Thus, strangers figure out their common ancestry, and thus their relationship to each other, by inquiring about similarities and differences in these rituals. Some major differences represent major historical divisions. For example, the funeral practice of covering gravesites with branches or with rocks distinguishes a traditional Hmong style from the traditional Chinese style that some Hmong adopted so that Chinese would not defile Hmong graves. Other ritual differences are minor, and more

### Table 1.1. Hmong Clan Names

| | | |
|---|---|---|
| Chang, Cheng, or Cha | Kong | Tang |
| Chu | Kue | Thao or Thor |
| Fang | Lor or Lo | Vang or Va |
| Hang | Ly, Le, or Lee | Vue |
| Her or Heu | Moua or Mua | Xiong or Song |
| Khang | Phang | Yang or Ya |

specific, such as whether a pig is released when it squeals and replaced with a chicken during the *ua nyuj dab* ceremony.

In addition to the lineage divisions, there is a societal distinction between types of Hmong. The major types are White Hmong (Hmoob Dawb) and Green Hmong (Moob Leeg or Moob Ntsuab, which is sometimes translated "Blue Hmong"). The labels refer to styles of women's clothes. White Hmong women wear pleated white hemp skirts and Green Hmong women wear pleated and batiked hemp skirts that are dyed in a dark blue indigo bath. But more than differences in women's skirts distinguish the two divisions: they have different language dialects, housing structures, and animistic rituals. Other people include the Striped Hmong [Hmoob Quas Npab] in Laos and the Black Hmong [Hmoob Dub] in Vietnam.

As a description of Hmong traditional society, patrilocal means that Hmong people live with their father's side of the family. When a woman marries, she leaves her father's household to join her husband's household and kin group. Members of one patrilocal household share living space and subsistence fields of crops such as rice, corn, and vegetables. They do not necessarily share cash crops; fathers and sons might have their own cash fields and manage their own money. Generally, however, the male head of household manages the money for the household (Cooper, 1984; Yang, 1993). Some families live together under one roof, building additional rooms as the family grows, and sharing food and eating together in groups of up to a hundred people. Other families separate when the original house becomes too crowded or brothers' wives do not get along or the land is too infertile to support everyone. Then, the older sons and their nuclear families move into new houses nearby or move into newly forming villages (with connections from relatives) in distant fertile lands, leaving the youngest son and his wife to care for his aging parents.

## Men

In this patriarchal society, Hmong men have more status and power than women (Cooper, 1984; Donnelly, 1994). Clearing the forest for their fields, men claim the land for themselves and their families. Men perform the ancestral and spirit rituals for their families, arrange marriage contracts between clans, and conduct funerals. Also, men settle disputes, informally within their families or between clans, or in formal court proceedings *(hais plaub)* between different families. Men gain power as they progress into middle age and lose power as they decline into old age. Men are given an adult name during a *tis npe laus* ritual, a rite of passage that denotes their respected new social status. This ritual usually occurs when a married man has two to three children and increased familial responsibilities. However, some Green Hmong families give men their adult names at the time of marriage. Old men are honored in the sense that their wishes are respected and their counsel is sought, but their decision-making power is slowly passed to their married sons, who manage the households and take care of their aging parents. (See Chapters 6 and 10.) Hmong use the term "elderly" to refer to respected men whose wisdom and counsel are sought; the term does not necessarily relate to advanced age, for many "elders" are in their forties and fifties.

## Women

Women have more private than public power (Cooper, 1984; Cooper, Tapp, Lee, & Schworer-Kohl, 1995; Donnelly, 1994; see also Schein, 2000). Generally, they influence events within their households directly and outside their households indirectly, through their husbands. Women gain power as they age. Young, newly married daughters-in-law *(tus nyab)* have no power in their husbands' families; they are open to criticism from their elders and must work hard to please members of their new family, especially their mothers-in-law. (See Chapter 3.) By middle-age, when they have married sons and daughters-in-law of their own, women exercise considerable influence over household and intra-familial events, such as decisions involving money, farming, cooking, animals, children, marriages, and how to respond to sick family members. Elderly women, like their husbands, are respected, but after their husbands die or relinquish household leadership, their married sons and daughters-in-law have decision-making power. In their old age, women depend on their sons for support, especially since their daughters have married, moved away, and joined other households and economic units.

Women work in the fields of their natal or their marital families; they have no separate fields of their own, and thus no way of supporting themselves outside of the family setting. A widow either stays with her husband's family, remaining single or marrying her deceased husband's younger brother, or marries a man from another clan and moves to his household. Her children, however, particularly boys and nonsuckling infants, usually stay with their father's family, since this is their social and spiritual home. (See Chapter 9.) The fate of divorced women and their children vary, depending upon the divorce agreement and the determination of guilt. Divorced women may or may not keep their children. Divorced women may be given their own land, but often they return to live with their fathers or brothers, who may see them as a burden. Unmarried women (as well as men) stay with their natal families, and those with physical or mental impairments are cared for by their parents and siblings.

## Marriages

Marriages generally come about in one of five different ways (Bertrais, 1978). Parents can arrange marriages *(nqis tsev hais poj niam)* between their children for the benefit of their children and the two families. An ideal arranged marriage unites a man's daughter and his sister's son (a cross-cousin marriage), because parents prefer to send their daughter to live with her aunt rather than with strangers and face the possibility of a cruel mother-in-law. Negotiations for an arranged marriage often involves consideration of the families' reputations, social connections, political histories, and health histories (whether any family members have, for example, congenital defects, mental retardation, or physical disabilities) and the reputations of the potential bride and groom, as well as approval from extended family members on both sides. In many instances, personal choice and the opinions of the two individuals involved, especially the bride, are secondary or not considered at all. Marriages also occur by mutual consent *(xav sib yuav)*, with two attracted people asking their parents for permission to marry, or by elopement *(caum txiv)*, with two people running away and sleeping together in the man's house. In forced marriages *(yuam sib yuav)*, families compel a pregnant woman and the father of her baby to marry. In bride capture *(txhom poj niam yuav)* a man, with the help of his male relatives or friends, physically captures the woman he wants and takes her to sleep in his house.

The traditional wedding ceremony begins with the ritual *lwm qaib,* when the woman enters the man's house through the spirit door and her soul is welcomed while a chicken is whirled above her head. A marriage could begin, however, when the couple sleeps together in the man's house or in his relative's house, without anyone conducting the ceremony. In bride capture and elopement situations, the new bride is confined to the man's house for three days, and the groom's family notifies the bride's family of the events. Even if the bride's family strongly disagrees with the marriage, they have few avenues of recourse to reverse these events. Regardless of how a marriage starts, on the third day, the groom's family performs a soul-calling ceremony to welcome the new bride's soul into the family and to inform their house spirits that a new person has joined them. Then, the entourage walks to the bride's parents' home to make arrangements for the rest of the rituals.

At the wedding ceremony *(ua tshoob)*, the two families negotiate the bride-price with the assistance of four men *(mej koob)*: two men representing the groom's family and two men representing the bride's family. The groom's family pays the agreed-upon bride-price *(nqe mis nqe hno)* to the bride's family and the bride's family gives dowry gifts to the bride *(nyiaj thiab khoom phij cuam)*. During the negotiations, any unsettled matters—including marital disputes—that took place between the two clans prior to the current marriage may be discussed and settled with a monetary fee. Also, any acts of disrespect to the bride's family by the groom or his family members during the courtship or initial marriage process must be healed with apologies and a monetary fee. These settlements are made to ensure that the groom's family will not abuse or take advantage of the bride, the bride's family is respected, and the two families will have good relations in the future. In contrast to the Western tradition, in Hmong marriages male family members—rather than the bride and groom—exchange marital "vows" and formally accept their new social titles of kinship. The groom's male family members profess their desire to take good care of the bride and the bride's male family members accept the bride-price as a symbol of the groom's family's commitment to take good care of their daughter (Bertrais, 1978). (See Chapter 11.)

The practice of polygyny (one man has more than one wife) is not uncommon. In one Laotian village in the 1960s, for example, 17 percent of men had more than one wife (Yang, 1975, 1993). Most polygynous men have two wives, but some men have as many as five wives. The decision to marry another woman could be made by a man and his first wife, a man and his male family members, or the man himself, for several reasons. The family may want help in the fields and in the house or they may want more sons. Or the man may want to expand his kinship connections or may have fallen in love with another woman. (See Chapter 12; see Plate 15.)

## Children

Adult household members take collective responsibility for raising children (Cooper, 1984; Geddes, 1976). Boys and girls learn many of the same life skills—agricultural, horticultural, and culinary—as well as social values, including respecting their elders. They also learn gender-differentiated skills. Girls learn to weave hemp cloth, embroider clothes, and raise animals in their own family compounds; they are not allowed to venture out into other people's compounds or the forest. Boys learn to make wooden tools, build houses, play musical instruments *(qeej* and *ncas)*, fell trees, and hunt with crossbows in the forests. Generally, while some boys learn some girls' skills, most girls do not learn boys' skills.

Storytellers—often grandparents—teach children about Hmong culture by relating family stories, folktales and myths *(dab neeg)* around evening fires after the work is done or during rainy days when people stay home or during the dry-season months when there is less field work (Johnson & Yang, 1992).

Generally, young children grow up in a permissive environment, with caregivers— adults and older siblings—responding quickly to their needs. Older children are treated more strictly, with an "attitude more one of critical guidance than of praise for the sake of encouragement" (Bliatout, Downing, Lewis, & Yang, 1988) and if necessary, parents use physical discipline. Children obtain life skills and take on responsibilities so that by the time they are in their mid-teens, they can function as an adult and can marry. (See Chapter 2.)

## Literacy

Hmong traditional society is nonliterate, but according to oral histories once upon a time Hmong had a written language, books, land, and a Hmong emperor *(Huab Tais)*, which they lost during their conflicts with the Chinese. In the past hundred years, several writing systems have been developed using Chinese characters; the Laotian, Thai, and Roman alphabets; a system of hieroglyphics called the Pollar Script; and a uniquely Hmong script. The romanized script (Romanized Phonetic Alphabet or RPA) was devised by Christian missionaries William Smalley, G. Linwood Barney, and Yves Bertrais in the 1950s and is the most widely used. The Hmong script, also called Pahawh (or Pahauh) Hmong script (Phaj Hauj Hmoob) or Chaofa script (Cob Fab or Lords of the Sky) is attributed to the messianic leader Shong Lue Yang (Bliatout et al., 1988; Tapp, 1989; Vang, Yang, & Smalley, 1990).

In Laos, few children were able to attend Lao primary schools until the United States Agency for International Development (USAID) set up primary schools in Hmong villages throughout Laos in the 1960s. Some of these students were able to continue their secondary education in the only high school in Vientiane, Laos (Weldon, 1999). In 1971, 340 Hmong high school students left Laos to study in Australia, Canada, France, and the United States (Bliatout et al., 1988).

## Health Status

There is limited data about health statistics for Hmong in Southeast Asia. Reports from Laos (Yang, 1993) and Thailand (Kunstadter, 1985, 1986) suggest that infectious diseases were the main health problem, related to high infant mortality rates and low life expectancy. Yang Dao speculates that malaria, dysentery, and tuberculosis in particular caused many deaths and reports 1968 death rates of 17/1000 in Sayaboury Province (which had some fighting) and 20–25/1000 in Xieng Khouang Province (which had heavy fighting). He states the birth rate before the war in the 1960s was estimated as 45–53/1000, which decreased during the war in 1970 to 37/1000. Population data from Xieng Khouang Province in 1970 revealed that 50 percent of the population was under the age of fifteen (Yang, 1993). A 1984 survey of Hmong villages in Thailand revealed a crude birth rate of 49.8/1000 and a crude death rate of 8.9/1000; extrapolating from histories, the infant death rate before 1951 was 13/1000, with infectious diseases accounting for 89 percent of the deaths (Kunstadter, 1986). The situation may have been similar for Hmong villagers in Laos.

## The Secret War in Laos and Its Aftermath: 1940s to 1990s

In the 1960s, the U.S. Central Intelligence Agency (CIA) recruited Hmong men to fight against the Vietnamese and Laotian communists and rescue U.S. pilots downed in Laos. When the United States ended its involvement in the Vietnam War in 1975, and the Pathet Lao communists took over Laos, Hmong people felt persecuted by the communist government because of their affiliation with the Americans. Between 1975 and 1995 almost 140,000 Hmong people fled Laos, seeking safe haven in Thailand. They expected that the CIA would keep its promise to help them after they had helped the United States. Beginning in 1975 and for the next twenty years, Hmong refugees in Thailand were relocated to the United States and other countries.

The refugee flight of Hmong people from Laos to Thailand and their subsequent resettlement far from Laos were the culmination of a long history of political, economic, and military events. This section briefly describes some of the complex historical events, including the role of the United States in the annihilation of Hmong people's traditional life in Laos, the massacre of Hmong people, and the creation of a Hmong diaspora. Understanding these events will help health care providers understand the source of Hmong people's mental anguish and distrust of Americans. (For more in-depth accounts, see Castle, 1992; Garrett, 1974; Goldfarb, 1982; Hamilton-Merritt, 1993; Pfaff, 1995; Robbins, 1979; Robinson, 1998; Rolland & Moua, 1994; Warner, 1995; Weldon, 1999; Yang, 1982.)

### The Secret War in Laos

During the early 1900s, French colonial Indochina was made up of Laos, Vietnam, and Cambodia. After World War II, communist Laotian and Vietnamese forces fought their respective colonial governments for independence. Vietnamese forces defeated the French at Dien Bien Phu, Vietnam, and the French signed the 1954 Geneva Accords of Indochina and withdrew from Laos and Vietnam. The accords stipulated that the Royal Lao Government would govern an independent Laos, although the country remained a member of the French Union, and Vietnam would be split into two countries, the communist-controlled North Vietnam and the independent—but still French influenced—South Vietnam.

Despite the accords, fighting between the communists and the noncommunists continued in both countries. Eventually, France pulled out of Vietnam completely, and the United States entered what had become a civil war between the South and the North Vietnamese forces, first with military advisers, and later with troops. A main military target was the Vietnamese communists' supply line, the Ho Chi Minh Trail, which wound its way from North Vietnam, across neighboring Laos, and into South Vietnam. The Vietnam conflict, having begun in the 1950s, escalated throughout the 1960s and into the 1970s.

The Hmong in Laos who did not remain neutral were divided in their loyalties between the communists and the royalists. Political ideology, familial affiliations, personal or familial power, geographical location, circumstances out of people's control, and a conflict between branches of the Lo and Ly clans affected decisions to join one side or the other. (The Lo-Ly family feud allegedly started when Lo Faydang's sister—who was also Touby Lyfoung's mother—committed suicide after her husband, Ly Foung, beat her [Cooper, 1984; Tapp, 1989; see also Lyfoung, 1996].) Some Hmong families sided with the Pathet Lao communists and joined the Lao People's Liberation Army, including followers of Lo Faydang Bliaya, who became the vice chairman of the Pathet Lao. Other families supported the Royal Lao Government, including followers of Touby Lyfoung, who had held an important administrative position in the Royal Lao Government and who became the minister of justice in the neutralist government.

In 1961, the CIA recruited Vang Pao, a Hmong lieutenant colonel in the Royal Lao Army, to enlist and train Hmong men to fight North Vietnamese and Pathet Lao communist armies. Later, he became a general and would command the eastern region, which included the provinces of Xieng Khouang, Sam Neua, and Phong Saly, where the fighting was the heaviest. Fighting also occurred in Luang Prabang province, while many western provinces, such as Bokeo, Nam Tha, and Sayaboury, were mainly unaffected by the war.

At first the vast majority of Hmong villagers were politically neutral. But as fighting became more intense and moved into their own villages and fields, more joined General Vang Pao or the communists. In their recruiting efforts, the CIA "promised that the United States would provide arms and supplies, and that in victory or defeat, the Americans would take care of them [the Hmong who fought against the communists]" (Pfaff, 1995, p. 39). There were also promises of better political and educational opportunities for the Hmong in Laos when the communists were defeated.

The fighting in Laos led to the 1962 Geneva Accords of Laos, which designated Laos as neutral; the signatories, including China, France, Laos, the Soviet Union, the United States, and Vietnam, agreed to halt all military operations in Laos. Although the United States removed its military personnel from Laos, it continued military operations there, as did the other parties. The U.S. Airforce struck at the Ho Chi Minh

Trail from airbases in Thailand. The CIA supported the Royal Lao Government against the Laotian communists with money, advisers, and equipment. USAID hired private airlines to provide essential food and other supplies to villagers and refugees, and set up schools and clinics in villages. To avoid the appearance of violating the 1962 accords and U.S. law, these war activities were kept secret from the U.S. Congress and the American public; hence, it became known as the "Secret War in Laos."

## Disrupted Hmong Lives in Laos

Between 1961 and 1975, U.S. airplanes dropped more than two million tons of bombs on northeast Laos, making it the most heavily bombed area in the world (Warner, 1995). By 1964 some thirty thousand Hmong and by 1967 almost forty thousand Hmong were serving as ground troops in the Royal Army, as guerrilla fighters in Special Guerrilla Units, and as support personnel, navigators, and pilots for the Royal Lao Airforce (Robinson, 1998). These soldiers fought against the Laotian communists, ambushing Vietnamese supply lines on the Ho Chi Minh Trail, guarding strategic U.S. radar installations, rescuing downed U.S. pilots, attacking Pathet Lao positions, and protecting their own villages and people. By 1975 between eighteen thousand and twenty thousand Hmong soldiers died and fifty thousand Hmong civilians died or were wounded (Robinson, 1998, p. 13).

The fighting, shelling, and bombing from U.S. planes so disrupted village agricultural life that families—older men, women, and children—fled to the jungle. From 1963 to 1973, an estimated one million people were displaced from their homes at least once, and in northeast Laos, half a million people were displaced from two to six times (Weldon, 1999, p. 51). In 1973, an estimated 890,000 Laotians were counted as displaced people by the Laotian government (Robinson, 1998, p. 7). Rather than leave Laos, these internal refugees sought temporary refuge in jungles and then returned to their villages or built new villages. USAID hired airplanes to fly in food and medical supplies. The planes and pilots came from allegedly private organizations, such as Air America, that were paid for by the CIA (Robbins, 1979). Also, families settled at Long Cheng (or Long Tieng), General Vang Pao's headquarters and airstrip; with a population of 50,000, it was the largest Hmong city in the world.

During these years, Hmong people also came in contact with biomedical personnel. USAID supplemented the country's meager biomedical services with hundreds of village dispensaries staffed by USAID-trained medics and with a hospital at Sam Thong staffed by a few American providers and USAID-trained medics and nurses. Although some people were reluctant to consent to invasive procedures (Westermeyer, 1986) and there were reports of Hmongs' distrust of medical practitioners (Yang, 1975), many people seemed willing to accept medicines, operations, and vaccinations (Weldon, 1999; personal communications in 1988 from J. Westermeyer, M.D., Choua Thao, R.N., Chue Vang, R.N., and Mai Lee Kong Vang, R.N., all of whom worked in Laos during the war).

## The End of the Secret War

After the 1973 Paris Peace Treaty ended the fighting in Vietnam, the U.S. and Laotian governments signed the Agreement on the Restoration of Peace and Reconciliation in Laos. In April 1974, three sides formed a coalition government, comprising the Royal Lao Government, the Pathet Lao, and the Neutralists. With the withdrawal of the U.S. forces from South Vietnam in 1975, the Pathet Lao acquired more power in Laos. When General Vang Pao attacked Pathet Lao troops, the prime minister criticized him and he resigned on May 5, 1975. Within days, the United States arranged to evacuate Vang Pao, his family, and Hmong residents out of Long Cheng. For four days, cargo planes lifted twenty-five hundred Hmong people out of Long Cheng to Thailand, while thousands of others scattered to the hills (Robinson, 1998; Warner, 1995).

At the end of May 1975, communist government forces fired on several hundred Hmong people crossing a bridge at Hin Heup on their way to Thailand, killing between five and eight people. The new government, increasingly dominated by the communist Pathet Lao, described those killed as "mercenaries in the employ of the CIA." The prime minister said to a foreign diplomat, "They [Hmong] were good soldiers. It's a pity that peace will mean their extinction" (Warner, 1995, p. 366).

## Aftermath of the Secret War

On December 2, 1978, the Pathet Lao took control of the government and formed the Lao People's Democratic Republic. The fate of the approximately 350,000 Hmong in Laos varied. Some actively supported the Pathet Lao government and gained administrative positions. Lo Faydang, for example, became vice president of the Supreme People's Assembly. Others continued their lives in their villages, unaffected by the war and its political changes. Still others returned to their villages and restarted their lives. Some Hmong people continued to live in the jungle, afraid of reprisals by the communists. In 1977, the Laotian government launched Sam Kieng, or Complete Destruction, "to wipe out the vestiges of Hmong resistance." Hmong deaths in Laos from 1975 to 1980 were estimated to range from fifty thousand to one hundred thousand (Robinson, 1998, p. 107). Hmong administrators, officers, and their wives were among the ten thousand Laotians arrested and interned in "seminars" or concentration camps. There they suffered punishment in the form of hard manual labor, little food, mental anguish, and physical torture—many died, including Touby Lyfoung (Warner, 1995).

Other Hmong people, believing that General Vang Pao would return, continued to fight against the Pathet Lao government. The Hmong resistance against the Laotian communist government was (and probably still is) supported by the Laotian Hmong in Thailand and in the United States. The resistance fighters are called the Chao Fa (or Cob Fab) or Lords of the Sky and are affiliated with either General Vang Pao's Laotian Liberation Front (Neo Hom) or Pa Kao Her's Democratic Chaofah Party (Pfaff, 1995; Panasuwan, 2000).

And many people fled to Thailand; by the end of 1975, forty-five thousand Hmong people entered hastily created refugee camps in Thailand and an equal number of people may have joined their relatives in Thai villages.

*Refugee Flight to Thailand*

Between 1975 and 1997, a total of 347,978 Laotian people left Laos, including 153,562 highland Lao, as counted by the United Nations High Commissioner for Refugees (UNHCR) (Robinson, 1998, p.294). (Ninety percent of the highland people were Hmong, and others were the Mien, Thai Dam, Khmu, Lao Theung, Lao Lue, and Htin.) Through the 1970s and the 1980s, people fled to escape the Complete Destruction policy, re-education camps, reprisals from the resistance, and loss of freedoms. Through the 1980s and 1990s, people fled for economic reasons as well as political reasons. In northeastern Laos, the extensively bombed and mined land could not be cultivated; in the south a prolonged drought decreased the national rice production; and throughout the country, the communist policies resulted in impoverished areas (Robinson, 1998).

People's refugee flights were varied. Families living in western Laos with education, political connections, and money crossed easily into Thailand, while others faced arduous journeys. The majority of the Hmong trekked through the jungle and hid from communist soldiers by sleeping during the day and walking at night. Along the way, some were ambushed by troops or ran into mine fields. They lived on what food they could forage. Some reported being bombed with "yellow rain" from airplanes. (These reports have not been substantiated and health consequences have not been medically clarified, but many people include the "yellow rain" attacks among their tragedies and blame it for health problems.)

When they arrived at the Mekong River, the Hmong made flimsy flotation devices or paid Laotian and Thai people to ferry them across on overcrowded boats or makeshift rafts. All along the way, death and disaster accompanied them. Families were separated; some were never reunited. People suffered from malnutrition, injuries, diseases, thefts, and rapes. People died from gunshot wounds, starvation, diseases, exposure, drownings, and accidental opium overdoses (opium was administered to keep infants and children from crying and giving away their presence to soldiers). (See Chapter 8.)

Most Hmong refugees found safe haven in refugee camps. The major camp was Ban Vinai, or Village of Discipline, which housed forty-five thousand Hmong people on four hundred acres of land, until it closed in December 1992. Chiang Kham held the nonpolitical arrivals after 1985 until it was closed in 1993. In 1992, Ban Napho became a camp for those who chose repatriation to Laos, were denied refugee status, or were rejected for resettlement, until it closed in December 1999. The Thai Department of Interior created these camps, in conjunction with the UNHCR, and staffed them by international voluntary relief agencies and nongovernment organizations that coordinated their efforts through the Coordination of Services for Displaced People in Thailand (CSDPT). (For an analysis of gender roles in camp activities, see Cha & Small, 1994.) Some refugees never entered the camps but just settled in Hmong villages throughout northern Thailand; if discovered, however, they were sent to the official refugee camps (Robinson, 1998). The number of people arriving from Laos, being captured in Thai villages, and being born equaled the number of people leaving by resettlement and death; this constant population led one analyst to call Ban Vinai "The Never Ending Refugee Camp" (Wright, 1986).

Initially, Laotian refugees were given formal refugee status by a group screening process, since they were considered to have a "well-founded fear of persecution for reasons of race, religion, nationality, [or] membership of a particular social group or political opinion" (Robinson, 1998, p. 6). In 1985, because the Thai government was concerned about the never-ending refugee camps (for Cambodians and Vietnamese, as well as Laotians), the Ministry of Interior unilaterally initiated an individual screening process. From 1985 to 1989, 31,001 people were screened, with 90 percent being recognized as political refugees. However, an uncounted number (perhaps several thousand) of Hmong people were "pushed back" into Laos, some with disastrous results. In 1989, the internationally agreed upon Comprehensive Plan of Action (CPA) resulted in an individual screening process; this stricter process resulted in 45 percent of Hmong people being denied refugee status (Robinson, 1998).

## Health and Health Care in Refugee Camps

Life in the refugee camps was difficult. The amount of space allotted to each family was generally quite small; sanitation facilities were limited; water supply was limited; and allotments of food were less than the international standard because of local corruption (Long, 1993; Robinson, 1998). Death rates and birth rates were high. In Ban Vinai in 1988, for example, half the population was under fifteen years of age and a quarter of the population was under five years of age (Robinson, 1998). While mortality figures are generally not available, Nongkhai camps' mortality rate was reported to be 33/1000 in March 1976 (Bliatout et al., 1988).

Many people had their first extensive contact with allopathic medicine—from preventative immunizations and contraception to curative medicines and minor operations—in the camps. Refugees were often suspicious of physicians' methods and motives: religious proselytizing was connected with health care, and Hmong refugees associated illnesses, deaths, and medical complications with the unfamiliar health care practices (Wright, 1986).

## Resettlement Choices and Repatriation

Despite the hardships of life in the camps, many Hmong political refugees were slow to volunteer for resettlement, for a combination of reasons. For one thing, refugee camp life was not much harder than village life had been, and, as Robert Cooper, the UNHCR field director in Chiang Kham Camp, speculated, the Hmong could be "more Hmong" in the camps than they had been able to be in their small and separated villages; the proximity of relatives allowed them to live their social lives and perform their spiritual rituals with extended relatives (R. Cooper, personal communication, 1990). Second, the refugees hoped they could someday return to their Laotian villages with a noncommunist Lao government. This dream was kept alive by the resistance war activities of General Vang Pao's United Lao National Liberation Front (or Neo Hom), which used the refugee camps as its base to fight in Laos (Pfaff, 1995). Third, refugees hoped that the Thai government would allow them to settle with their relatives in the Thai mountains. Fourth, people were reluctant to face the difficulties in resettling. Resettled family members sent back reports of difficulties with language, jobs, housing, and dealing with mainstream people, some of whom attacked and ate refugees. And finally, people were waiting to hear about their relatives, those not yet arrived from Laos or in other camps or with nonrefugee status or in resettled countries so they could be reunited (Long, 1993; Robinson, 1998; Tapp, 1989).

By the end of 1999, the last Laotian refugees left Thailand, over twenty-four years after the first Laotian refugees had arrived. Everyone was either resettled to third countries (see below) or was repatriated to Laos. Twenty-nine thousand Laotian lowland and highland people were repatriated to the Lao People's Democratic Republic (Robinson, 1998). (For an assessment of women's needs in repatriation, see Cha & Chagnon, 1993). About 80 percent of these were certified political refugees who chose to return to Laos or who were rejected by third countries. Only about 20 percent were not eligible for resettlement because they were not officially recognized as refugees. Provided with financial and material assistance (including land, tools, seeds, and housing materials) people could choose one of three options: individual families could return to their villages or small groups of families could join existing villages or large groups of people could start their own village (Robinson, 1998). About 60 percent of Hmong chose to start new villages (E. Kirton, personal communication, February 2000). Some Hmong organizations in the United States have protested against the repatriation process, accusing the Laotian government of killing repatriated peoples. The UNHCR directors in Laos, who monitored the process, denied that any deaths occurred and certified that the majority of repatriated refugees were doing well (E. Kirton, personal communication, February 2000).

## Resettlement in the United States

A total of 108,000 Hmong refugees were resettled in the United States. Most Hmong were destined for Australia, France, and the United States, but some went to Argentina, Canada, French Guyana, and New Zealand. The people who resettled first tended to have more formal education, French- or English-language skills, literacy, and experience in government and military authority positions than those who resettled later. Some extended families were resettled together, and others were separated and sent to different countries on different continents. For settlement to the United States (but not to all countries) men with multiple wives had to decide which wives and children to claim and which wives and children to disavow. Some sons went first to pave the way and other sons remained behind to take care of their parents, many of whom refused resettlement.

The refugees destined for resettlement in the United States spent twenty weeks in Phanat Nikom camp outside of Bangkok, where they attended educational sessions designed to help them adjust to American life. The International Organization for Migration (IOM) also conducted physical exams, immunizations, and chest X rays. People had to be cured if they had tuberculosis, venereal disease, or leprosy before they and their families could enter the United States. People were rejected if they were found to be mentally retarded, mentally ill, an opium addict, a communist, a criminal, or a polygamist, or if they had lied on their application (Robinson, 1998).

U.S. resettlement agencies—such as the U.S. Catholic Conference, Lutheran Immigration and Refugee Service, International Rescue Committee, and Church World Service—settled Hmong families with individual or organizational sponsors in cities and small towns across America. Hmong refugees who arrived in 1980 received thirty-six months of federal funds to help them adjust to their new lives, and their states received funds for language and job-training programs. In 1982, the cash assistance was reduced to eighteen months, and later all federal funds to support states' refugee assistance programs were rescinded.

Resettled people could also sponsor their family members, so that by 1982, 56 percent of all Hmong refugees in Minnesota were sponsored by their families. Over the years, resettled Hmong families relocated in different cities and states so they could be with their families. Partly as a result of this "secondary migration," the state that housed the largest number of Hmong refugees was California (where most people live in Fresno, Merced, and Sacramento), followed by Minnesota (where most people live in St. Paul and Minneapolis), and Wisconsin (where most people live in urban communities). Further migration as a result of changing social and economic conditions has brought many Californian Hmong to Minnesota and North Carolina, among other states.

## Health-Related Consequences

Monumental geopolitical forces far beyond the control of the Hmong dramatically influenced their lives. They faced death and disability; they lost some of their family members and saw some killed; they were bombed in their homes and fled to the jungle repeatedly; they faced possible death, capture, torture, rape, and imprisonment and risked drowning in the Mekong River as they fled Laos, as well as harassment and robbery by Thai people as they made their way to refugee camps in Thailand. Their sufferings occurred because of ideological conflicts in the aftermath of French colonial rule in Indochina, the U.S. political goal of containing communism in Southeast Asia, the CIA scheme to recruit Hmong men and boys as soldiers, and the U.S. military decision to drop two million tons of bombs on northeastern Laos, more than on any other area in the world.

The aftermath of these events is profound. Today, many Hmong suffer from depression, posttraumatic stress disorder, and culture shock. They share a sense of alienation, vulnerability, and powerlessness—which often translate into a self-protective mistrust of others' intentions. The experiences Hmong people carry with them from war and its aftermath, perhaps especially because of their experiences as refugees, are powerful influences in their interactions with health care providers. For this reason and for the sake of basic human compassion, health care providers need to have some sense of the traumatic historical context out of which their Hmong patients have emerged.

## Changing Lifestyle in the United States

Life changed drastically for Hmong refugees who came to the United States. When people fled war and persecution in their homeland, they had no idea what changes they would have to face. They moved from small self-sufficient agricultural villages without electricity, toilets, or vehicles to modern cities, where they had neither the resources nor the knowledge to be self-sufficient. For most people, it was a hundred-year leap in a twenty-four-hour plane ride. Transplanted Hmong society is still largely patrilineal, patrilocal, and patriarchal, though kinship relations and gender roles are changing on American soil. (For more information on changing life-styles, see Anderson, 1996; Bliatout, 1986; Bliatout et al., 1988; Corlett, 1999; Culhane-Pera, Naftali, Jacobson, & Xiong, 2002; Dana, 1993; Danes, O'Donnell, & Sakulnamarka, 1993; DeOca et al., 1994; Detzner, 1996; Donnelly, 1989; Downing & Olney, 1982; Duchon, 1997; Dunnigan, 1982; Faderman & Xiong, 1998; Foo, 2002; Hall, 1990; Hendricks, Downing, & Deinard, 1986; Hmoob Thaj Yeeb, 1998; Koltyk, 1998; Kroll, Habenicht, & Mackenzie, 1989; G. Y. Lee, 1986a; S. J. Lee, 2001, 2002; Ly, 1993; Mattison, Lo, & Scarseth, 1994; M. N. Moua, 2002; X. Moua, 2001; Olson, 1999; Parker, 1996; Peterson, 1990; Spring, 2001; Trueba, Jacobs, & Kirton, 1990; Vandeusen, 1982; Vang, 1994; Westermeyer, 1986, 1988; Westermeyer, Lyfoung, & Neider, 1989; Westermeyer, Neider, & Vang, 1984; and Xiong, 2000; for more information on acculturation, see Clark & Hofsess, 1998.)

### Elders

Elders, no longer repositories of wisdom based on relevant experience, are less respected in the United States. They suffer from culture shock, not knowing how to live or what to do. They want and need to contribute to the family but are unable to be gainfully employed, and so they do what they can. They may, for example, contribute their government checks to their families, baby-sit for their grandchildren while their children work, or embroider *paj ntaub* for New Year's clothes. Nonetheless, these activities can feel inconsequential in comparison to the contributions of the elders in Laos. Intergenerational conflicts too often end with elders losing self-esteem, exacerbating their feelings of worthlessness, depression, and rejection (see Chapters 6, 9, 10, 14, and 15). Ridden with the infirmities of old age, some elders are placed in nursing homes, despite the long-standing cultural norm that children should care for their parents until death, because family members are not able to take care of them and meet the demands of U.S. society (see Chapter 15). Alone, taken care of by strangers, they feel rejected and abandoned. Depression and posttraumatic stress disorder from the war compound their struggles to adjust to a new society (see Chapters 6, 8, and 10).

### Adults

Adult men and women have had to learn English and get jobs to support their families. While some adults have done well in school and have obtained jobs or started their own businesses, many have had difficulty adjusting to U.S. society. Also, people face discrimination as minorities in a majority society (Hein, 2000). Many people who served in the war carry physical and emotional scars and suffer from depression, chronic pain, or posttraumatic stress disorder (see Chapter 10). Not surprising, the stress of acculturation increases depression and anxiety (Nicholson, 1997), while adjusting to society by learning English and obtaining employment decreases mental distress (Westermeyer et al., 1984; Westermeyer, 1988; Westermeyer & Her, 1996).

Many adults have difficulty providing for the financial needs of their families. In 1996, 71 percent of Hmong in one St. Paul neighborhood were on public assistance and 80 percent of Hmong children in St. Paul were eligible for free or reduced school lunches (Anderson, 1996). The "Welfare to Work" laws passed by the U.S. Congress in the late 1990s increased the economic pressures on Hmong refugee families, making adjustment to a new life more difficult. Some people became more depressed, and some even committed suicide when removed from welfare programs (Chung & Bemak, 1996).

Gender roles are changing. Women are more active outside the home: they attend school, hold jobs, drive cars, and have leadership roles in community events. Even young women and daughters-in-law have more influence inside homes: managing money, participating in family conferences, and making decisions independent of men (see Chapters 2 and 9). Women's sides of the family *(neej tsa)* are becoming more important in the household's day-to-day events, and in family's problems. These changes may contribute to women's increased power within their families but they produce a lot of stress between men and women as both genders seek to make sense of their new relationships, roles, and responsibilities.

Marriages still can occur in five ways, but arranged marriages and bride capture are less common and less widely accepted. Some men have faced kidnapping and rape charges in U.S. courts for abducting women to be their brides. And some polygynous relationships do occur, although they are not legal marriages in the United States. Extramarital affairs and divorces, however, seem to occur with greater frequency than they did in Laos (see Chapters 3, 4, 11, and 12). While most marital disputes are still handled within the family, more people are turning to the U.S. judicial and social service systems for assistance and for legal documentation (see Chapter 11).

Domestic abuse and violence are on the rise in recent years as people find it more and more difficult to meet the challenges of raising well-disciplined children, surviving economically, and satisfying the emotional, spiritual, and physical needs of families. The Hmong community and mainstream social service agencies are working hard to find ways to help people who are struggling with domestic abuse. In the mid-to-late 1990s, shocking news of women killed by their husbands or lovers, men who took their own lives, and children killed in violent relationships outraged many helpless-feeling Hmong across the nation (Hmoob Thaj Yeeb, 1998).

Other societal problems—such as addictions to tobacco, alcohol, opium, and gambling—have increased, placing further burdens on families (Anderson, 1996; Hmoob Thaj Yeeb, 1998; Minnesota Department of Human Services, 2002; Westermeyer et al., 1989; Zander, 2002; Zander & Xiong, 1996). These problems are due to cultural disintegration, economic deprivation, and impaired mental health, particularly depression and posttraumatic stress disorder. Efforts to counter the problems are numerous and have been undertaken by groups as diverse as independent Hmong organizations and mainstream societal organizations with bicultural personnel. Some people see these efforts as successful, for "even though there are many changes, the value of preserving the strengths in the Hmong community is strong" (Hmoob Thaj Yeeb, 1998, p. 4).

## Adolescents

Adolescents have more influence in the family in the United States than they did in Southeast Asia. Their English-language skills are often superior to their parents' and equip them to take an active role in negotiating the relationships between their families and U.S. institutions. This role upsets the traditional relationship of elders and young people. Elders are losing respect and face while adolescents are losing the guidance of their elders. Adolescents and young adults feel the pressure to be good Hmong sons, daughters, and daughters-in-law and at the same time to be successful students and workers (see Chapters 6, 9, and 15). These roles are frequently experienced as culturally contradictory. Conflicts between the generations have generally heightened tensions in the family. Some children born in this country grow up disillusioned, angry, and rebellious. And some parents, fearing child protection authorities because they know parents have been jailed for administering physical discipline, are reluctant to discipline their teenagers. Also, many parents feel ill equipped to reach out to children who may be engaged in drugs, gangs, and risky sexual behaviors (see Chapter 10). Concerned their teenagers will choose unwisely, parents are reluctant to grant them freedom to make their own decisions or travel by themselves. These restrictions in turn can increase adolescents' anger and resistance to parents' cultural expectations.

## Children

Children present so many challenges in this new society that some parents feel they have failed as parents. While still desiring many children (see Chapter 2), parents have become acutely aware of the cultural and economic pressures to provide adequately for their children—not just basic food, clothing, and shelter but also costly educations and material possessions. When children speak directly, use vulgar language, and do not follow their directives, parents feel that children have learned from the society at large to be disrespectful. The traditional ways of responding to disobedient and disrespectful children included hitting; but in this country, Child Protective Services has investigated children's bruises, with the result that parents are fearful and uncertain how to respond to unruly children (see Chapters 5, 6, 7, and 10). Some parents may feel powerless and inadequate, not knowing how to raise children in this new society.

Both boys and girls have educational opportunities in the United States that far exceed their parents' opportunities in Southeast Asia. Over the past twenty-five years, many young adults have graduated from technical, baccalaureate, professional, and doctorate programs throughout the country. These educated men and women are fast becoming leaders and spokespersons for the Hmong community and they take pride in their careers.

## Health Status

While there is limited data about health statistics for Hmong in the United States, there is evidence that while child mortality has declined dramatically, adult health is deteriorating. (For data on Southeast Asian health status, see Takada, Ford, & Lloyd, 1998; Collins et al., 2002.) Reproductive histories collected from Hmong women in Merced, California, in 1987 suggest that the infant mortality rate was around 120/1000 in Laos, 90/1000 in Thai refugee camps, and about 9/1000 in the United States (a rate similar to that for the entire U.S. population) (Kunstadter & Kunstadter, 1990).

Results of health history questionnaires of adults over forty years of age in northern Thailand and Fresno, California, reveal that adult health is worse in California than in Thailand, with twenty times the amount of diabetes and hypertension, thirteen times the amount of mental distress and depression, and twice as many respiratory complaints (Kunstadter, 2001). Physical examinations during health fairs of volunteer adults in Fresno indicate that 79 percent of adults were overweight (>25 body mass index or BMI), 31 percent were obese (>30 BMI), and 24 percent had hypertension. All of these problems increase with length of time in the United States (Lee et al., 2000). Furthermore, many children are overweight and are becoming obese (Gjerdingen, Ireland, & Caloner, 1996).

Analyses of death certificates in Fresno from 1980 to 1999 reveal a decrease in deaths from infectious diseases and an increase in deaths from injuries and cardiovascular and metabolic diseases (Kunstadter & Vang, 2001). Nonetheless, infectious diseases are not absent; about 18 percent of the population are Hepatitis B carriers (Gjerdingen & Lor, 1997), some people have noncommunicable parasites (such as strongyloides and liver flukes), and some people's latent tuberculosis infections have become active.

Hmong people have higher rates of cervical, nasopharyngeal, stomach, hepatic, and pancreatic cancers, as well as higher rates of leukemia and non-Hodgkin's lymphoma, but lower rates of breast, prostate, and colorectal cancers than other people in central California (Mills & Yang, 1997). Hmong children have higher rates of dental caries than white children (Lemay et al., 1998). Hmong have more complications from appendicitis and have more operations with large incisions than with a laparoscope, in comparison with others in Fresno (Hu, 2000, 2001). Hmong have more uric acid stones, larger renal stones, and more renal impairment from their kidney stones, with less optimal treatment over longer periods of time than non-Hmong in St. Paul (Portis, 2002).

But all health statistics are not worse for Hmong people, when compared with majority Americans. In the 1980s, Hmong women had lower rates of high-risk pregnancies, lower complications of labor and delivery, and lower rates of cesarean-section (Edwards, Rautio, & Hakanson, 1987). Whether these rates have increased, as has occurred for other immigrant women, has not been evaluated.

Indeed, refugee flight and resettlement have brought profound challenges in a short time, with some failures and some successes in responding to those challenges. Nonprofit organizations founded by Hmong for the Hmong are finding ways to respond to the community's needs. And Hmong professionals are working with mainstream society to find creative ways to serve the Hmong in all aspects of life: social, medical, legal, educational, and economic. Hmong are making their homes in the United States, from Alaska to Florida. Reaching across the oceans, Hmong Americans are maintaining a strong sense of identity with Hmong in Southeast Asia and China and are continuing their relationships with Hmong throughout the world by letters, audiotapes, videotapes, newsletters, e-mail messages, and visits. In fact, the post-1975 Hmong diaspora seems to have broadened and strengthened the worldwide sense of Hmong identity, while the societal changes have challenged their cultural integrity.

## Traditional Spiritual Concepts

Hmong traditional religious beliefs are animistic. Beliefs about spirits, souls, birth, and death are similar to those of other animistic cultures around the world. This section describes general Hmong animist beliefs and subsequent sections focus on specific spiritual concepts about health, illness, and healing. The reader must be cautious about the English words that are used to translate Hmong concepts. While the English words "souls" and "spirits" can be used interchangeably, Hmong concepts of souls and spirits are distinct. To deal with the confusion, we consistently translate *ntsuj plig* as "soul," the energy inside people, and *dab* as "spirits," including evil spirits, good spirits, ancestral spirits, household spirits, ghosts, and nature spirits, although a few *dab* are better translated as "god." (For more information on traditional Hmong spiritual concepts, see Bliatout, 1983, 1993; Cha, 2000; Chindarsi, 1976, 1983; Conquergood, Thao, & Thao, 1989; Cooper, 1984; Cooper et al., 1995; Ensign, 1994; Geddes, 1976; Johnson & Yang, 1992; Lemoine, 1986; Morechand, 1968; Plotnikoff, Numrich, Wu, Yang, & Xiong, 2002; Siegel & Conquergood, 1985; Symonds, 1991, 2002; Tapp, 1989; Xiong, 1998b.)

### The Life Circle

The Hmong believe that the physical world and the spiritual world co-exist. The physical world is the Land of the Light (Yaj Ceeb): the world of the living, palpable and visible. The spirit world is the Land of the Dark (Yeeb Ceeb): the world of the dead and the supernatural, invisible and impalpable. Interactions occur between these co-existing worlds. Gods and spirits in the spirit world interact with human souls in the physical world, and humans interact with spirits in the spirit world.

Since life and death are joined in a continuous circle—the life circle—humans travel between these two worlds. Birth and death are doorways into these two worlds; birth is the door into the physical world and death the door into the spirit world. A person's reincarnated soul (see below) will be born again and again to live in the physical world. A reincarnated being is a direct result of the kind of life that soul previously lived in the physical world. A person who steals or murders, for example, may be reborn as an animal to be hunted by others, while a person who is noble may be reborn with a good fate and into a family of good fortune. When reborn, the soul carries with it a paper or mandate of life *(daim ntawv los ua neej)* that designates its luck or fate *(txoj hmoov)*, including its date of death.

## Gods

Hmong people conceive of multiple gods or supreme beings in the sky and on the earth who have important roles in the functioning of the natural world. We summarize some of the most common beliefs here and refer the readers to other texts for more details. (See Bliatout, 1983; Chinadarsi, 1976; Cooper et al., 1995; Johnson & Yang, 1992.)

Saub is a benevolent god who lives in the sky and who was the creator of all people. (Christian Hmong conceive of him as God.) Ntxwv Nyoog is a malevolent god who guards the gates to the dark afterlife. (Christian Hmong conceive of him as the devil.) Nyuj Vaj Tuam Teem sits behind a large desk and writes licenses for rebirth. Four gods hold up the four corners of the earth *(plaub tug tim tswv nyob plaub ceg kaum ntuj)*.

There are many gods of natural phenomenon, such as Lady Sun (Nkauj Hnub), Lord Moon (Nraug Hli), and the Dragon King (Zaj Laug). The Dragon King lives at the bottom of the sea and controls the water. He can appear as the rainbow (Zaj Sawv). Certain bodies of water are believed to house male or female dragons *(zaj)* who can steal the souls of those who play in or around the water. Yaum Xob is a god of thunder and lightning who can frighten and harm people for their misdeeds, especially lactating women who let breast milk drip onto the ground where animals could consume the milk. *Vij sub vij sw* are gods of accidents and disasters, who may be attracted to places where people have been injured or to people who have been injured.

## Spirits

Spirits *(dab)* are divided into two main types: wild spirits *(dab qus)* and tame spirits *(dab nyeg)*. Wild spirits include spirits of animate beings and inanimate objects in nature, such as rivers, trees, rocks, mountains, and river valleys. Tame spirits include healers' helping spirits *(dab neeb, dab tshuaj, dab khawv koob)*, ancestral spirits *(dab niam dab txiv, dab txwv zeej txwv koob)*, and house spirits *(dab vaj dab tsev, such as dab ncej tas, dab xwm kab, dab roog, dab kaum vaj kaum tsev, dab qhov cub, dab qhov txos, dab thab, dab txhiaj meej, and dab qab vag tsib taug)*. Helping spirits nurture, guide, and help healers cure people; healers maintain their own relationships with these spirits and nonhealers have nothing to do with them. Male heads of household are responsible for maintaining the relations and meeting the obligations that household members have with their ancestral spirits and their house spirits. In some Hmong families women take care of the spirit of the door *(dab roog)* that resides in the bedroom; but in other Hmong families, each married man takes care of his own *dab roog* that resides in his bedroom.

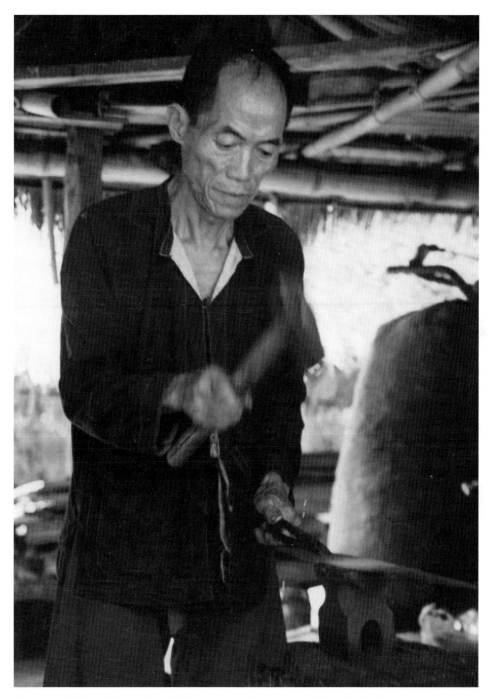

Plate 1. A blacksmith works at his forge. He makes ceremonial tools for shaman, such as metal hoops, knives, and bells, and metal necklaces and bracelets for others to wear for protection from spirit-caused illnesses. Thailand 2000. (Kathleen A. Culhane-Pera [KCP])

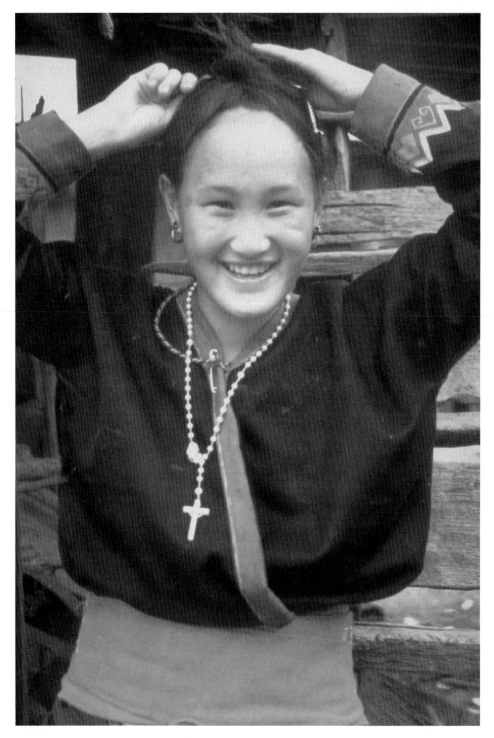

Plate 2. A young woman wears both a twisted metal necklace from a spiritual healing ceremony and a rosary from her family's conversion to Catholicism. Most people are affiliated with only one religion. Thailand 1990. (KCP)

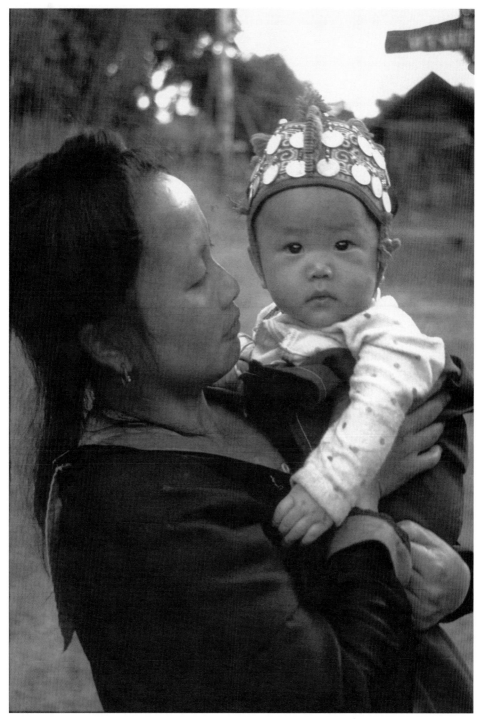

Plate 3. A White Hmong baby girl wears her traditional hat to keep her soul happy. Silver necklaces are also given to children to please their souls. Children's amulets ward off spirits and can be twisted plant fibers or cloth necklaces or cloth pouches containing herbal medicines. Thailand 1990. (KCP)

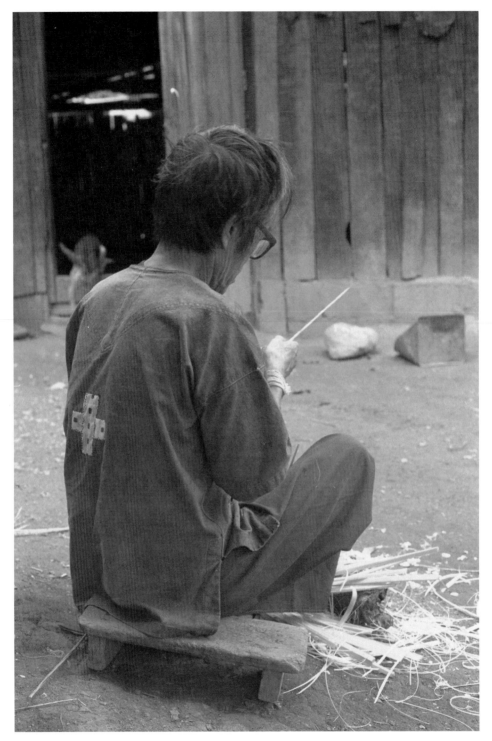

Plate 4. An older man wears a shirt with a white fabric cross. It was placed on his shirt during a ritual to extend his life *(ua neeb tiam ntawv)*. Thailand 2000. (KCP)

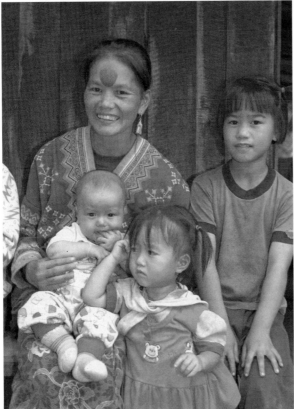

Plate 5. A woman has a circular bruise on her forehead from cupping *(nqus)*, a traditional healing method to treat illnesses such as headaches and colds. Thailand 1999. (KCP)

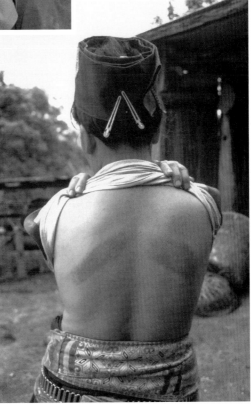

Plate 6. A woman shows her linear bruises from vigorous coin rubbing *(kav)* that treated her cold. Thailand 1990. (KCP)

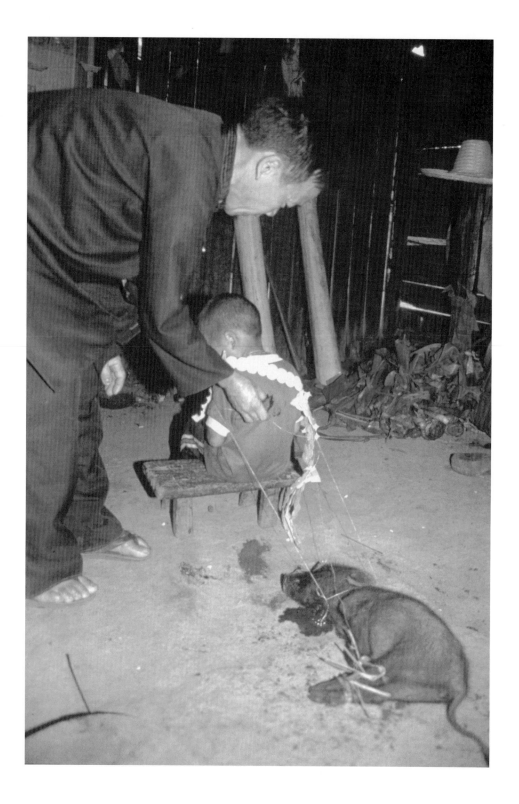

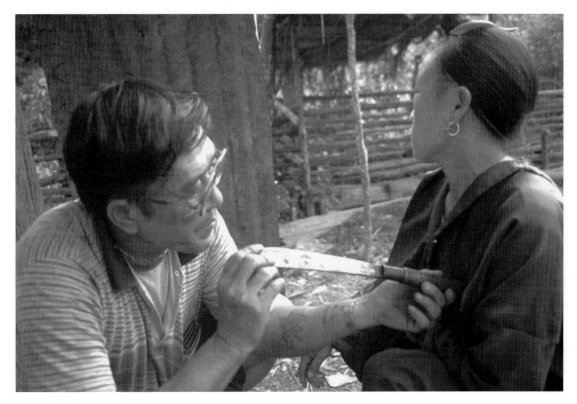

Plate 8. A man blows along a knife's metal blade to ease a woman's chest pain, during traditional magical healing *(khawv koob)*. Thailand 1990. (KCP)

Plate 7. (Opposite) A shaman places blood from a sacrificed pig on a boy's shirt during a curing ceremony *(ua neeb kho)*, thus directing the pig's soul to guard the boy for one year. The boy sits on the stool before the altar, with spirit money draped over his shoulder and back, and is connected to the pig with hemp strings. The spirit money will be burned, paying the pig's soul for its obligation. Thailand 1989. (KCP)

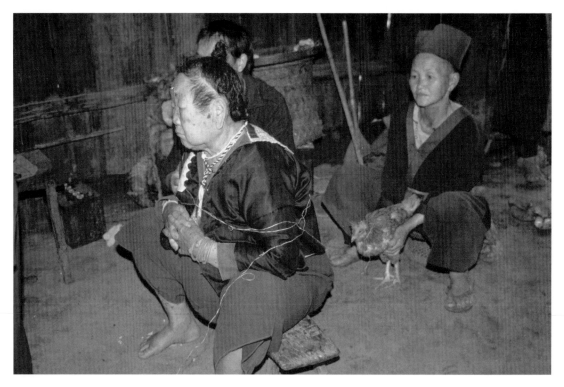

Plate 9. A woman sits during a shaman's healing ceremony *(ɯa neeb kho)*, with spirit money over her right shoulder and under her feet. Hemp strings around her body connect her to the chicken held by her daughter-in-law. The chicken will be killed and its soul directed to protect the sick woman's soul for one year. Thailand 1991. (KCP)

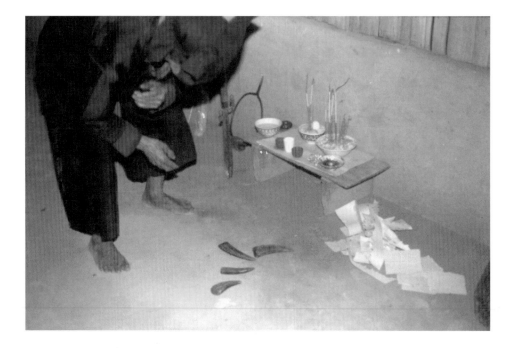

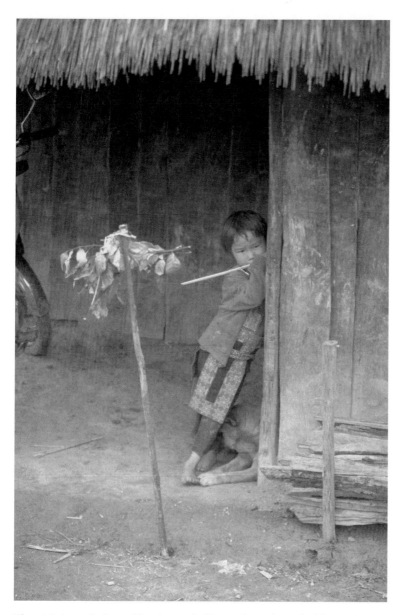

Plate 11. A symbol outside a home indicates that a household member is following a prohibition *(caiv)* for physical and spiritual health reasons. The common greeting when approaching a house is, *"Nej puas caiv?* [Are you following any prohibitions?]" The symbols may also be made of woven bamboo. Thailand 1989. (KCP)

Plate 10. (Opposite) A shaman communicates with spirits about a person's illness. He wears a black veil over his head and studies the positions of the thrown horns *(khov kuam)*. On the floor nearby is a shaman's metal hoop and dagger, spirit money, and a makeshift altar with essentials for the ceremony: two bowls of rice with incense—one of which holds an egg—a bowl of spirit water, three cups containing alcohol, and a plate for burning spirit money. The cement floor reflects new construction methods for Hmong homes that traditionally had dirt floors. Thailand 1992. (Prasit Leepreecha)

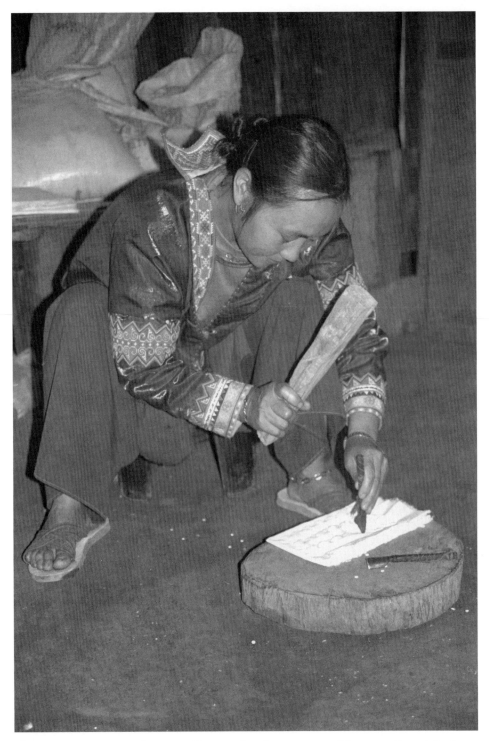

Plate 12. A woman pounds paper with a metal tool to prepare spirit money for spiritual ceremonies *(txaug ntawv)*. Thailand 2000. (KCP)

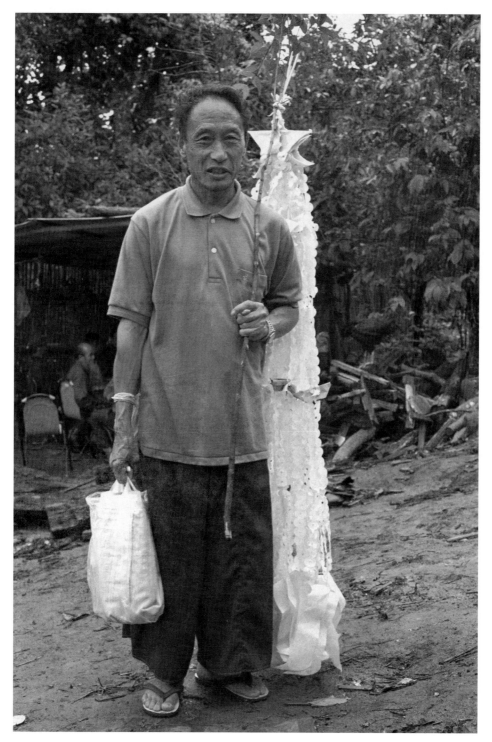

Plate 13. An in-law carries spirit money on a pole to participate in part of a funeral *(qhua txws)*. Men who are married to aunts, sisters, or daughters of the dead person will burn the spirit money to show their respect for the deceased, who will use the money to buy materials in the spirit world *(dab teb)*. Thailand 1999. (KCP)

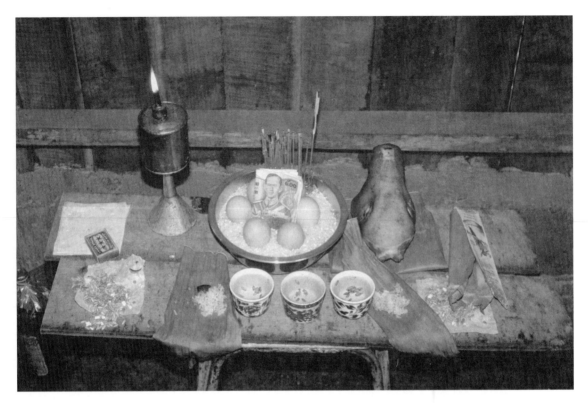

Plate 14. A New Year spirit table is situated below the household spirit altar *(dab xwm kab)*. On the table are a bowl of uncooked rice with boiled eggs, incense, Thai paper money, a pig oil lamp, puffed rice on spirit money, cooked rice on bamboo leaves, three cups of whiskey, paper money with rice kernels, and a grilled pig head on a bamboo leaf. Thailand 1990. (KCP)

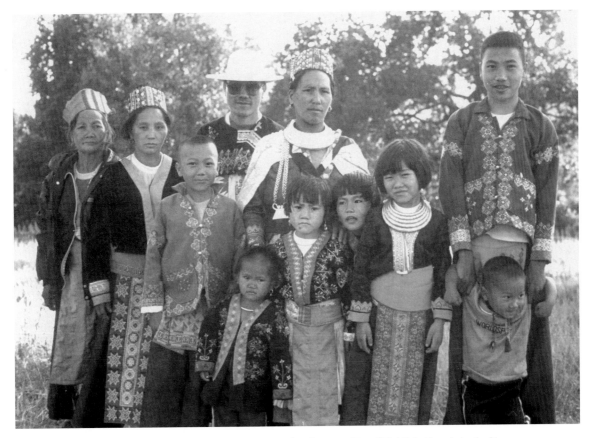

Plate 15. A White Hmong family dresses up for the New Year (Noj Peb Caug), including
husband, two co-wives, seven children, and the elder wife's mother. Thailand 1992. (KCP)

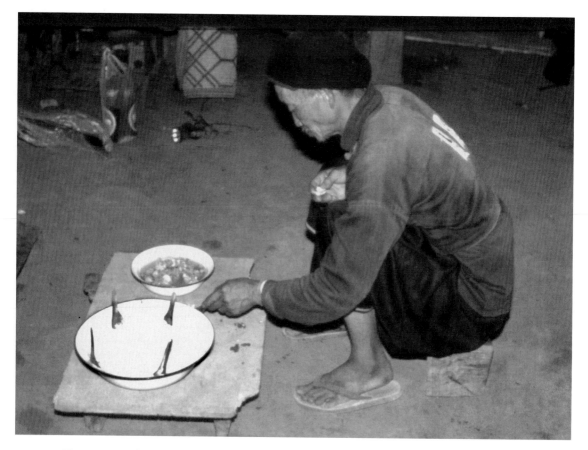

Plate 16. A male household head fulfills his obligations to communicate with his ancestral spirits *(laig dab)*. Before him is a large bowl of rice with four spoons and a bowl of meat stew for the spirits to eat. Thailand 1998. (Prasit Leepreecha)

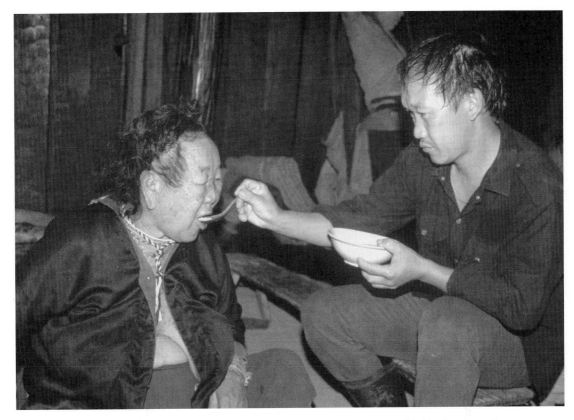

Plate 17. A son feeds his sick mother to express his love or filial piety *(hlub)*. She is wearing amulets around her neck and wrist to protect against spirits and soul loss. Thailand 1991. (KCP)

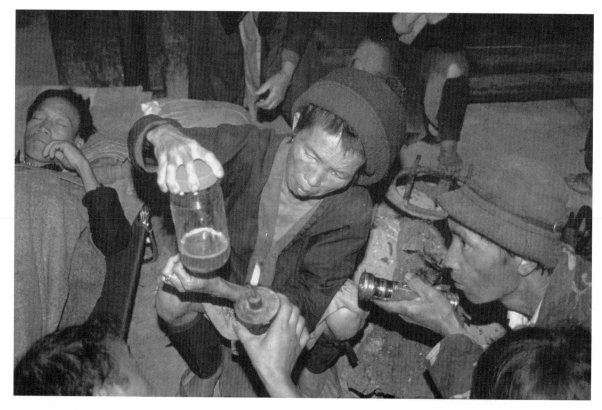

Plate 18. A woman shows the bone and hide fragments she sucked from a sick man's stomach to heal black magic spells. A man with a flashlight and a man with a pig oil lamp examine the contents while the sick man rests. Thailand 1990. (KCP)

## Souls

Animists believe that each person has several souls *(ntsuj plig)*. While there is disagreement about the exact number of souls (one, three, seven, twelve, thirty-one, or
more) and their specific names, one frequent description is that each person has three
major souls, each of which has three minor souls.

One major soul, the residing soul or shadow *(ntsuj duab* or *plig zov ntxa)*, remains
with the body at all times. After death, this soul will stay with the body as it disinte-
grates. This is the soul that living descendants revere and invite to eat and drink with
them during specific spiritual rituals *(laig dab)*. (See Plate 16.)

Another major soul is the wandering soul *(ntsuj vaj, ntsuj nyuj, ntsuj plig loj leej,* or
*yawm saub tus ntsuj duab)*, which leaves the body and goes to the spirit world when
the person dreams or is frightened, or it may wander off to play and interact with
other souls or spirits. At death, the wandering soul goes to the land of the spirits,
where life continues much as it does on earth; souls live in houses, plant fields, and
raise animals.

The third major soul, the reincarnation soul *(ntsuj plig thawj thiab* or *ntsuj qaib)* is
reborn into another being, a human or an animal; this soul carries the fate from the
previous life to the next existence. After the dead person has been buried thirteen
days or more, relatives will perform special ceremonies *(xi plig* and *tso plig)* to release
this soul to be reincarnated.

## Changing Spiritual Concepts

### Animism

In traditional Hmong communities, all aspects of life—marriages, births, illnesses,
deaths, funerals, harvests, disputes, kinship relations, and appropriate relationships
between people—were intertwined with animistic beliefs and values. In the United
States, all aspects of Hmong society, including animistic beliefs about cosmology, are
being challenged. When people first arrived, they wondered about the wild land spirits. Where do these spirits reside? Which are friendly and which are evil? How are they
offended? How do they expect to be appeased? Over the years, some answers have
become apparent: the dragon in one lake claims unsuspecting swimmers; and the
failure to make offerings to the land spirits causes illnesses. Other answers remain
hidden, and people wonder whether Americans have driven the spirits from their
land. (For more information, see Capps, 1991, 1994; Hammand, 1984; Plotnikoff, et
al., 2002; Siegel & Conquergood, 1985.)

One speculation—that spirits are frightened by electrical wires and lights—is related to the knowledge that spirits are frightened by the blacksmith's fire. The fire can
twist strands of silver, copper, and iron into necklaces, bracelets, or anklets; placed
appropriately during a shaman's ceremony, these amulets can ward off spirit attacks.
Since most people now do not have access to a blacksmith forge, they substitute necklaces, bracelets, or anklets made of twisted strands of white, red, and black cloth that
represents the three metals. (See Plates 1, 2, 17, and 19.)

Some animists are extremely concerned about the danger to health of neglecting the spirits. They believe that the spirits, enraged at the neglect, lack of reverence, and even outright disrespect shown them, have communicated their displeasure and have punished people by making them sick (see Chapter 4). For example, shaman and community leaders were concerned that the deaths of young healthy people in their sleep (which doctors called Sudden Unexpected Nocturnal Death Syndrome or SUNDS) were caused by vengeful spirits (see Chapter 10). (For more information on SUNDS, see Adler, 1994; Bliatout, 1983.) In response, in 1986, animists in St. Paul conducted a community healing ceremony to make amends to the offended spirits. Many in the community interpreted this ritual as successful: the number of sleeping deaths diminished—a perceived decline that was consistent with epidemiological data.

On many fronts American society is a challenge to the practice of animism. In general, housing is not friendly to ceremonies: apartment doors connect living spaces to inner corridors rather than to the outdoors; multiple apartments mean that different families' household spirits must share one roof; and close, nonanimist neighbors may object to the noise that accompanies the rituals. Fire laws impede the burning of spirit money or animal bones during ceremonies. Public health laws prohibit the killing of animals inside city limits. Public noise ordinances limit the noise from shaman's gongs, rattles, and chanting. Drug laws prohibit the cultivation of hemp plants, which are necessary to make the hemp cloth used in funeral ceremonies (even though Hmong use a non-pharmacologically-active species of marijuana to produce their cloth) (see Morgan & Culhane-Pera, 1994). Indeed, shaman and community leaders have been arrested for breaking the law while conducting their ceremonies.

In response to these challenges, people have made changes. Shaman perform their rituals in houses rather than apartments. Animals are brought into houses in cages and are placed behind the shaman's bench during the shamanic ritual. Chickens are brought into funeral homes but are carried away to be slaughtered elsewhere. Sometimes cows stand outside funeral homes, with strings connecting them to the corpse. White cotton cloth, yarn, and string replace bleached hemp in weddings, healing ceremonies, and funerals. Burning is limited, and fire permits are obtained. People have bought farms to raise animals and provide a space where ceremonies can occur. And some rituals have been dropped because the challenges are insurmountable (such as burying placentas under floors in houses).

The most profound challenge to animism is that fewer people are learning the rituals. As young adults struggle to fit into American society, they must spend time learning skills and knowledge that will help them adjust to current challenges. And some young adults doubt the relevance of old beliefs to their current lives. In short, while elders conduct the rituals, young people study their school assignments, go to work, watch videotapes, play computer games, or talk with their friends. In addition, some people are converting to Christianity.

## Christianity

Hmong people in southern China first came into contact with Christianity in the 1800s, and some people in Laos met Catholic missionaries in the early 1900s and others met Protestant missionaries in the 1940s. Many conversions occurred in groups of hundreds or thousands in short periods, as whole villages followed their leaders' decisions to become Christian. Explanations for these mass conversions, in addition to following leaders, include belief in an oral history that predicted foreigners would return their lost book to them and belief in a messiah that would liberate them from their difficult life conditions (Capps, 1994; Tapp, 1989).

The vast majority of Hmong Christians have converted in the United States, for additional reasons. Here Hmong have converted to please church resettlement sponsors, receive scholarships to private Christian schools, join other Christian relatives, and find unity with nonrelated Hmong community members. Some have converted because of the difficulty of finding traditional healers and ritual specialists, the difficulty of performing rituals prohibited by local laws, and or the need to protect themselves from spirit-caused illnesses. (See Chapters 4 and 9.) People have severed their relationship with their traditional spirits, or "thrown away the spirits" *(lawb dab)* through a prayer ceremony with a minister or a ritualistic burning of their spiritual affects. Some Christian Hmong have rejected Jesus and returned to their traditional religion; one reason to return to animism is a desire to use shamanic healing methods for chronic, recurring, or life-threatening illnesses, especially if prayer has not been effective (see Chapter 8). Generally, both the Christian and the animist communities tell people they should choose and follow one path, rather than following both at once or changing paths repeatedly. Also, Christian and animist leaders warn against the lack of religious commitment, for unprotected souls are more vulnerable to illness, out of the protection of either God or animist spirits. (See Plate 2.)

Although all Christian denominations reject shamanic healing rituals, they respond to other traditional animistic rituals in different ways. Hmong Catholics continue to use traditional rituals and symbols but give them new meanings. The traditional ceremony to welcome a three-day-old baby, for example, includes naming the child *(tis npe)*, calling the baby's soul *(hu plig)*, and tying strings around the baby's wrists *(khi hlua tes)* (Rice, 2000a). Hmong Catholics welcome the three-day-old baby by praying to Jesus and blessing the baby, while tying strings around the baby's wrists. One part of an animist funeral includes sending the soul to the land of the ancestors by a song *(qhuab ke)*. In Hmong Catholic funerals, people sing a new version of the song, which sends the person's soul to heaven and to Jesus. It may be that more Catholics than Protestants use traditional healing methods or try to blend both religions (see Chapter 13).

Hmong Protestants use traditional American and European songs, rituals, and texts translated into Hmong language. Unlike Catholics, they do not generally incorporate animistic concepts, rituals, or language, but they do build ideas about the devil on the traditional ideas of evil spirits, and they promote Jesus as savior on the animist understanding of life as difficult and full of suffering.

Conversions to Christianity often include everyone living under the same roof because families generally believe that animists and Christian spirits cannot peacefully co-exist in the same household. Household spirits occupy specific places and do not tolerate other spirits in their space; therefore, Christian spirits cannot live in animist homes. When families convert to Christianity, they may place the cross where the *dab xwm kab* used to rest, across from the spirit doorway into the house. Because men have primary responsibility to perform the animist rituals in patriarchal Hmong homes, they have the primary role in deciding whether to abandon the spirits and join the Christians. Brothers, fathers and sons, or uncles and nephews may consider the issues and convert together, either as individuals or as family units. When people from different religions marry, they often decide to follow one path; usually the bride changes to fit with the religion of her husband's household. Nonetheless, some individuals—especially women and teenagers—become Christian even if the whole household does not "throw away the spirits," and in some households the women influence the family's religious choices. When the whole household does not convert, animist spirit shrines remain in their places in the house, and the cross is a private symbol.

Families feel the division between animism and Christianity most acutely when brothers or uncles are on different paths; in some families the issue is extremely divisive and painful. Some Christian Hmong believe that the traditional way of the spirits is the way of the devil, and that the pagan ancestral worshipers will burn in hell for eternity. Accordingly, they are reluctant to attend animist family rituals, such as shaman ceremonies and funerals. In contrast, some animist Hmong perceive Christianity and animism to be compatible: Jesus and Siv Yis (the original shaman) were both great healers, and the Christian God and Saub or Huab Tais Ntuj (the major god in the heavens) are the same being. Animist Hmong are generally more willing to attend Christian family rituals, such as weddings and funerals, than their Christian family and friends are to attend animistic ceremonies. Others are unwilling because, they say, the songs and prayers take too long. Similarly, Christian Hmong say they cannot spend an entire day observing a shaman ceremony and therefore prefer to arrive only when the shaman ceremony is over and the feast is prepared and ready to eat. Disagreements within the same family over issues of health, illness, and appropriate healing actions may stem from different religious orientations (see Chapters 4, 9, and 15).

## Traditional Beliefs about the Causes of Illness

Traditional Hmong beliefs about the causes of illness can be described in many different schemas. We describe their beliefs in four categories: natural, supernatural, social, and personal etiologies (see Table 1.2). (For more information about causation, see Bliatout, 1986, 1990; Cha, 2000; Chindarsi, 1976; Culhane-Pera, 1989; Kirton, 1985; Symonds, 1991; Thao, 1986; Xiong, 1998b.) What people believe about the causes of their illnesses can affect their choices for treatments and can influence their emotional reactions to their discomfort. Since the concept of interconnectedness is central to the Hmong idea of health, any illness episode can be interpreted as having more than one etiology. For example, a natural etiology—such as a contagion or bad weather—or a concurrent supernatural etiology can be used to explain why many people are sick at the same time with the same problem (*ib phaum mob* or *ib phaum khaub thuas*).

## Table 1.2. Traditional Hmong Beliefs about Illness Causation

*Natural Etiologies*
Metaphysical imbalance
Contagion and germs
Heredity
Bodily constitution

*Supernatural Etiologies*
Souls
Shaman-helping spirits
Spirits or ghosts
Sorcery

*Social Etiologies*
Stressful social interactions
Curses

*Personal Etiologies*
Habits
Accidents
Reckless behaviors
Failure to follow cultural proscriptions

*Natural Etiologies*

Hmong ideas about natural etiologies can be described in terms of metaphysical characteristics similar to the Chinese concept of yin/yang. The balance of various elements in nature and in the body is essential to health: hot/cold, wet/dry, female/male, and dark/light. Imbalance in these natural and bodily forces can result in illness. Hmong believe that weather—hot or cold, dry or wet, windy or calm, but particularly a change in weather and a build-up of wind or pressure *(cua)*—can cause illness. Cold rainy weather can cause colds. If wind blows on a woman in her postpartum month, she will get arthritis and headaches in her old age (see Chapters 3 and 13). Foods, whether thermally or metaphysically hot or cold, can cause illness. If hot and sweaty people drink cold water or take cold baths, they will get sick *(lub cev ceeb)*. If menstruating women drink or eat anything ice cold, they will have premenstrual and menstrual cramping and "bad" or irregular periods or both, and they can become infertile *(lub cev khub)*. If sick children with fevers and rashes smell fried foods, they will get sicker *(phiv mob)* (see Chapter 5).

Contrary to what some Western health care workers think, the germ theory is not new to Hmong people. Ear infections, diarrhea, chicken pox, small pox, tuberculosis, and other diseases are associated with contagious germs. Some germs *(kab mob)* are observable (parasites, mites, lice, scabies, etc.) and some are not, but their existence is recognized. And as a response to contagion, affected people can be avoided or isolated; during small pox epidemics in Laos, whole villages were quarantined.

The concept of inherited disorders *(muaj caj ceg mob li)* is part of Hmong traditional knowledge. It is similar to the biomedical concept of genetically transmitted diseases, but it is not just a biological etiology, since women who marry into a family can be susceptible to that family's diseases and the disorder may be understood as caused by a curse *(khaum)*. Also, a pregnant woman's behavior can cause congenital defects. This concept is similar to the biomedical concepts of the effects of maternal behaviors on pregnancy outcomes, such as smoking tobacco, drinking alcohol, and using street drugs.

People's ability to resist illness is described in terms of their bodily constitution: healthy bodies can resist diseases better than weak bodies can. A healthy body has good fat and blood *(roj ntshav zoo)*, light and strong bones *(pob txha sib)*, and firm muscles *(nqaij nruj)* and is fat *(pham pham* for babies and *rog* for adults*)*. A sickly body has bad fat and blood *(roj ntshav tsis zoo)*, heavy and weak bones *(pob txha hnyav)*, and flabby muscles *(nqaij muag muag)*, and is skinny or emaciated *(soob soob* for babies and *yuag yuag* or *ntxaug ntxaug* for adults*)*.

## Supernatural Etiologies

The Hmong distinguish between supernatural problems caused by souls, shaman-helping spirits, spirits or ghosts, and sorcery.

### SOULS

Souls *(ntsuj plig)* can make people sick in many ways; soul loss *(poob plig)* is probably the most common. Lost souls must be retrieved for the person to be healthy or eventually the person will die. The wandering soul may wander off by itself and not be able to find its way back to the body; it may be caught in the dream world if the person wakes up too quickly; or it may leave after an emotional trauma, such as being frightened by a fall or an attack or by the sight of someone dying. Also, the reincarnation soul may leave the body if it is enticed by seductive spirits or stolen by evil spirits, or if it has chosen to be reincarnated. This reincarnation soul may inhabit a human or animal fetus while the person is alive, but once its new form is born, its prior body will die (see Chapter 14).

Since children's bodies and souls are less well-integrated than those of adults, children are particularly vulnerable to soul loss. When a child falls, the wandering soul or residing soul might not get up. When the child is running around playing, the wandering soul might be separated from the child. Hence, when parents see a child fall or when they take a child home, the adult will call the soul to come along too *(paiv tsev)* to prevent soul-loss. If the child later gets sick, a formal soul-calling ceremony must be performed (see Chapter 6). If a person falls or is frightened during a funeral, a soul-calling ceremony or a shaman ceremony will be performed immediately, before the dead person's soul can take the person's soul away to the spirit world (see Chapter 14).

There are other types of soul problems that cause illnesses. A child's soul may be unhappy with its name, its clan, or its parents (especially if they have made disparaging remarks about the child or if they are having marital conflicts). A child's soul may be angry about something that occurred in a previous life; it may want the grievance remedied or the debt paid *(tshuav nqe)*. In these situations, a healer will have to call the soul, offer it riches, make apologies, pay the debts *(them nqe)*, rename the child, or give the child a new clan name to entice the soul to stay. Souls stolen by spirits are considered a type of spirit-caused illness (see below).

## SHAMAN-HELPING SPIRITS

When shaman-helping spirits *(dab neeb)* choose someone (usually a man but sometimes a woman) to become a shaman, that person becomes sick; the shaman who treats the sick person reveals the spirits' choice *(dab neeb los thawj)*. Only if the chosen person accepts the responsibility of becoming a shaman will he physically recover. As a healer, he can use his personal knowledge of the path of sickness and death to help others (see Chapter 8). When a shaman dies, the shaman-helping spirits tend to choose someone, particularly one of the shaman's children, to take his place. A shaman must maintain a constantly healthy relationship with his helping spirits. If a shaman offends his helping spirits by not thanking them or by performing rituals not consistent with their wishes, the helping spirits may show their anger by making the shaman sick. Some shaman observe a special diet prescribed by their helping spirits.

## SPIRITS

Many types of spirit can cause spirit illnesses *(raug dab)*, including ancestral spirits *(dab niam dab txiv)*, household spirits *(dab nyeg)*, evil wild spirits *(dab qus)*, and unsettled ghosts *(dab tsis tau chaw mus)*. Ancestral spirits and household spirits protect the family; in return, families revere the ancestors and house spirits, include them in ceremonies, periodically send them spirit money and food by burning special ritual paper, and once in a lifetime send a cow *(ua nyuj dab)* to the deceased mother and the deceased father. If the family members neglect their responsibilities, or if the spirits need something from the family members, then spirits communicate their need by making someone sick. When the shaman divines the reasons behind the illness, the ancestor spirits or household spirit's message is revealed, and a ceremony is arranged to appease the spirits (see Chapters 4, 12, 13, and 15).

Wild spirits bring illnesses and death to people in various ways. *Piv nyus vaim* are Laotian jungle spirits that can transform shapes into animals, usually monkeys. When humans disturb the spirit's land, *piv nyus vaim* respond by stealing their souls. People usually die, because a shaman's power cannot match this spirit's power. If a village is built on the spirit's land, the spirit will steal their souls one at a time until everyone in the village is dead. If a hunter walks through the land, he may hear the spirit's distinct sound and try to leave before the spirit steals his soul; often his attempt is futile and he will be stricken with an illness and die within several days.

*Dab tsog* and *poj ntxoog* are malevolent wild spirits that can cause illness or death by taking away or tampering with people's souls. *Dab tsog dej* live by waterfalls and *dab tsog qhuab* live on land during the day, visiting their victims in the night. While people are sleeping, the spirits sit on top of them and squeeze the breath out of them *(tsuam)*. Thus, some people believe that these evil spirits cause Sudden Unexpected Nocturnal Death Syndrome (Adler, 1994; Bliatout, 1983; see Chapter 10). Hmong people say that when a woman crosses the stream where *dab tsog dej* lives, he has intercourse with her soul and can cause a miscarriage, stillbirth, or infertility. *Poj ntxoog* live by streams and often take the form of little girls with long hair; however, they can also transform into other human and animal forms. When they fall in love with a person, they will take that person's soul, and the person becomes sick.

People who are stricken with seizures are thought to be caught by spirits *(raug dab peg)*. The spirits will cause a person to fall to the ground, with clenched fists, stiffened arms and legs, eyes rolled back, unresponsive to verbal stimuli, and foaming at the mouth. This illness may be remedied by shaman. If shaman can bring only temporary relief, people may be susceptible to spirit capture throughout their lives.

The souls of the dead may cause illness also. During a funeral ceremony, a man sings a song *(qhuab ke)* that takes the wandering soul of the dead person into the spirit world to reunite with the ancestors. After burial, the living family members release the reincarnation soul *(tso plig)* so it can be reincarnated. Many people who died during wartime and refugee flight did not receive proper funerals and burials, and so their souls are forever lonesome, forced to roam about the physical world in an endless and futile search for their ancestors. These forlorn souls may make people sick as a way to communicate their distress and plea for assistance (see Chapter 13). In rare circumstances, a person may have been killed to guard hidden treasure; this soul cannot be reincarnated until it kills someone else to take its place, such as an unsuspecting treasure hunter.

SORCERY

People who are motivated by hate or revenge can make other people sick through sorcery *(raug pob zeb,* or *nyuj ciab)*, which can take various forms. The most common black magic practiced by the Hmong is *tso pob zeb tom,* literally, "casting stones to bite." People hire black magic specialists who send stones or other objects into people's bodies to make them very sick. To remove the stones, one must either hire the person who cast the stones or hire someone who has higher knowledge and power than the person who sent the stone (see Chapter 12). Some people say that Hmong people learned black magic from Lao and other ethnic groups. Many people are hesitant to talk about sorcery; if thought to be knowledgeable, they may be accused of being black magic specialists themselves.

## Social Etiologies

Social etiologies of illness involve human-human interactions as well as human-human-spirit interactions. When people mistreat each other in their day-to-day lives, the stress and anxiety can cause illness. A person who mocks *(qog)* a sick or disabled person may be cursed with that same illness or have children born with that same disability. And when people curse each other, serious illness can result. Words are powerful: gentle words can bring a blessing *(foom koob hmoov)* and harsh words can bring illness or misfortune *(foom lus phem)*. For example, an older woman who has suffered maltreatment or verbal abuse by a younger person can utter words in her anger and suffering that will bring misfortune on the younger person. Saub, the major god in the sky, hearing their dispute, will make the guilty person sick.

*Personal Etiologies*

Personal behaviors, too, can affect a person's health. Using tobacco, opium, and alcohol, suffering an accidental injury, engaging in reckless behavior, and not following health-promoting proscriptions can make people sick. Addiction to opium may cause weight loss, constipation, infertility, and general debilitation (Westermeyer, 1982). Accidental injuries may cause pain and impediments immediately after their occurrence, as well as years later in the form of muscle aches, joint pains, or an array of illnesses *(mob laug)*.

Not following health promotions can result in a wide range of difficulties. According to Hmong custom, food should be boiled with very little spice in order to avoid the strong odors that may aggravate a child's illness; hence, parents feel responsible if their sick children become worse *(phiv mob)* after they fry foods with garlic and chilies (see Chapter 5). Women are expected to revere their parents-in-law; if a woman has a difficult time delivering a baby, the family may interpret the difficulty as a result of the woman's inappropriate thoughts, words, or deeds against her husband's family. After deliveries, women are expected to follow specific restrictions *(caiv)* in eating, sex, and physical activities during their postpartum month. If they suffer from headaches, pains in their joints, back, and muscles *(mob laug)* or prolapsed uterus *(hlaus duav)* later in their lives, they may connect these problems with their failure to observe the postpartum proscriptions (see Chapters 3 and 13).

## Changing Beliefs about the Causes of Illness

Most Hmong in the United States continue to conceive of health holistically, in terms of an integration of the body and its souls. However, science classes in primary and secondary schools, advanced studies in nursing and medicine, and health care providers in medical facilities are influencing Hmong people's ideas about diseases, causations, and bodily functions and malfunctions. Among natural etiologies, the Hmong now include environmental chemicals, such as pesticides, fertilizers, and medicines given to animals. These environmental poisons are closely linked with a social etiology, because people blame Americans for putting poisons in their food (see Chapter 13). Germs and contagion may be figuring more prominently in concepts of natural disease, such as colds and sexually transmitted diseases. Spiritual etiologies now include ideas about spirits in the United States and the concept of Christian sin (see Chapters 4, 9, and 13). Social etiologies include the stress of being a refugee and of being caught in generational conflicts, as the generations adjust differently to American society (see Chapters 5, 10, and 15). (For more information on beliefs about the causes of illness, see Bliatout, 1988; Cha, 2000; Kirton, 1985.)

## Traditional Therapeutic Practices

Traditional therapeutic practices include home therapies, medicine doctors with herbal medicines, ritual or magical healers, soul callers, and shaman. (For more information on traditional healing, see Ahrens, 1994; Bliatout, 1988, 1990, 1993; Capps, 1991,

1994; Cha, 2000; Cheon-Klessig, Camilleri, McElmurry, & Ohlson, 1988; Chindarsi, 1976, 1983; Cooper et al., 1995; Culhane-Pera, 1989; Culhane-Pera, Cha, & Kunstadter, 2003; Ensign, 1994; Fadiman, 1997; Geddes, 1976; Johnson & Yang 1992; Kirton, 1985; Lemoine, 1972a, 1986; Morechand, 1968; Nuttall & Flores 1997; Spring, 1989; Symonds, 1991; Thao, 1986; Vang, Vang, Simmons, Tashima, & Ramirez, 1985; Xiong, 1998b.)

## *Home Therapies*

Traditionally, family members perform a vast array of healing modalities, including coining, cupping, divining, soul calling, ritual healing, and administering herbal medicines. Throughout their lives, men and women learn about illnesses, causations, and treatments. Women particularly know about medicinal plants—for example, fresh herbs *(tshuaj ntsuab)* and dried barks and roots *(tshuaj qhuav)*—that are made into teas for internal ailments or poultices for skin and musculoskeletal problems. And both men and women know how to release an illness caused by a natural etiology, such as a build-up of air, a change in the weather, germs, or spoiled food. They can vigorously rub specific areas of the body with silver coins *(kav* or coining); exert a negative pressure on the skin *(nqus* or cupping with a glass cup or *txhuav* or sucking with a horn); vigorously massage the abdomen and the arms, legs, and fingers *(zaws)*; and then poke the area with a needle or a knife *(hno)* to release the wind, illness, or bad blood. Finally, to diagnose the ailment, they examine the color, consistency, and movement of the patient's blood in a glass of water. These therapies are performed for the relief of many types of common ailments, such as colds, coughs, abdominal pains, and diarrhea. If, however, the problem is unusual, seems to be serious, or does not respond to home therapies, then family members seek out the assistance of folk specialists. (See Plates 5, 6, 23–26.)

## *Medicine Doctors*

A medicine doctor *(kws tshuaj)*, usually a woman but sometimes a man, examines the patient's body, diagnoses the condition, and gives medicinal treatments she has harvested from the forest or from her own medicinal garden. Her knowledge comes from apprenticing with an older medicine doctor and from her helping spirits *(dab tshuaj)*, whose wisdom guides her as she examines, diagnoses, and prescribes. Some medicinal healers have special areas of knowledge, and some are generalists. People may consult them for a wide range of physical ailments, including fevers, headaches, wounds, abdominal pains, menstrual irregularities, infertility, impotence, prolonged labor, fetal malpositions, and many others. People usually pay a nominal fee for their services, although the medicine doctors may give free treatments to those who ask graciously. In cases of treatment for infertility, medicine doctors may expect payment only if the medicine proves effective. And if the treatment is effective and the couple does not keep their end of the bargain, the medicine doctor may curse them, for their action is interpreted as cunning, dishonest, and disrespectful to both the medicine doctor and her helping spirits. And some doctors would say that their helping spirits could make them sick if they were not paid, since the clients and doctor were being disrespectful to the helping spirits.

## Ritual or Magical Healers

A ritual healer *(kws khawv koob)*, sometimes referred to as a magical healer, performs healing rituals *(khawv koob)* to cure various types of ailment, depending on specific knowledge. This healer, who is usually a man, learns his craft from other healers who pass along their knowledge, healing power, and helping spirits *(dab khawv koob)*. He calls the spirits with incense and communicates with them using ancient Chinese and Laotian words. The healer directs his helping spirits toward the person's ailment through different media, including a bowl of water with silver coins, a metal knife, or his own breath. Families consult healers with expertise in specific problems, such as burns, broken bones, eye problems, startled children, childhood fevers with rashes, hemorrhage, recurrent spontaneous abortions, and headaches (see Chapters 5 and 14). Some ritual healers gain their power through Laotian spirits that unveil solutions to the many forms of physical, psychological, and spiritual suffering that humans face on earth. (See Plate 8.)

## Soul Callers

Some illnesses may be caused by soul loss and thus require a soul-calling ceremony *(hu plig)* (see Chapters 6 and 14). Many types of evidence indicate that soul loss has occurred: historical events, such as being frightened or falling at a funeral; physical symptoms, such as fatigue or failure in children to thrive; divination procedures, such as breaking an egg into water; or physical signs observed by family members, such as pallor, sunken eyes, or dry lips, or interpreted by healers, such as the pattern of blood vessels behind the ear lobe. If no household member knows how to call the soul or if the family's attempt is not successful or if the patient's condition is serious, then a revered soul caller *(tus hu plig)* is consulted. While variations exist, the basic soul-calling ritual starts where the fright or fall occurred and then moves to the spirit door of the sick person's house. To entice the soul back home, the healer holds a live chicken while chanting sweet words, burning incense, and offering whiskey and food to the soul. The healer divines the soul's response by interpreting the pattern of split animal horns (or makeshift wooden pieces to resemble horns) that he throws on the floor. After the chicken is cooked, the caller examines the chicken's feet, tongue, and skull for evidence that the soul has returned and to interpret its condition. If the ceremony is unsuccessful, a shaman will have to retrieve the wayward soul. (See Plates 27–29.)

## Shaman

The supreme folk healers are the shaman *(tus txiv neeb)*, who have varying levels of abilities. Low-level healers choose to learn some shamanic healing rituals; they are called white-faced shaman *(tus txiv neeb muag dawb)* because they conduct their healing rituals without going into a trance as chosen shaman do. They can call wayward souls and strengthen people's spiritual health. However, shaman who have the ability and skill to go into a trance have been chosen by shaman-helping spirits *(dab neeb los thawj)*. With the help of an experienced shaman, the shaman-in-training learns to enter into a trance with either a black or red cloth over his face *(tus txiv neeb muag dub* or *muag liab)*, speak the spirit language, travel between the spirit and physical worlds, fight offending spirits, and negotiate settlements with the spirits so sick people can get well (see Chapters 8 and 13). (See Plate 10.)

Although anyone from the sick person's family may initially ask a shaman to perform a ceremony, usually it is male family members and not the sick person (see Chapter 10). Male family members must be present, however, to bow to the shaman at the beginning and end of the ritual. Initially, the shaman may throw goat or cow horns *(khob kuam)* at the base of the shaman's shrine *(thaj neeb)* or perform other divination procedures to gain a general idea of the reasons for the illness. The position of the horns conveys the spirits' responses to the questions posed. Usually the shaman does not examine the sick person's body to diagnose the illness or discover its cause. Next, the shaman performs a diagnostic ritual *(ua neeb saib)* to determine more specifically what spiritual problem is causing the illness. He sits astride a bench in front of his shrine, a cloth over his face, a bell on his finger, and a rattle in his hand. A male assistant bangs the gong behind him, and the shaman enters into a trance. The bench becomes a winged horse carrying him into the land of the rain and clouds to fight and negotiate with the spirits causing the illness. Having won the battle, the shaman convinces the defeated spirits to relinquish their hold on the person within a specified time. The shaman returns from his dangerous trip and comes out of the trance. He tells the family that he won the battle and assures them that if the spirits keep their promises, do not lie, or do not change their minds, the sick person will recover within the specified number of days *(teem caij)*.

If the sick person does recover, the family commissions the shaman to do the curing ceremony *(ua neeb kho)*. During this ritual, the cured person sits behind the shaman, who goes into a trance; at specific points, the shaman's assistants burn spirit paper money, kill the designated animals (usually chickens or pigs), and dab the cured person's shirt with the animals' blood. The shaman commands the animals' souls to stay either with the spirits in exchange for the sick person's soul or with the sick person and guard his soul. The animals' souls thus commissioned must stay at their jobs until the following New Year's ceremony, at which time they will be released from their bondage when the shaman burns the lower jaws of the sacrificed animals so they can be reincarnated *(mus thawj thiab)*. In addition, strings may be tied around the sick person's wrist to keep the wandering soul in the body; three types of metal strand may be twisted into amulets to ward off evil spirits; or strips of white or white, red, and black cloth may be sewn onto the back of the sick person's shirt to symbolize that the mandate of life (or the predetermined date of death) has been extended *(ntxiv ntawv)*. (See Plates 4, 6, 9, 12, 14, 17, 19, and 21.)

After the shaman has determined the cause and won the battle with the spirits, further ceremonies might have to be performed. For example, a cow might be sacrificed to a deceased parent *(ua nyuj dab)*. A grave disturbed by animals or overgrown with plants may be repaired *(kho lub ntxa)*. A reincarnated soul that is going to be born in the body of another being might have to be captured and returned *(tsis pub mus thawj thiab)*. The souls of a pregnant woman and her fetus might have to be separated so they do not both die from complications in labor and delivery *(faib thiab)*. If a family is bothered by spirits, a shaman may call all their souls together as they stand as a group encircled with hemp strings *(koos plig)* or a shaman may confine them to the house *(caiv)* for a specific number of days in order to hide their souls from evil spirits. (See Plate 11.)

## Changing Therapeutic Practices

Traditional Hmong therapies persist in the United States today. Families across the country practice coining, cupping, massage, soul calling, ritual healing, and use of herbal medicines. Since tropical plants are often difficult to obtain or to grow, women grow what they can in their summer gardens or in their winter greenhouses. They send fresh plants from warmer to colder parts of the country, send for dried plants from Laos and Thailand, and barter or sell what they have to their community. The knowledge of ritual healing and soul calling is being passed on. New shaman are being chosen and are apprenticing. Time will tell whether enough young people are learning these skills to keep them alive after the elders are gone.

Some Hmong people bring their traditional healing modalities—particularly massage, medicines, and ritual healing—to hospitalized family members. After initial uncertainty, concern, and even fear, some hospitals have come to accept these practices. Rituals that involve burning incense have required hospitals to make accommodations. Some hospitals allow burning incense only in special rooms, while a few allow it anywhere, including intensive care units, as long as there is no open flame. Shaman ceremonies are not conducted in hospitals, however, since shaman spirit shrines must be located in houses where there are household spirits. Sometimes a shaman may perform the necessary ritual at home, while the patient remains in the hospital; but at other times the sick person must be present for the ceremony to be effective. (For other changes in shaman practices, see above, Changing Spiritual Concepts.)

Christian prayer groups led by ministers and priests gather in hospitals, churches, and homes on behalf of those who need healing. For many Christian Hmong families, these groups seem to substitute for the healing function of the shaman, generating feelings of well-being, hope for speedy recoveries, and confidence that there will be a cure. Almost all Christians continue to use traditional herbal medicine *(tshuaj ntsuab)*. Some may use ritual or magical healing. Other Christians do not, convinced that these traditional healers have connections with spirits that are inconsistent with their Christian beliefs. Nonetheless, when serious or chronic illnesses do not respond to prayer or Western medicines, some Christians turn to traditional healing practices, including shaman rituals, and some people convert back to animism (see Chapters 4 and 8). (For more information on changing therapeutic practices, see Ahrens, 1994; Bliatout, 1988, 1990, 1993; Capps, 1991, 1994; Cha, 2000; Cheon-Klessig et al., 1988;

Culhane-Pera, 1989; Ensign, 1994; Fadiman, 1997; Kaptchuk, 1997; Kirton, 1985; Lemoine, 1986; Moua, 1996; Nuttall & Flores, 1997; Putsch, 1988; Spring, 1989; Xiong, 1998a.)

## Traditional Beliefs and Practices
## Regarding Disease Prevention and Health Promotion

Traditional Hmong concepts of health promotion and disease prevention correspond to Hmong concepts of disease causation. To prevent children's illnesses, parents must cover their children's heads with hats to protect them from the wind; make them beautiful silver necklaces to please their souls; attach dried herbal amulets to their hats, necklaces, or bracelets to ward off evil spirits; refrain from washing their fontanels, where a soul resides; call them ugly so that spirits who steal beautiful children will not be alerted to a child's beauty; and please their children so that their souls do not get angry and leave (see Chapters 5 and 6). To avoid the house spirits' anger, women must not touch the ancestral post. In some families, daughters-in-law cannot climb up to the loft above the fireplaces or else their fathers-in-law will become blind because of a curse *(tsawm thiab foom)* placed generations ago. Women must not be physically above their husbands, such as on roofs while changing the thatch or uphill while planting corn or harvesting crops, or else their husbands will lose sexual power.

Pregnant women must refrain from raising their arms above their heads or carrying heavy objects to avoid a miscarriage and from cutting cloth in their bedrooms to avoid causing their child to have a cleft palate. They must refrain from rearranging their bed during pregnancy to avoid a second or third trimester miscarriage or premature birth. To ensure a healthy pregnancy and easy delivery, women should eat what they crave and must think welcoming thoughts about their baby and have pleasant relationships with their parents-in-law. (see Chapter 3). In their postpartum month, new mothers must follow the traditional cultural prescriptions and prohibitions in order to regain their health, ensure breast-milk production, maintain fertility, and enjoy old age without rheumatism. Also, a new mother must avoid pregnant women because an unborn child's soul may take away a new mother's milk, depriving her newborn of sufficient milk supply. (For more information on prenatal and postpartum health, see Morrow, 1986; Rice, 1997, 1999, 2000b, 2000c; Spring, 2001; Spring, Ross, Etkin, & Deinard, 1995; Spring, Davis, & Rode, 1997.)

To preserve their health, men must not enter households that have been placed under restrictions to appease the spirits *(caiv)*, in order to prevent the spirits from attacking them; must avoid making love immediately after sweating from hard labor in a hot sun, to preserve their sexual strength; and must not walk under women's pants on a clothesline, to protect against impotence. If men fail to conduct marriage, funeral, and household spirit rituals correctly or fail to thank land spirits after harvesting rice crops, the spirits can make them and their family members sick. If men weave hemp cloth, animals will not enter their traps. Men of certain clans may have specific taboos; for example, men of the Yang clan cannot eat beef hearts or they will die. And animist families must have a shaman ceremony performed annually to protect their souls from harm, disaster, and illness.

When children are sick, parents prepare boiled bland foods and avoid cooking odiferous foods to prevent their children from becoming sicker (see Chapter 5). When people are ill from soul loss or spiritual causes, restrictions may be placed on them and their families, such as not leaving their home or not having others visit for several days; if these restrictions are not followed, the sick people may not recover. Also, a cloth human figurine *(moj zej)* may be sewn on the back of a sick person's shirt to fool evil spirits who might want to take his or her souls away.

While most of these actions seem foreign to Western health care providers, they illustrate the richness and complexity of the Hmong traditional concepts of disease prevention, as well as the connection between ideas about disease causation and actions to prevent disease.

## Changing Beliefs and Practices
## Regarding Disease Prevention and Health Promotion

Both animist and Christian Hmong continue to practice some traditional measures of prevention in the United States. As Hmong become more aware and knowledge-able about Western concepts of illness and the Western medical system, their beliefs and practices are changing. Nonetheless, biomedical practices to detect or prevent diseases, such as cancer screening and vaccinations, present challenges. Many people have been unwilling to undergo Pap smears, sigmoidoscopies, and other embarrassing or risky procedures to look for asymptomatic diseases (see Chapter 4). Despite the modest success of special programs to increase rates of Pap smears and mammograms, resistance persists, particularly among older women who have poor English-language skills and no formal American education.

In the 1980s and 1990s many parents and grandparents were reluctant to inject dead or weakened germs into their children to prevent diseases they may not catch because the adults were concerned the shots would cause fright, fevers, swollen pain-ful limbs, paralysis, and death. Parents were most reluctant to vaccinate children whom they believed were most vulnerable to the side effects, such as young infants, skinny children, and heavy-boned children. Out of their love *(hlub)* for their children, some parents delayed vaccinations until their children were older (Xiong & Culhane-Pera, 1995; see Chapter 5). Low rates of measles vaccinations were linked with a measles outbreak in St. Paul (Henry, 1999). Resistance to vaccinations is decreasing as people become more familiar with them and as side effects are seen less often. Some parents report that vaccinated children are sick less often or sick less severely than non-vaccinated children. Generally, family members assess both the risks of the procedures to prevent diseases and the risks of the diseases before deciding whether to obtain vaccinations.

## Concepts of Anatomy and Bodily Functions

Traditional concepts of anatomy and bodily functions are difficult to ascertain. No historical texts exist, and present-day descriptions of traditional concepts seem to have been influenced by modern medical concepts. Nonetheless, while Hmong people's concepts of the human body may be similar to Western concepts, the cultural associations and social implications of bodily functions are very different. The following descriptions come from interviews with Hmong men and women and from professional clinical experience with Hmong patients and their families in the United States from 1994 to 1999 (Xiong, 1998a). (For more information on Hmong concepts of anatomy and bodily functions, see Fang, 1995; Wausau Area Hmong Mutual Association, 1995.)

Every part of the human body, from head to toe, is essential to the whole. Many Hmong animists believe that each body part has a "soul" existence, which is so important that if one body part is sick, deprived, or saddened, the whole body will eventually become affected. One man explained, "If the mouth thought, 'The stomach is too greedy; I will not eat so the stomach will have no food,' then it too will be deprived. For if there is no food, the body dies and when the body dies, the mouth dies."

The brain *(lub hlwb)* is the thinking center. The soul that governs the head and protects the body resides on the baby's soft spot (the anterior fontanel). Hence, the soft spot is a sacred place, and some parents do not wash this area until the soft spot closes. Similarly out of reverence, people do not touch each other's heads, particularly adults' heads. Touching the head of an adult is disrespectful and degrading.

The heart *(lub plawv)* is the central organ of the body, providing it blood and life. According to one shaman, the reincarnation soul resides in the heart. Of the souls that a shaman is called upon to retrieve, this is the fastest; it is described as *tus ntsuj rag huab pag*—the fastest central soul. If this soul has left the body to be reincarnated, the shaman must exercise tremendous strength and power to capture and return it. If the shaman cannot catch the soul, the shaman has no choice but to say, "Good-bye and good luck." Once this soul is born into another being, the body it previously occupied dies, because its life center is gone.

Westerners associate emotions with the heart. The Hmong, however, locate emotions in the liver *(nplooj siab)* (see Table 1.3). People's personalities, attitudes, and certain behaviors are described in terms of the liver (see Table 1.4).

Some people believe the liver's two halves represent two parts of a person's per-

## Table 1.3. Liver as the Seat of Emotions

| Emotion | White Hmong Expression | Literal Translation |
|---|---|---|
| happy | *zoo siab* | good liver |
| stress free | *kaj siab* | light liver |
| encouraged | *muaj siab* | have liver |
| satisfied | *txaus siab* | done liver |
| angry | *chim siab* | angry liver |
| lonely | *kho siab* | longing liver |
| jealous | *mob siab* | pained liver |
| frustrated or worried | *ntxhov siab* | clouded liver |
| depressed | *nyuaj siab* | troubled liver |
| deeply wounded | *tu siab* | broken liver |

sonality. One side is the seat of goodness *(daim nplooj siab zoo)* and the other side is the seat of badness *(daim nplooj siab phem)*. A person who has a larger good lobe tends to be good-hearted, and vice versa. The two lobes often battle within an individual; sometimes the good lobe wins and sometimes the bad lobe wins. In good-natured people, the good lobe wins more often and in bad-natured or evil people, the bad lobe wins most of the time.

The lungs *(lub ntsws)* are the breathing organs. While the biomedical concept of the lung acting to oxygenate hemoglobin in red blood cells is not part of people's understanding of lungs and blood, people do recognize that entry of air or wind *(cua)* into the body is essential for life.

Blood *(ntshav)* is the sustainer of life, strength, and color; the quantity of each person's blood is finite and is not rejuvenated. If people lose too much blood, they become weaker and sicker. This is why patients might oppose blood draws, especially if they are bleeding, pale, fatigued, or weak (see Chapter 3). People recognize the presence of red blood and dark blood in the body, interpreting bright red blood as alive and good *(ntshav ciaj* or *ntshav liab)* and dark black blood as dead and bad *(ntshav tuag* or *ntshav dub)*.

The stomach *(lub plab)* and the intestines *(hnyuv)* are understood to be digestive organs; the stomach is as important as the intestines. Patients are more willing to let surgeons remove part of their intestines than part of their stomachs because intestines are larger than stomachs. The gallbladder *(lub tsib)* contains green or bitter fluid. Patients may be willing to allow surgeons to remove a diseased gallbladder because they view gallbladders as being less than essential. The functions of the spleen *(po liab)* and the pancreas *(po dawb)* are not clear to most people; in fact, some people do not distinguish the two organs, or are not familiar with the pancreas (see Chapter 8). The kidney filters blood *(lub nraum lim ntshav)* in order to make urine, which is stored in the bladder.

Now that the Hmong have been in contact with Western ideas of biology and

## Table 1.4. Liver as Character Type

| Character Type | White Hmong Expression | Literal Translation |
|---|---|---|
| brave, confident | *siab loj* | big liver |
| easily frightened | *siab me* | small liver |
| generous | *siab dav* | wide liver |
| stingy, judgmental | *siab nqaim* | narrow liver |
| good person | *siab zoo* | good liver |
| selfless person | *siab dawb* | white liver |
| bad person | *siab phem* | bad liver |
| malicious person | *siab dub* | black liver |
| hardworking, efficient | *siab sib* | light liver |
| slow, inefficient | *siab hnyav* | heavy liver |
| patient | *siab ntev* | long liver |
| impatient | *siab luv* | short liver |

medicine for twenty to thirty years, they are adopting English words for some concepts and adapting Hmong words to clarify others. The variations in words can result in confusion with interpretation and communication errors. To date, there is no Hmong medical terminology book available that is agreed upon by Hmong health care professionals, traditional healers, community leaders, and elders.

Certain phrases in Hmong do not directly correspond to the same organs as the English equivalent. For example, *siab* means liver, but *hauv siab* means chest and not the literal translation, "inside the liver." If a Hmong person describes pain as *mob hauv siab,* the pain may be located in the chest or in the epigastrium, next to the liver. Thus, the assessment of a Hmong person with chest pain must include a careful history and examination with the assistance of a medically trained interpreter.

## Traditional Illness Decision Making

Caring for sick family members is an expression of love *(hlub),* a strong social value of devotion toward family members. Because Hmong people measure love in actions rather than in words, caring for sick people is an important expression of love. People assume the sick role when they are weak and infirm. Unable to eat, drink, perform social tasks, or fulfill social responsibilities, sick people take to their beds. Family members then take care of them, feeding, clothing, and grooming them, and making medical decisions about the appropriate healers and necessary therapeutic modalities. Because sickness impairs the ability to think clearly and make correct decisions, people expect that healthy family members are the best people to make decisions about the sickness. Sick people experience this caring in a loving manner. While they may not participate in the discussions, their best interests and desires are considered. In general, this is true whether the sick person is a child, an adult, or an elder, though sick adults may be more involved than sick children and elders in the decision-making process. (See Chapters 9, 13, and 15; see Plate 17.)

While certain people—particularly male family elders, clan leaders, or community leaders—are highly respected and have more power *(muaj kev cai* or *hwj chim)* to influence the process, usually there is no one decision maker who tells everyone what to do. Rather, family members talk at length about risks and benefits, consequences of action and inaction, and alternative approaches. Families value working together to arrive at a consensus. A shared family-based decision ultimately means family-based shared responsibility for the consequences of actions or inactions. If a patient or a patient's parent or spouse makes an independent decision, then he or she is solely responsible for the outcome and could be socially reprimanded for any negative consequences of the decision. (See Chapters 3, 5, 7, 9, and 11.)

As a decision-making unit, families value their traditional knowledge about illness and their abilities to heal many ailments. Most healing happens within the extended family. Traditional adults are confident of their abilities to call souls, give medicines as teas or poultices, or make offerings to household and ancestral spirits. They know whom to consult, how to evaluate the results of the consultation, and how to decide whether to follow the healer's recommendation. When in their collective judgment specific expertise is warranted, families will seek out trusted specialists.

They value the respect that traditional healers show them, as they fulfill their social duty to their sick family member, and they value treating the healer with a concordant amount of respect. If healers treat them disrespectfully, they may no longer feel required to be respectful to the healer, and their trust of the healer and the healer's specific recommendations decrease.

As consulted healers and providers lay out their recommendations, family members weigh the pros and cons of all the options before deciding which is the best route of care for the sick patient. If the risks of the intervention are great, then family members may decide not to use that approach. After treatments, family members evaluate their effectiveness. If the expected or desired result does not ensue, then family members may try other alternatives. If treatments fail, family members are comforted by the cultural interpretations of the sufferings or death: perhaps fate determined the length of the person's life or the soul wanted to be reborn or evil spirits succeeded in their goal or germs arrived from other villages.

Family members' beliefs about an illness—its cause, the meaning of the signs and symptoms, the severity, and the diagnosis—influence their decision to seek care and to respond to recommendations for diagnostic tests or therapeutic modalities. Family members determine possible etiologies by considering the sick person's symptoms, bodily signs, and historical events, as well as conducting divination procedures. While any sickness could have a natural or a supernatural etiology, generally signs and symptoms that are acute and discrete tend to be caused by natural etiologies. But diseases that have protracted courses and general debilitating symptoms, such as fatigue, weight loss, and loss of appetite, tend to be caused by supernatural etiologies. Bodily signs that indicate a supernatural etiology include feverish heads with nonfeverish bodies, erratic pulses that stop when attacking spirits are named, and blood that is flowing backward in an ear. Since interpreting signs and symptoms can be confusing, people turn to historical events and divination procedures to assist them. If a baby has been startled, a child has fallen at a funeral, or an adult has had an accident, family members will be more convinced about an underlying soul loss. Divination procedures help people identify the offending spirits, diagnose soul loss, determine where the soul has gone, and determine which spiritual healers have the power to heal the situation.

Etiology may be considered concurrently with the meaning of signs and symptoms, including illness severity. If the illness is considered common or nonserious (such as a cold or watery diarrhea), people may do nothing. If specific symptoms or bodily signs indicate that the illness is serious, people are more motivated to spend resources—time, energy, money, and animals—on addressing the illness. Determining etiology and seriousness and diagnosis is not always straightforward; people's evaluations can change, and any given illness episode can be understood to have more than one etiology, severity, or diagnosis.

The suspected etiologies, severity, and diagnoses influence treatment choices. For natural etiologies, people turn to natural treatments (herbs, massage, coining, cupping, ritual healing, or even Western medical providers); for soul loss, families arrange for soul-calling ceremonies; and for supernatural problems, they consult shaman. Many illnesses are assumed to be due to natural etiologies, and so natural treatments are often attempted first. If the treatments are not effective, if the illness changes or worsens, or if biomedical providers cannot find anything wrong, then family members may pursue possible supernatural etiologies.

In addition, family members have to consider logistical issues as they make their decisions, including the accessibility of healers, the availability of transportation, the costs of the healers and travel, and the competing demands on their time, money, and other resources.

## Changing Illness Decision Making

Health care decision making is changing in the United States. The process is highly variable and is in flux; there is no single decision-making path that fits all sick people, all illnesses, or all families. General elements are presented here, and a sampling of the range of decision-making practices are represented in the stories in this book.

Many of the traditional Hmong ideas and activities about sickness, disability, infirmity, and families' responsibilities to care for infirm people continue in the United States. When most people—particularly middle-aged and older adults—are unable to work or carry out their household duties, they stop working and allow their families to care for them, including making medical decisions for them. Families are still active in making decisions for members who are sick, and they are as responsible for adults as they are for children. Thus, Hmong families are perplexed when health care providers intervene on the behalf of minors, for the families see themselves solely responsible for the welfare of their children, as they are for adult family members (see Chapters 5 and 7).

Some sick individuals—particularly American-educated young adults—are taking more active decision-making roles. They may voice their opinions at family conferences or make their own decisions without asking for family assistance or make decisions that go against their family's wishes. Nonetheless, they may still experience social displeasure with their decisions, particularly if there are negative consequences of their actions (see Chapters 2, 3, and 9).

Who participates in family-based decision making is changing. Although the husband's side of the family *(kwv tij)* still has the main responsibility for medical decision making, the wife's side of the family *(neej tsa)* may join the husband's side of the family in the deliberations, with women's sisters and maternal grandparents speaking their opinions and voicing their desires more often than in the past (see Chapters 3, 4, and 15). More women speak at family conferences, whether they sit in or behind the inner circle of discussants. Some sick women make their own final decisions after hearing the entire family's opinions, wishes, and desires. Family members also consider advice from a wider community of people, including extended family, friends, interpreters, church members, community members, Hmong professionals, and American friends. Other people's experiences hold considerable weight, particularly when dealing with life-threatening illnesses or dangerous therapies that are new for patients and their families.

People's characteristics—including their age, gender, religious beliefs, amount of formal education, and extent of acculturation—influence their preferences. In general, older people who were born in Laos, follow the traditional religion, and do not speak English are more comfortable with traditional Hmong therapies and more concerned about adverse effects of allopathic medicine and surgery than young adults educated in the U.S. school system. Family members still evaluate the risks and the benefits of care as they make decisions for their sick loved ones, whether about examinations, diagnostic procedures, or treatments. While their understandings and evaluations of risks and benefits are changing, they may refuse care that is dangerous or has serious side-effects, even when providers believe the therapy may be lifesaving. For example, people are more willing to consent to appendectomies now than in 1979, but many people are still fearful of radiation and chemotherapy for cancer. Generally, Hmong people are more willing to accept the risks of the intervention if they feel the potential benefits are worth the risks. (See Chapters 13 and 15.)

Likewise, family member's feelings of trust and distrust toward specific healers, medical care providers, interpreters, and institutions influence their reactions to suggested actions. These reactions are influenced by personal past experiences and stories from the community, as well as from interactions with providers and healers in the current illness. The more patients and family members feel respected the more trusting of specific providers and therapies they are. (See Chapters 4 and 12.)

Healers and doctors are more numerous and accessible in urban areas of the United States than in rural mountainous Laos. Here, in addition to traditional Hmong healers, there are Cambodian, Vietnamese, and Chinese healers, medicines, and modalities; in addition to medical doctors, there are acupuncturists, chiropractors, naturopaths, nurse practitioners, psychologists, and midwives. Nonetheless, there are fewer Hmong healers, and noise ordinances and the lack of herbal medicines limit their practices. Other barriers to care include poor transportation, distant facilities, limited hours of operation, and lack of trained medical interpreters. Also, the direct costs (fees for doctors, diagnostics, and therapies) and the indirect costs (lost pay because of lost work and fees for baby-sitters and transportation) can impede people's choices. If people lack medical insurance, do not have money for the necessary animals, or cannot afford to lose work, they will likely postpone their visits to doctors or shaman.

## Hmong Experiences with Western Medicine

### Western Biomedicine in Laos

Hmong people in Laos had little access to Western-trained health care providers until the CIA-sponsored medics and the USAID-sponsored medical relief efforts were established in the 1960s (Weldon, 1999) and until the nongovernment agencies provided care in Thai refugee camps in the 1970s and 1980s (Wright, 1986). According to Hmong women who were nurses in Laos and men who were medics in Laos and Thailand, Hmong people had mixed reactions to Western medicine. They were impressed with the efficacy of intravenous fluids, blood transfusions, antibiotics, and operations that repaired war wounds. But they also were concerned about the adverse effects of Western therapies. They witnessed limb paralysis after immunizations and deaths after lumbar punctures and operations. They speculated that inadequately trained people were learning on them and that improper medicines were being given to them. And they passed on the horrific rumor that Hmong people's flesh was being packaged into cans and sent to the United States for Americans to eat.

## Western Biomedicine in the United States

### DIAGNOSTIC PROCEDURES

In the United States, Hmong people generally are willing to allow physicians to examine their bodies and diagnose their problems; perhaps they are at ease because traditionally, medicine women and ritual healers performed physical exams. If people have symptoms, or fear diseases, they may even allow physicians to examine genital areas. Cancer screening of genitals, breasts, and colons in asymptomatic people, however, tends to be less accepted. (See above, Changing Beliefs and Practices about Disease Prevention and Health Promotion; see Chapters 3 and 4.)

One of the most common concerns is that physicians draw too much blood. This concern is based on the Hmong perception that blood is a nonrenewable life fluid; when too much is lost, people die. When blood is drawn from the inner arm, moreover, people complain of lightheadedness and weakness in that arm or on the same side of the body, which they relate to disturbed blood flow. To deal with these concerns, providers may offer other options, such as using finger-sticks, drawing less blood, postponing blood tests, and prescribing iron supplements that will help the patient's body recover from the blood loss (see Chapter 3). People seem to be more willing to have their blood drawn when they perceive that testing their blood is essential to their getting the help they desire, or when they feel that they have too much blood, which is making them weak, and they want one or two tubes of blood withdrawn so they will feel better.

While Hmong patients generally accept giving urine or stool samples, they are likely to resist the more invasive diagnostic procedures, such as lumbar punctures (see Chapter 5). Ordinary X rays, ultrasounds, CT scans, and MRI scans are generally accepted, since there are no perceived harmful side effects, while invasive X rays, such as barium enemas, retrograde pyelograms, and angiograms draw resistance. Nuclear medicine scans are usually accepted. (However, if people understood more about the radioactivity, they might be less willing, given the extent of their fear about cancer radiation therapy [see Chapter 15].)

### WESTERN MEDICATIONS

Generally, Hmong people want and are willing to take medicines to relieve symptoms from acute illnesses. People generally have difficulty, however, with taking medicines for chronic illnesses, such as arthritis. They expect to have their symptoms improve, and if the medicine does not cure their problem, they do not want to continue taking it. Also, they do not expect to continue medications if they have no signs or symptoms in "silent" chronic diseases, such as hypertension (see Chapter 8). Among the concerns many people express about medicines, two stand out: that physicians do not give the best medicines to Hmong people but instead keep them for Americans and that Western medicines are too strong for Asian people. They are disturbed by side-effects of medicines, and even if the side-effect is mild, they may discontinue taking the medicine. Because of the side-effects of anti-hypertensive medicines, chemotherapy drugs, or birth control pills, for example, people may be resistant to starting or continuing the medications (see Chapters 2 and 13).

## OPERATIONS

While some people accept operations, and some even ask for operations to relieve their ailment (see Chapters 13 and 15), operations give rise to both physical and spiritual concerns. People are concerned about the long list of physical complications described on the consent form—among them hemorrhage, infection, anesthetic reaction, and death. They also wonder whether after the operation they will be able to fulfill their social roles as parent, breadwinner, wife, or daughter-in-law. Some are under the impression that, in order to protect themselves from long-term disability, they must avoid physically demanding work and sexual intercourse for one year after an operation. Indeed, stories abound about chronic postoperative pains (see Chapters 2, 3, 4, 7, 9, 13, 14, and 15).

Operations (and autopsies) have deleterious short- and long-term effects on the three major souls. Even decades later, the residing soul will object if metal fillings, prosthetics, or staples are not removed before the person is buried and will express the displeasure by make living descendents sick (see Chapter 13). The reincarnation soul may have to carry a defect from its physically altered body into the next life (see Chapter 4). A defective wandering soul may not be able to find his ancestors in the spirit world. In addition, soul loss can occur. The wandering soul may be frightened away by the fearful anticipation of an upcoming operation and it may not return from the anesthetic-induced sleep. If soul loss does occur during an operation, family members will consult hospital personnel for permission to initiate the soul-calling rituals in the operating room. Adversely affected, any one of the three major souls can express its anger by making living family members sick.

Since organs in the body have different values, operations are likely to be seen differently, according to the part of the body that is operated on. The Hmong are less likely to consent to operations on the major organs, such as the liver, lung, kidney, brain, and heart, than on minor organs, such as the gall bladder and appendix. While some people are willing to consent to the destruction or removal of these relatively less important organs, others are resistant. Whether an amputation is accidental or surgical, people may want their digits and limbs kept until they die so the body can be buried whole (see Chapter 13).

Finally, there are also issues of distrust of surgeons. People are concerned that the surgeons want to operate on them because they want to learn, experiment on, or purposely harm Hmong people. Stories about surgeons taking advantage of Hmong people abound. These fears are influenced by their experiences: a recent study showed that a surgeon performed more abdominal than laparoscopic appendectomies on

Hmong children, who had longer hospitalizations than white children (Hu, 2000, 2001). (See below, Relationships with Health Care Providers; see also Chapters 7, 9, and 13.)

## TRANSFUSIONS, ORGAN DONATIONS, AND ORGAN TRANSPLANTATIONS

In the late 1970s and 1980s, many people resisted blood transfusions and organ transplantations because they were concerned about the unseen dangers of mixing blood and body parts, particularly diseased blood and organs. Some accepted blood transfusions only in life-and-death situations, while others declined even in such situations. As Hmong people have become more acquainted with the U.S. health care system and have had experiences with life-saving procedures, more people are willing to accept blood transfusions and liver or kidney transplants. However, few people donate blood and even fewer people have donated organs, because they are concerned about the adverse effects on their own body. Those who participate in blood drives are those who were born in the United States, seem to be more acculturated, and have fewer spiritual concerns (see Chapters 9 and 14).

### Relationships with Health Care Providers

Hmong place great value on trusting relationships with healers, whether traditional healers or U.S. health care providers. But there are many barriers to developing a trusting relationship with U.S. health care providers, including different languages, differences in body language and style of communication, and the inherent imbalance of power. These barriers are compounded by historical and personal experiences Hmong have had with Americans and by their social, economic, and political situations, such as their being poor and on medical assistance. Many Hmong who are on public assistance feel that U.S. doctors and hospital personnel provide suboptimal care and prescribe ineffective treatments to people on welfare (see Chapters 5, 7, and 13).

In large part, Hmong patients desire to trust their providers but many question whether providers can be trusted. Many Hmong make decisions about providers' trustworthiness based on providers' language style, tone of voice, body language, patience in answering questions, open-mindedness, willingness to listen, willingness to compromise, and reputation within the community. Hmong patients prefer providers who are experienced and fear inexperienced providers who may be more likely to make life-threatening mistakes. Hmong patients also prefer to work with interpreters so they can adequately communicate with non-Hmong-speaking providers.

Interactions between Hmong patients, their families, and U.S. health care workers often do go well. Health care workers with the aid of health care interpreters may effectively reach across language barriers and cultural differences to offer assistance with multiple health problems. But many interactions do not go well, as some stories in this book demonstrate. Different beliefs about the body; different decision-making practices; different perspectives about appropriate treatments; different evaluations of the risks and benefits of diagnostic procedures, medicines, and operations; and different expectations of the doctor's role all contribute to disagreements and conflicts. Varying degrees of conflict occur; probably the greatest amount of conflict occurs in pediatric cases when physicians feel a special obligation to be an advocate for patients' medical needs over families' specific desires (see Chapters 5, 6, and 7). Disagreements and serious conflicts are often about roles and responsibilities and who has the power to implement his or her view of what is right.

Doctors have more power than Hmong patients, given their respected social position, high socioeconomic class, and professional licensure by the state and given that their views of health, disease, and treatment are aligned with the judicial system. Thus, doctors can usually turn the conflicts in their favor, especially when the conflicts about appropriate life-saving treatments for minors lead to court-ordered therapies (see Chapters 5 and 7).

Hmong families have less power. Many of their characteristics contribute to their lower position. They are refugees scarred by attacks during their flight from Laos to Thailand, minority members in a society prone to discrimination and prejudice, non-English speakers in a society that speaks English-only, and welfare recipients in a society that degrades welfare recipients. Furthermore, when they are sick, the health care institutions that are available to them often focus on health care providers' needs more than patients' needs. In health care settings, Hmong patients too often feel powerless to get their needs met and to protect themselves from powerful providers who could harm as well as help them. Thus, families usually are on the "losing" end of their disagreements or differences with providers.

The consequences of serious value conflicts between Hmong families and U.S. providers are felt throughout the Hmong community and contribute to people's suspicion and distrust of the health care system. Families tell stories that pass through the community with warnings.

> Don't go to this hospital, they will suck your brains out.
> Don't go to those doctors because they will call the police and force your
>     child to be tortured.
> Don't go to that clinic or they will experiment on you.
> Don't go to that hospital or they will take out your body parts and give them
>     to Americans.

Some families keep sick members at home away from the doctors as long as possible, in order to keep them safe. Other people implore doctors to give the best health care to their sick family members. They try to obtain "100 percent guarantees" from surgeons for good outcomes or threaten doctors with violence if their family member is harmed. Whether people feel personally vulnerable in health care settings or not, they have heard these stories and are vigilant against possible abuse and neglect by providers.

Through these experiences, Hmong families are learning about the power of allopathic health care to heal sick bodies with medicines and save dying people with invasive procedures and machines. They are also learning about the disappointing limits of biomedicine, its inability to relieve suffering from chronic pains related to depression, stress, and alienation, or to cure chronic silent killers, such as diabetes and hypertension, or to provide holistic care for the body, mind, and soul. Hmong families are learning how to interact with professionals of higher social status and authority: when to ask or answer questions, when to listen or ignore "patient education," and when to comply with or refuse orders. And, they are learning limits about when they can make decisions for their children and when doctors, judges, and police will force them to conform.

(For more information about biomedicine in the United States, see Barrett et al., 1998; Bliatout, 1988, 1990; Cha, 2000: Culhane-Pera, 1987, 1988, 1989; Culhane-Pera & Vawter, 1998; Deinard & Dunnigan, 1987; Ensign, 1994; Fadiman, 1998; Finck, 1984; Haga, 1995, 1997; Henry, 1996, 1999; Hoang & Erickson, 1985; A. E. Johnson, 1996; S. Johnson, 1996; S. K. Johnson, 1995; Kirton, 1985; Kraut, 1990; Kunstadter, 1995; E. Lee, 1997; P. Lee, 1991; Minnesota Center for Health Care Ethics, 1995, 1997; Morrow, 1986; Mouacheupao, 1999; Muecke, 1983; Nuttall & Flores, 1997; O'Connor, 1995; Osborn, 1992; Parker & Kiatoukaysy, 2001; Rairdan & Higgs, 1992; Rice, 1997; Schauberger, Hammes, & Steingraeber, 1990; Schultz, 1982; Spring et al., 1995; Spring et al., 1997; Spring, 2001; True, 1997; Vawter & Babbitt, 1997; Waters, Rao, & Petracchi, 1992; Westermeyer & Thao, 1986; Wittet, 1983; Xiong, 1998a, 1998b.)

## Conclusion

Successful cross-cultural healing relationships between Hmong families and U.S. health care providers require that professionals and institutions have insight into the nature and depth of the divergent cultural and health beliefs of traditional animist Hmong families and U.S. health care professionals. The recent history of the Hmong and the relationship between the Hmong and Americans during the Secret War in Laos and their resettlement in the United States as refugees is crucial to understanding the source and depth of distrust that many Hmong have for Americans, especially Americans in positions of authority. The traditional beliefs about what causes sickness and what techniques heal are deeply rooted in animist beliefs, just as today's health beliefs are related to traditional cosmology, Christian ideology, and biomedical perspectives. Health care practitioners, administrators, and policy makers can use the information in this chapter to gain familiarity with key elements of traditional culture, traditional health beliefs and healing practices, and health-related decision-making practices, as well as changes in these beliefs and practices in the United States. This type of cultural knowledge about the cultural groups served is essential for health care personnel, administrators, and policy makers committed to providing culturally responsive care.

## References

Adler, S. R. (1994). Ethnomedical pathogenesis and Hmong immigrants' sudden nocturnal deaths. *Culture, Medicine, and Psychiatry 18,* 23–59.

Ahrens, L. (1994). *Traditional health care practices of the Hmong.* Unpublished master's thesis. University of Wisconsin, Oshkosh.

Anderson, B. K. (1996). Frogtown/Summit-University Hmong Community Assessment. Minneapolis, MN: Hmong American Partnership.

Barrett, B., Shadick, K., Schilling, R., Spencer, L., del Rosario, S., Moua, K., & Vang, M. (1998). Hmong/medicine interactions: Improving cross-cultural health care. *Family Medicine, 30*(3), 179–184.

Bertrais, Y. (1978). *The traditional marriage among the White Hmong of Thailand and Laos.* Chiangmai, Thailand: Hmong Centre.

Bliatout, B. T. (1983). *Hmong sudden unexpected nocturnal death: A cultural study.* Portland, OR: Sparkle Enterprises.

Bliatout, B. T. (1986). Guidelines for mental health professionals to help Hmong clients seek traditional healing treatment. In G. L. Hendricks (Ed.), *The Hmong in transition.* New York: Center for Migration Studies of New York, Inc., Southeast Asian Refugee Studies of the University of Minnesota, 349–363.

Bliatout, B. T. (1988, March 5). *Hmong refugees: Some barriers to some Western health care services.* Paper presented at conference on Southeast Asians in the United States, Arizona State University, Tempe, AZ.

Bliatout, B. T. (1990). Hmong beliefs about health and illness. *Hmong Forum, 1,* 40–45.

Bliatout, B. T. (1993). Hmong death customs: Traditional and acculturated. In D. P. Irish, K. F. Lundquist, & V. Jenkins-Nelsen (Eds.), *Ethnic variations in dying, death, and grief: Diversity in universality.* Washington, D.C.: Taylor & Francis, 79–100.

Bliatout, B. T., Downing, B. T., Lewis, J., & Yang, D. (1988). *Handbook for teaching Hmong-speaking students.* Folsom, CA: Southeast Asia Community Resource Center, Folsom Cordova Unified School District.

Capps, L. L. (1991). *Concepts of health and illness of the protestant Hmong.* Unpublished doctoral dissertation, University of Kansas, Kansas City.

Capps, L. L. (1994). Change and continuity in the medical culture of the Hmong in Kansas City. *Medical Anthropology Quarterly (new series), 8*(2), 161–177.

Castle, T. (1992). *At war in the shadow of Vietnam: U.S. military aid to the Royal Lao Government, 1955–1975.* New York: Columbia University Press.

Cha, D. (2000). *Hmong-American concepts of health, healing, and illness, and their experience with conventional medicine.* Unpublished doctoral dissertation, University of Colorado, Denver.

Cha, D., & Chagnon, J. (1993). *Former war-wife, refugee, repatriate: A needs assessment of women repatriating to Laos.* Washington, DC: Asia Resource Center.

Cha, D., & Small, C. A. (1994). Policy lessons from Hmong and Lao women in Thai refugee camps. *World Development, 22*(7), 1045–1059.

Cheon-Klessig, Y., Camilleri, D., McElmurry, B., Ohlson, V. (1988). Folk medicine in the health practice of Hmong refugees. *Western Journal of Nursing Research, 10,* 647–660.

Chindarsi, N. (1976). *The religion of the Hmong Njua.* Njua, Bangkok: Siam Society.

Chindarsi, N. (1983). Hmong shamanism. In J. McKinnon & W. Bhruksasri (Eds.), *Highlanders of Thailand.* London: Oxford University Press, 187–193.

Chung, R. C., & Bemak, F. (1996). The effects of welfare status on psychological distress among Southeast Asian refugees. *Journal of Nervous and Mental Disease, 6,* 346–353.

Clark, L., & Hofsess, L. (1998). Acculturation. In S. Loue (Ed.), *Handbook of immigrant health.* New York: Plenum Press, 37–59.

Collins, K. S., Hughes, D. L., Doty, M. M., Ives, B. L., Edwards, J. N., & Tenny, K. (2002, March). *Diverse communities, common concerns: Assessing health care quality for minority Americans.* Findings from the Commonwealth Fund 2001 health care quality survey. Available from *www.cmwf.org/publist/publist2.asp?CategoryID=11*

Conquergood, D., Thao, P., & Thao, X. (1989). *I am a shaman: A Hmong life story with ethnographic commentary, South East Asian refugee studies project* (Occasional Papers No. 8). Minneapolis: Center for Urban and Regional Affairs, University of Minnesota.

Cooper, R. (1984). *Resource scarcity and the Hmong response: A study of settlement and economy in northern Thailand.* Singapore: Singapore University Press.

Cooper, R., Tapp, N., Lee, G. Y., & Schworer-Kohl, G. (1995). *The Hmong* (2nd ed.). Bangkok: Artasia Press.

Corlett, J. L. (1999). *Landscapes and lifestyles: Three generations of Hmong women and their gardens.* Unpublished doctoral dissertation, University of California, Davis.

Culhane-Pera, K. A. (1987, April). *Hmong people's reactions to surgery.* Paper presented at the annual meeting of the North American Primary Care Research Group, Minneapolis.

Culhane-Pera, K. A. (1988, April). *Hmong beliefs about blood and their impact on blood drawing.* Paper presented at the national meeting of the Society for Applied Anthropology, Tampa.

Culhane-Pera, K. A. (1989). *Analysis of cultural beliefs and power dynamics in disagreements about health care of Hmong children.* Unpublished master's thesis, University of Minnesota, Minneapolis.

Culhane-Pera, K. A., & Vawter, D. E. (1998). A study of health care professionals' perspectives about a cross-cultural ethical conflict involving a Hmong patient and her family. *Journal of Clinical Ethics, 9*(2), 179–190.

Culhane-Pera, K. A., Naftali, E. D., Jacobson, C., & Xiong, Z. B. (2002). Cultural feeding practices and child-raising philosophy contribute to iron-deficiency anemia in refugee Hmong children. *Ethnicity and Disease, 12*(2), 199–205.

Culhane-Pera, K. A., Cha, D., & Kunstadter, P. (2003). Hmong in Southeast Asia and the United States. In C. Ember & E. Ember (Eds.), *Encyclopedia of medical anthropology: Health and illness in the world's cultures.* Boston, Kluwer/Plenum.

Dana, A. F. (1993). *Courtship and marriage traditions of the Hmong.* Unpublished master's thesis, California State University at Fresno.

Danes, S., O'Donnell, K., & Sakulnamarka, D. (1993). *Middle generation Hmong couples and daily life concerns.* Minneapolis: Minnesota Agricultural Experiment Station.

Deinard, A. S., & Dunnigan, T. (1987). Hmong health care: Reflections on a six-year experience. *International Migration Review, 21*(3), 857–865.

DeOca, J., Friou, J., Kunstadter, P., Kunstadter, S., Lazarus, M., Shreeniwas, S., et al. (1994). *Determinants and consequences of Hmong age at marriage in Sacramento.* Sacramento: Department of Demography, University of California.

Detzner, D. F. (1996). No place without a home: Southeast Asian grandparents in refugee families. *Generations, 20*(1), 45–48.

Donnelly, N. D. (1989). *The changing lives of refugee Hmong women.* Unpublished doctoral dissertation, University of Washington, Seattle.

Donnelly, N. D. (1994). *The changing lives of refugee Hmong women.* Seattle: University of Washington Press.

Downing, B. T., & Olney, D. P. (1982). *The Hmong in the West: Observations and reports.* Minneapolis: Southeast Asian Refugee Studies Center, Center for Urban and Regional Affairs, University of Minnesota.

Duchon, D. A. (1997). Home is where you make it: Hmong refugees in Georgia. *Urban Anthropology, 26*(1), 71–92.

Dunnigan, T. (1982). Segmentary kinship in an urban society: The Hmong of St. Paul-Minneapolis, MN. *Anthropological Quarterly, 55*(3), 126–134.

Edwards, L. E., Rautio, C. J., Hakanson, E. Y. (1987). Pregnancy in Hmong refugee women. *Minnesota Medicine, 70*(11), 633–637.

Ensign, J. S. (1994). *Traditional healing in the Hmong refugee community of the California Central Valley.* Unpublished doctoral dissertation, California School of Professional Psychology, Fresno.

Faderman, L., & Xiong, G. (1997). *I begin my life all over: The Hmong and the American immigrant experience.* Boston: Beacon Press.

Fadiman, A. (1997). *The spirit catches you and you fall down: A Hmong child, her American doctors, and the collision of two cultures.* New York: Farrar, Straus, and Giroux.

Fang, T. (1995). *Basic human body and medical information for Hmong speaking people (Tuabneeg lubcev hab kev mobnkeeg rua cov haslug Hmoob).* Pinedale, CA: Chersousons.

Finck, M. S. (1984). Southeast Asian refugees of Rhode Island: Cross-cultural issues in medical care. *Rhode Island Medical Journal, 67,* 319–321.

Foo, L. J. (2002). Hmong women in the US: Changing a patriarchal culture. In L. J. Foo, *Asian American women: Issues, concerns, and responsive human and civil rights advocacy.* New York: Ford Foundation. Retrieved January 8, 2003, from *www.aapip.org/jag.html*

Garrett, W. E. (1974). The Hmong of Laos: No place to run. *National Geographic Magazine, 143* (January), 78–111.

Geddes, W. R. (1976). *Migrants of the mountains: The cultural ecology of the Blue Miao (Hmong Njua) of Thailand.* Oxford: Clarendon Press.

Gjerdingen, D. K., Ireland, M., & Chaloner K. M. (1996). Growth of Hmong children. *Archives of Pediatrics and Adolescent Medicine, 150*(12), 1295–1298.

Gjerdingen, D. K., & Lor, V. (1997). Hepatitis B status of Hmong patients. *Journal of the American Board of Family Practice, 10*(5), 322–328.

Goldfarb, M. (1982). *Fighters, refugees, immigrants: A story of the Hmong.* Minneapolis, MN: Carol Rhoda Books.

Haga, C. (1995, May 21). Mother and daughter fight for common ground when kidneys fail and folk medicine won't do. *Minneapolis Star Tribune,* A1, A8.

Haga, C. (1997, August 30). After transplant, woman looks to future. *Minneapolis Star Tribune,* A1, A12.

Hall, S. E. (1990). Hmong kinship roles: Insiders and outsiders. *Hmong Forum, 1,* 25–39.

Hammand, R. (1984, September 15). Religion complicates Hmong choice. *St. Paul Pioneer Press,* 1H, 4H, 6H, 8H.

Hamilton-Merritt, J. (1993). *Tragic mountains: The Hmong, the Americans, and the secret wars for Laos, 1942–1992.* Bloomington: Indiana University Press, 1993.

Heimbach, E. E. (1979). *White Hmong-English dictionary.* Ithaca, NY: Southeast Asia Program Publications, Cornell University.

Hein, J. (2000). Interpersonal discrimination against Hmong Americans: Parallels and variation in microlevel racial inequality. *Sociological Quarterly, 41*(3), 413–429.

Hendricks, G. L., Downing, B. T., & Deinard, A. S. (Eds.). (1986). *The Hmong in transition.* New York: Center for Migration Studies of New York, Inc., Southeast Asian Refugee Studies of the University of Minnesota.

Henry, R. R. (1996). *Sweet blood, dry liver: Diabetes and Hmong embodiment in a foreign land.* Unpublished doctoral dissertation, University of North Carolina at Chapel Hill.

Henry, R. R. (1999). Measles, Hmong, and metaphor: Culture change and illness management under conditions of immigration. *Medical Anthropology Quarterly (new series), 13*(1), 32–50.

Hmong Cultural Center. (n.d.). *Hmong zodiac (Tsiaj nres xeem).* Retrieved April 23, 2002, from *www.hmongcenter.org/hmongzodiac.html*

Hmoob Thaj Yeeb. (1998). *Taking a public stand: Completing the journey from war to peace through the ending of violence.* St. Paul, MN: Initiative for Violence-free Families and Communities.

Hoang, G. N., & Erickson, R. V. (1985). Cultural barriers to effective medical care among Indochinese patients. *Annual Review of Medicine, 36,* 229–239.

Hu, J. (2000) *Under the knife: Medical "non-compliance" in Hmong immigrants.* Unpublished doctoral dissertation, Emory University, Atlanta, GA.

Hu, J. (2001). Increased incidence of perforated appendixes in Hmong children in California [Letters to the editor]. *New England Journal of Medicine, 344*(13), 1023–1024.

Johnson, A. E. (1996). *Hmong patient and family interviews.* St. Paul, MN: United Hospital & Children's Health Care.

Johnson, C., & Yang, S. (1992). *Myths, legends, and folk tales from the Hmong of Laos.* St. Paul, MN.: Macalester College, Department of Linguistics.

Johnson, S. (1996). Hmong. In J. G. Lipson, S. L. Dibble, & P. A. Minarik (Eds.), *Culture & nursing care: A pocket guide.* San Francisco: UCSF Nursing Press.

Johnson, S. K. (1995). *Diabetes in the Hmong refugee population.* Unpublished doctoral dissertation, University of California, San Francisco.

Kaptchuk, T. (1997). Consequences of cupping [Letters to the editor]. *New England Journal of Medicine, 336*(15), 1109.

Kirton, E. S. (1985). *The locked medicine cabinet: Hmong health care in America.* Unpublished doctoral dissertation, University of Santa Barbara, Santa Barbara, CA.

Koltyk, J. A. (1998). *New pioneers in the heartland: Hmong life in Wisconsin.* Needham Heights, MA: Allyn & Bacon.

Kraut, A. M. (1990). Healers and strangers: Immigrant attitudes towards the physician in America: A relationship in historical perspective. *Journal of the American Medical Association, 263*(13), 1807–1811.

Kroll, J., Habenicht, M., & Mackenzie, T. (1989). Depression and posttraumatic stress disorder in Southeast Asian refugees. *American Journal of Psychiatry, 146*(12), 1592–1597.

Kunstadter, P. (1985). Health of the Hmong in Thailand: Risk factors, morbidity, and mortality in comparison with other ethnic groups. *Culture, Medicine, and Psychiatry, 9,* 329–351.

Kunstadter, P. (1986). Ethnicity, ecology, and mortality in northwestern Thailand. In C. R. Janes, R. Stall, & S. M. Gifford (Eds.), *Anthropology and epidemiology: Interdisciplinary approaches to the study of health and disease.* Dordrecht, Holland: D. Reidell, 125–156.

Kunstadter, P. (1995). *Culturally appropriate health care: Hmong in Laos, Thailand, and the USA.* Paper presented at the Intercongress of the International Union for Anthropological and Ethnological Sciences, Florence, Italy.

Kunstadter P. (2001, March 12). *Health implications of globalization at the village level: The good, the bad, and the ugly: Some results of comparative research in Thailand and the US.* Paper presented at the Woodrow Wilson School of International Studies, Princeton University, Princeton, NJ.

Kunstadter, P., Chapman, E. C., & Sabhasri, S. (1978). *Farmers in the forest.* Honolulu: University Press of Hawaii.

Kunstadter, P., & Kunstadter, S. L. (1990). Health transitions in Thailand. In J. C. Caldwell, S. Findley, P. Caldwell, G. Santow, W. Cosford, J. Braid, & D. Broers-Freeman (Eds.), *What we know about health transition.* Canberra, Australia: Health Transition Centre, Australian National University, 213–250.

Kunstadter, P., & Vang, V. (2001). Mortality transition among Hmong refugees in Fresno County, California, 1980–2001. Unpublished.

Lee, E. (Ed.). (1997). *Working with Asian Americans: A guide for clinicians.* New York: Guilford Press.

Lee, G. Y. (1986a). Culture and adaptation: Hmong refugees in Australia. In G. L. Hendricks, B. T. Downing, & A. S. Deinard (Eds.), *The Hmong in transition.* New York: Center for Migration Studies of New York.

Lee, G. Y. (1986b). White Hmong kinship terminology and structure. In B. Johns & D. Strecker (Eds.), *The Hmong world I.* New Haven, CT: Yale Southeast Asia Studies.

Lee, P. (1991). *Health care systems utilized by the Hmong in California: A case study in Stanislaus County.* Unpublished master's thesis, California State University, Stanislaus.

Lee, S., Xiong, G., Vang, V. K., Comerford, M. (2000). *Hypertension rates increase with length of stay in the US among Hmong refugees in California.* Paper presented at the annual meeting of the American Public Health Association, Boston.

Lee, S. J. (2001). More than "model minorities" or "delinquents": A look at Hmong American high school students. *Harvard Educational Review, 71*(3), 505–528.

Lee, S. J. (2002). Learning "American": Hmong American high school students. *Education and Urban Society, 34*(2), 233–246.

Leepreecha, P. (2001). *Kinship and identity among Hmong in Thailand.* Unpublished doctoral dissertation, University of Washington, Seattle.

LeMay, W. R., Gonzalez, C. D., Henry, M., Frazier, P. J., & Hanrahan, L. (1998). Early childhood caries experience in a Hmong population. [Abstract]. *Journal of Dental Research, 77,* 708.

Lemoine, J. (1972a). L'initiation du mort chez les Hmongs: III. Les themes. *L'Homme, 12*(3), 84–110.

Lemoine, J. (1972b). *Un village Hmong Vert du Haut Laos: Milieu technique et organisation sociale.* Paris: Centre National de la Recherche Scientifique.

Lemoine, J. (1986). Shamanism in the context of Hmong resettlement. In G. L. Hendricks, B. T. Downing, & A. S. Deinard (Eds.), *The Hmong in transition.* New York: Center for Migration Studies of New York, Inc., and Southeast Asian Refugee Studies Project of the University of Minnesota, 337–348.

Long, L. D. (1993). *Ban Vinai: The refugee camp.* New York: Columbia University Press.

Ly, M. (1993). *Hmong women: Their roles and responsibilities.* Minneapolis: Association for the Advancement of Hmong Women in Minnesota.

Lyfoung, T. (1996). *Touby Lyfoung.* Fresno, CA: Touby Lyfoung Foundation.

Mattison, W., Lo, L., & Scarseth, T. (1994). *Hmong lives from Laos to LaCrosse: Stories of eight Hmong elders.* LaCrosse, WI: The Pump House.

Mills, P. K., & Yang, R. (1997). Cancer incidence in the Hmong of Central California, United States, 1987–94. *Cancer Causes & Control, 8*(5), 705–712.

Minnesota Center for Health Care Ethics. (1995). *Western medicine through Hmong voices* [videotape]. Minneapolis: Author.

Minnesota Center for Health Care Ethics. (1997). *Trading beliefs: Four Hmong families consider relinquishing their traditional health beliefs* [videotape]. Minneapolis: Author.

Minnesota Department of Human Services. (2002). *What's beyond: Cultural perspectives on problem gambling in the southeast Asian community* [videotapes, discussion guide, and facilitator's guide]. Available from Minnesota Department of Human Services. Compulsive Gambling Program, 651-582-1819.

Morechand, G. (1968). Le Chamanisme des Hmong. *Bulletin de l'Ecole Française d'Extrême Orient, 54,* 53–294.

Morgan, S., & Culhane-Pera, K. (1994). *Threads of life: Hemp and gender in a Hmong village.* Available from Hmong Arts, Books, and Crafts, 651-293-0019.

Morrow, K. (1986). Transcultural midwifery: Adapting to Hmong birthing customs in California. *Journal of Nurse-Midwifery, 31*(6), 285–288.

Mottin, J. (1980). *History of the Hmong.* Bangkok, Thailand: Rung Ruang Ratana Printing.

Moua, J. L. (1996). *The uses of herbal medicine in health care practices of Hmong refugees, and policy implications in Merced County, California.* Unpublished master's thesis, California State University, Stanislaus.

Moua, M. N. (Ed.). (2002). *Bamboo among the oaks: Contemporary writing by Hmong Americans.* St. Paul: Minnesota Historical Society Press.

Moua, X. (2001). *Hmong clan leaders' roles and responsibilities.* Unpublished master's thesis, California State University, Fresno.

Mouacheupao, S. (1999, April 17). *Attitudes of Hmong patients to surgery.* Paper presented at the annual spring research forum of the Minnesota Academy of Family Physicians, Minneapolis.

Muecke, M. A. (1983). Caring for Southeast Asian refugee patients in the USA. *American Journal of Public Health, 73*(4), 431–438.

Nicholson, B. L. (1997). The influence of pre-emigration and post-emigration stressors on mental health: A study of Southeast Asian refugees. *Social Work Research, 21*(1), 19–31.

Nuttall, P., & Flores, F. C. (1997). Hmong healing practices used for common childhood illnesses. *Pediatric Nursing, 23*(3), 247–251.

O'Connor, B. B. (1995). Hmong cultural values, biomedicine, and chronic liver disease. In B. B. O'Connor, *Healing traditions: Alternative medicine and the health professions.* Philadelphia: University of Pennsylvania Press.

Olson, M. C. (1999). "The heart still beats, but the brain doesn't answer:" Perception and experience of old-age dementia in the Milwaukee Hmong community. *Theoretical Medicine and Bioethics, 20*(1), 85–95.

Osborn, D. G. (1992). Conflict and collaboration in cross-cultural health care. *World Health Forum, 13,* 315–319.

Panasuwan, P. (2000). *Chao Fa: A history that could be true.* Chiang Mai, Thailand: Benya Publishing House.

Parker, M. K. (1996). *Loss in the lives of Southeast Asian elders.* Unpublished doctoral dissertation, University of Minnesota, St. Paul.

Parker, M., & Kiatoukaysy, L. N. (1999). Culturally responsive health care: The example of the Hmong in America. *Journal of the American Academy of Nurse Practitioners, 11*(12), 511–518.

Peterson, S. (1990). *From the heart and mind: Creating paj ntaub in the context of community.* Unpublished doctoral dissertation, University of Pennsylvania, Philadelphia.

Pfaff, T. (1995). *Hmong in America: Journey from a secret war.* Eau Claire, WI: Chippewa Valley Museum Press.

Plotnikoff, G. A., Numrich, C., Yan, D., & Xiong, P. (2002). Hmong shamanism: Animist spiritual healing in Minnesota. *Minnesota Medicine, 85*(6), 29–34.

Portis, A. (2002). [Differences between kidney stones in Hmong and non-Hmong in St. Paul, MN: A chart review.] Unpublished data.

Putsch, R. W. (1988). Ghost illness: A cross-cultural experience with the expression of a non-Western tradition in clinical practice. *American Indian and Alaska Native Mental Health Research, 2*(2), 6–26.

Rairdan, B., & Higgs, Z. (1992). When your patient is a Hmong refugee. *American Journal of Nursing, 92*(3), 52–55.

Rice, P. L. (1997). Giving birth in a new home: Childbirth traditions and the experience of motherhood among Hmong women from Laos. *Asian Studies Review, 20*(3), 133–148.

Rice, P. L. (1999). When the baby falls! The cultural construction of miscarriage among Hmong women in Australia. *Women and Health, 30*(1), 85–103.

Rice, P. L. (2000a). Baby, souls, name, and health: Traditional customs for a newborn infant among the Hmong in Melbourne. *Early Human Development, 57,* 189–203.

Rice, P. L. (2000b). *Hmong women and reproduction.* Westport, CT: Bergin and Harvey.

Rice, P. L. (2000c). Nyo dua hli—30 days' confinement: Traditions and changed childbearing beliefs and practices among Hmong women in Australia. *Midwifery, 16*(1), 22–34.

Robbins, C. (1979). *Air America.* New York: Putnam's Sons.

Robinson, W. C. (1998). *Terms of refuge: The Indochinese exodus and the international response.* New York: United Nations High Commissioner for Refugees.

Rolland, B. J., & Moua, H. U. (1994). *Trail through the mist.* Eau Claire, WI: Eagles Printing.

Savina, F. M. (1930). *Histoire des Miao.* Hong Kong: Société des Missions Etrangeres de Paris.

Schauberger, C. W., Hammes, B., & Steingraeber, P. H. (1990). Obstetrical care of a Southeast Asian refugee population in a midwestern community. *Journal of Perinatology, 10*(3), 280–284.

Schein, L. (2000). *Minority rules: The Miao and the feminine in China's cultural politics.* Durham & London: Duke University Press.

Schultz, S. (1982). How Southeast-Asian refugees in California adapt to unfamiliar health care practices. *Health and Social Work, 7*(2), 148–156.

Siegel, T. (Producer), & Conquergood, D. (Writer/Producer). *Between two worlds: The Hmong shaman in America* [Motion picture]. Available from Filmmakers Library, 124 East 40th Street, New York, NY 10016.

Spring, M. A. (1989). Ethnopharmacologic analysis of medicinal plants used by Laotian Hmong refugees in Minnesota. *Journal of Ethnopharmacology, 26,* 65–91.

Spring, M. A. (2001). *Reproductive health and fertility of Hmong immigrants in Minnesota.* Unpublished doctoral dissertation, University of Minnesota, Minneapolis.

Spring, M. A., Davis, K., & Rode, P. (1997). The Hmong community. In *Prenatal care among Southeast Asian women in St. Paul and Minneapolis.* St. Paul, MN: The Urban Coalition, 25–43.

Spring, M. A., Ross, P. J., Etkin, N. L., & Deinard, A. S. (1995). Sociocultural factors in the use of prenatal care by Hmong women in Minneapolis. *American Journal of Public Health, 85*(7), 1015–1017.

Symonds, P. V. (1991). *Cosmology and the cycle of life: Hmong view of birth, death, and gender in a mountain village in Northern Thailand.* Unpublished doctoral dissertation, Brown University, Providence, RI.

Symonds, P. V. (2002). *Calling in the soul: Gender and the cycle of life in a Hmong village.* Seattle: University of Washington Press.

Takada, E., Ford, J., Lloyd, L. (1998). Asian Pacific Islander health. In S. Loue (Ed.), *Handbook of immigrant health.* New York: Plenum Press, 303–327.

Tapp, N. (1989). *Sovereignty and rebellion: The White Hmong of Northern Thailand.* Singapore: Oxford University Press.

Thao, X. (1986). Hmong perception of illness and traditional ways of healing. In G. Hendrick, B. T. Downing, & A. S. Deinard (Eds.), *The Hmong in transition.* New York: Center for Migration Studies of New York and Southeast Asian Refugee Studies of the University of Minnesota, 365–378.

True, G. (1997). "My souls will come back to trouble you": Cultural and ethical issues in the coerced treatment of a Hmong adolescent. *Southern Folklore, 54*(20), 101–114.

Trueba, H. T., Jacobs, L., & Kirton, E. (1990). *Cultural conflict and adaptation: The case of Hmong children in American society.* New York: Falmer Press.

Vandeusen, J. (1982). Health/mental studies of Indochinese refugees: A critical overview. *Medical Anthropology, 6*(4), 231–252.

Vang, K., Vang, H. T., Simmons, C., Tashima, N., & Ramirez, D. T. (1985). *Hmong concepts of illness and healing with a Hmong/English glossary.* Fresno: Nationalities Services of Central California.

Vang, C. K., Yang, G. Y., & Smalley, W. A. (1990). *The life of Shong Lue Yang: Hmong "mother of writing"* (Southeast Asian Refugee Studies, No. 9). Minneapolis: University of Minnesota, Center for Urban and Regional Affairs.

Vang, M. M. (1994). *Hmong mothers and daughters: Cultural adjustment and conflict.* Unpublished master's thesis, California State University, Stanislaus.

Vawter, D. E., & Babbitt, B. (1997). Hospice care for terminally ill Hmong patients: A good cultural fit? *Minnesota Medicine, 80*(11), 42–44.

Warner, R. (1995). *Back fire: The CIA's secret war in Laos and its link to the war in Vietnam.* New York: Simon and Schuster.

Waters, D., Rao, R., & Petracchi, H. (1992). Providing health care for the Hmong. *Wisconsin Medical Journal, 91*(11), 642–651.

Wausau Area Hmong Mutual Association, Inc. (1995). *English-Hmong anatomy and medical phrase book.* (1st ed.). Wausau, WI: Author.

Weldon, C. (1999). *Tragedy in paradise: A country doctor at war in Laos.* Bangkok: Asia Books.

Westermeyer, J. (1982). *Poppies, pipes, and people: Opium and its use in Laos.* Berkeley and Los Angeles: University of California Press.

Westermeyer, J. (1986). Indochinese refugees in community and clinic: A report from Asia and the United States. In C. Williams & J. Westermeyer (Eds.), *Refugee mental health in resettlement countries.* Washington D.C.: Hemisphere, 113–130.

Westermeyer, J. (1988). A matched pairs study of depression among Hmong refugees with particular reference to predisposing factors and treatment outcomes. *Social Psychiatry and Psychiatric Epidemiology, 23,* 64–71.

Westermeyer, J., & Her, C. (1996). English fluency and social adjustment among Hmong refugees in MN. *Journal of Nervous and Mental Disease, 184*(2), 130–132.

Westermeyer, J., Lyfoung, T., & Neider, J. (1989). An epidemic of opium dependence among Asian refugees in Minnesota: Characteristics and causes. *British Journal of Addiction, 84,* 785–789.

Westermeyer, J., Neider, J., & Vang, T. F. (1984). Acculturation and mental health: A study of Hmong refugees at 1.5 and 3.5 years postmigration. *Social Science and Medicine, 18*(1), 87–93.

Westermeyer, J., & Thao, X. (1986). Cultural beliefs and surgical procedures. *Journal of the American Medical Association, 255*(23), 3301–3302.

Wittet, S. (1983). *Southeast Asian refugee concerns about health care in the U.S.* Unpublished master's thesis, University of Washington, Seattle.

Wright, A. (1986). *A never-ending refugee camp: The explosive birthrate in Ban Vinai.* Unpublished manuscript, Bangkok, Thailand.

Xiong, P. (1998a). *Hmong health concepts and understanding of human anatomy.* Unpublished manuscript, St. Paul, MN.

Xiong, P. (1998b). *Souls, shamans and medicine.* Unpublished manuscript, St. Paul, MN.

Xiong, P., & Culhane-Pera, K. (1995, April). *Hmong perceptions and attitudes about immunizations.* Paper presented at Hmong National Education Conference, St. Paul, MN.

Xiong, Z. B. (2000). *Hmong-American family problem-solving interactions: An analytic induction analysis.* Unpublished doctoral dissertation, University of Minnesota, St. Paul, MN.

Yang, D. (1975). *Les Hmong du Laos face au development.* Vientiane, Laos: Editions Siosavath.

Yang, D. (1982). Why did the Hmong leave Laos? Observations and reports. In B. Downing & D. Olney (Eds.), *The Hmong in the West*. Minneapolis: Southeast Asian Refugee Studies Project, Center for Urban and Regional Affairs, University of Minnesota, 3–18.

Yang, D. (1993). *Hmong at the turning point*. Minneapolis, MN: WorldBridge Associates.

Yang, K. (in press). Problems in the interpretation of Hmong clan surnames. In G. Lee, N. Tapp, C. Culas, & J. Michaud (Eds.), *Hmong/Miao studies: History, language, identity*. Chiang Mai, Thailand: Silkworm Press.

Zander, D. B. (2002, August 1). Loneliness and isolation may lead to casino gambling addiction among Hmong elders: Available resources and ways to prevent problems. *Hmong Times*, 3.

Zander, D. B., & Xiong L. P. (1998, March). The effects of problem gambling on Southeast Asian families and their adjustment to life in Minnesota. Paper presented at the conference on Hmong mental health, University of Wisconsin, Eau Claire.

## Further Hmong Resources

### Annotated Bibliographies

Pfeifer, M. E. (2002). *Annotated bibliography of Hmong-related works: 1996–2001*. St. Paul: Hmong Resource Center, Hmong Cultural Center.

Smith, J. C. (1996). The Hmong, 1987–1995: *A selected and annotated bibliography*. Minneapolis: University of Minnesota Refugee Studies Center.

### Web Sites

Asian & Pacific Islander American Health Forum home page. *http://apiahf.org/* [June 13, 2002].

Association of Asian Pacific Community Health Organizations home page (1999). *www.aapcho.org* [June 13, 2002].

Hmong Cultural Center, Inc. *Hmong subject bibliographies*. Available from *www.hmongcenter.org/hmonsubbib.html* [June 13, 2002].

Hmong Health Website. *www.hmonghealth.org* [February 6, 2003].

Hmong HomePage. *www.hmongnet.org* [January 31, 2003].

Hmong Language Institute home page. *www.hmonginstitute.org* [January 30, 2003].

Hmong Studies Internet Resource Center home page. *www.hmongstudies.org/* [June 13, 2002].

Hmong Studies Journal home page. *www.members.aol.com/hmongstudies/HSJ.html* [June 13, 2002].

Lao Community Health Web home page. *www.laofamily.org/health/index.html* [June 13, 2002].

*On-line Hmong-English dictionary*. Retrieved January 31, 2003, from McKibben Family Home Page at *http://members.citynet.net/brianm/hmdict/list.htm*

National Asian Women's Health Organization home page. *www.nawho.org/* [October 17, 2000].

Minnesota Department of Health. (2002). *Refugee health information*. Retrieved January 30, 2003, from *www.health.state.mn.us/divs/dpc/adps/refugee/refugeepub.htm*

Minnesota Department of Health. (2002). *Vaccine brochures*. Available from *www.health.state.mn.us/divs/dpc/adps/tran_lang.htm* [January 30, 2003].

## Motion Pictures

American Cancer Society. (1997). *Cancer: What you should know (Koj yuav tsum paub dab tsi txo)*. Available from American Cancer Society-Minnesota, 952–925–2772.

Haley, N. (1983.) *Great branches, new roots: The Hmong family.* Available from Hmong Film Project, 2258 Commonwealth Avenue, St. Paul, MN 55108.

Levine, K., & Levine, I. W. (1983). *Becoming American: The odyssey of a refugee family.* Available from *www.newday.com/films/Becoming_American.html*

Minnesota Department of Health. (1998). *Anemia prevention (Paab miv nyuas cov ntshaav lab kuam muaj zug)*. Available from Minnesota Department of Health WIC Program, 651-281-9912.

Siegel, T. (2001). *The split horn: Life of a Hmong shaman in America.* Available from *www.alchemyfilms.com*

Spring, M. A. & Deinard, A. (1989). *Pregnancy in America: Prenatal care for Hmong women.* In Hmong language with written English script. Available from Amos Deinard, MMC 85, 420 Delaware St. SE, Minneapolis, MN 55455.

Spring, M. A. & Deinard, A. (1992). *Contraceptive information for Hmong couples in America.* In Hmong language with written English script. Available from Amos Deinard, MMC 85, 420 Delaware St. SE, Minneapolis, MN 55455.

Spring, M. A. & Deinard, A. (1992). *Hmong family planning in America.* In Hmong language with written English script. Available from Amos Deinard, MMC 85, 420 Delaware St. SE, Minneapolis, MN 55455.

Spring, M. A. & Deinard, A. (1992). *Pap smear and colposcopy: Health-care for Hmong women in America.* In Hmong language with written English script. Available from Amos Deinard, MMC 85, 420 Delaware St. SE, Minneapolis, MN 55455.

Spring, M. A. & Deinard, A. (1997). *Adult dental care for Hmong in America.* In Hmong language with written English script. Available from Amos Deinard, MMC 85, 420 Delaware St. SE, Minneapolis, MN 55455.

Spring, M. A. & Deinard, A. (1997). *Preventing baby-bottle tooth decay in Hmong children.* In Hmong language with written English script supplied. Available from Amos Deinard, MMC 85, 420 Delaware St. SE, Minneapolis, MN 55455.

Spring, M. A. & Deinard, A. (2001). *Breast cancer awareness and screening methods for Hmong women.* Available from Amos Deinard, MMC 85, 420 Delaware St. SE, Minneapolis, MN 55455.

Vang, D. & Finck, J. (1983). *Peace has not been made.* Available from Office of Refugee Settlement, Cranston, RI, 401–464–2127.

Xiong, P. (2000). *Hmong Health Promotion Project. Nrhiav Kev Noj Qab Nyob Zoo.* English and White Hmong versions. Available from St. Paul Family Health Center, 962 University Avenue West, St. Paul, MN 55104.

PART II

# Women's Health

*Case Stories and Commentaries*

# 2

# Controlling Fertility

## *A Case Story*

Mrs. Pader Moua came to the United States when she was eight years old. She married when she was sixteen and her husband was twenty-eight. They have been married for eight years, have four children (two boys and two girls), and do not want any more children because of the high cost of raising children in this country.

During the month after the birth of their fourth child, Mrs. Moua took a Hmong herbal medicine to prevent future pregnancies. When she became pregnant six months later, she and her husband decided she would have an abortion. After the abortion, when the clinic staff asked the couple to choose a reliable Western type of contraception, they said they could not make a decision right then; they needed time to discuss it. In the meantime, they planned to continue to use the withdrawal method combined with natural family planning. They believed tubal ligation can cause chronic abdominal pain and interfere with a woman's ability to work. Also, men in the community have been known to ridicule the few Hmong men who have undergone vasectomy. They were uncertain about using other methods.

Six months later Mrs. Moua became pregnant again. She delivered a baby boy. Now, with five children, the Mouas agreed to try using condoms but refused to use any pills or injections. Having heard stories of Hmong women who experienced complications from contraceptive medications, they remained convinced that it would be unsafe for Mrs. Moua to take any Western medication to prevent pregnancy. The pills, they said, were made for Western women, not for Hmong women.

When Mrs. Moua saw her family physician for a routine visit and revealed that she and her husband were not using condoms—since the condoms caused irritation and were damaging her body—clinic staff, including a Hmong nursing assistant, urged Mrs. Moua to try Depo-Provera. Mrs. Moua refused, knowing that her husband believed the drugs were too dangerous and that it was unhealthy for a woman not to have menstrual periods.

A month later Mrs. Moua made an appointment to receive Depo-Provera. She asked the clinic staff not to tell her husband since she knew he would object. The clinic staff felt very relieved and assured her they would keep her secret.

## Questions for Consideration

### *Questions about Culture*

How do traditional Hmong beliefs and practices regarding preventing or postponing pregnancies differ from those of U.S. health care professionals?

What methods did Hmong couples use to control fertility in Laos?

What is known about how Hmong couples in the United States make decisions about controlling fertility, pregnancies, and the desired number of children?

What methods of controlling fertility are most readily accepted by Hmong couples in the United States? Why?

Why might the Mouas have decided to continue their second unplanned pregnancy?

What factors might have influenced Mrs. Moua's decision to receive Depo-Provera?

How is Mr. Moua's role in the decision making similar to or different from the role of U.S.-born husbands?

### *Questions about Cross-Cultural Health Care Ethics*

In what ways do risk/benefit assessments by the U.S. health care practitioners differ from those of Mrs. and Mr. Moua?

In what ways is protection of patient confidentiality understood differently by Hmong patients and U.S. health care professionals? What possible conflicts might these differences raise?

What ethical conflicts can exist for U.S. health care professionals involved in assisting couples like the Mouas to find an acceptable option to prevent pregnancy?

### *Questions about Culturally Responsive Health Care*

How can U.S. health care practitioners convey information about fertility and contraception that is most helpful to traditional Hmong couples?

In what ways is this case an example of a good cross-cultural health care relationship?

*Commentary*

# Hmong Preferences for Natural Family Planning

*Marline A. Spring, Ph.D., and Mayly Lyfoung Lochungvu*

Hmong-American couples who want to limit their number of births frequently find it difficult to select and use reliable contraception. They fear invasive scientific contraceptive methods and lack understanding about current Western knowledge of human fertility (Spring, 2001). In this commentary we review the Hmong-American ideals of family composition and discuss the health concerns that influence their decision making about using modern contraceptives. We then examine actions taken by the Mouas in their efforts to limit family size and analyze the intercultural miscommunication illustrated in the case. Finally, we suggest how clinicians can better meet the needs of people like the Mouas.

## Hmong Patterns of Family Building

The Hmong social organization evolved in an Asian environment that favored large, self-sufficient families in which people fostered the well-being of other family members. People relied on and promoted siblings first, then cousins, and finally other clan members. Toward this end, women gave birth to and raised as many children as was their destiny to have. Limiting the number of children born in a family was generally not considered desirable because large families were regarded as more resourceful and successful.

A concept central to Hmong cosmology is that a woman's luck *(hmoov)* or destiny *(ntawv)* determines the number of children she will bear. Husbands and wives may not discuss family planning or contraception because they rely on their destiny to determine the number of their children. These families are frequently larger than those in Laos because infant mortality rates in the United States are lower. Further, the near-universal change from breast-feeding in Southeast Asia to bottle-feeding of infants in the United States has eliminated the contraceptive effect of breast-feeding.

A growing number of Hmong couples are adapting to the U.S. economic environment by having fewer children than their parents had in Laos. In general, couples who have more intercultural contact tend to discuss and plan their desired completed family size and take decisive actions to effect it. These couples often have regular jobs outside of the home and may also have established relationships with American people through educational, religious, or civic organizations. Frequently, husbands are the first to favor smaller families and to encourage their wives to use modern contraceptives. The empirical and theoretical explanations for these demographic changes are beyond the scope of this commentary (see Kunstadter, Kunstadter, Podhisita, & Ritnetikul, 1989).

Although Hmong people are making adjustments, couples try to attain certain cultural ideals. Hmong couples feel obliged to have sons who can care for their elderly parents, reproduce the lineage, and preserve the memory of the deceased by performing rituals in which they venerate ancestors. Daughters cannot serve in these capacities because they become members of the lineages and the clans into which they marry and for whom they produce members (Symonds, 1991). Couples who have only daughters frequently continue to have children until they have at least one son, and often they try for two. Those who have only sons may try for a daughter, but in these cases, couples are increasingly willing to forgo a daughter.

A second goal is to have at least two children of each sex so that each child has a same-sex sibling on whom to rely and in whom to confide. Many couples feel compelled to have more children than they consider economically prudent in attempts to have another boy for their only son or another daughter for their only daughter. They consider it cruel to leave a child without providing a same-sex sibling because the child will be lonely. Some believe that it is difficult to be a Hmong woman in the United States and that each needs a sister for emotional and social support. Similarly, a Hmong man can ask his brother for help any time, but he will stop and consider the obligation before asking a cousin or others for help. Further, while siblings can be counted on for support, same-sex siblings know each other more intimately, so they are in a better position to have the best interest of the other in mind at all times.

Preferences of family composition are changing among highly educated Hmong women and men. Like many Hmong Americans, they frequently begin child-bearing at an early age (Dunnigan, Olney, McNall, & Spring, 1997), but they indicate that they will have only two or three children. The women want to devote time to their careers, and men anticipate that they cannot support more children. They submit that daughters are as able as sons to care for their parents in the United States. Some point out that daughters are more gentle and caring toward parents. These women are currently in their early child-bearing years, and it is too soon to evaluate this trend.

The Mouas are in a good position to be resolute about having no more children. First, each child has a same-sex sibling, and the parents may feel fortunate that their fifth child was a son. Second, they are in the segment of the Hmong population in which couples discuss family size. Third, they agree on limiting births, and Mr. Moua demonstrated his support of this goal when he accompanied Mrs. Moua to the abortion.

## Western Methods of Limiting Births

Most Hmong American couples are aware of Western pharmacological, technological, and surgical methods of limiting births. While some use Western contraceptives successfully, the unpleasant or adverse experiences that others have had with these methods are recounted in the Hmong community, and many, like the Mouas, are afraid to try them.

## Abortion

Mrs. Moua is among the minority of Hmong women who have undergone abortion for the purpose of controlling family size. Hmong people more commonly favor restricting the use of abortion to other situations, such as poor maternal health, poverty, fetal defect, rape, and a need to preserve the reputation of an unwed woman. Some favor banning all abortions. Among those who choose abortion, many voice preference for the medical abortion technique, rather than a surgical procedure. Although many do favor the availability of abortion to all women, they would not elect to have an abortion or want their wife to have one. They believe that the surgical abortion procedure is dangerous and unpredictable because the uterus is subject to injury when it is "scraped." People have heard of women who became infertile or developed cancer following an abortion, and many attribute these conditions to uterine damage incurred during the procedure. Others fear that a spirit of the fetus may return and punish the woman in this or future lives by causing infertility, fetal or infant deaths, deaths of other loved ones, irreversible losses such as blindness or disfigurement, or other hardships (see Chapter 13). Some Hmong women suffer from chronic burning abdominal pain after one abortion, while others develop the condition after two or more abortions. These accounts lead many Hmong to believe that a medical abortion can be less risky than a surgical procedure, and that having one abortion may be safe, but more than one can cause permanent physical damage. These stories may have prompted the Mouas to decide against a second abortion.

## Surgical Sterilization

To many Americans, Mrs. Moua would appear to be a good candidate for surgical sterilization because she and her husband do not want to have more children. However, this procedure is not popular in the Hmong community. First, many women are reluctant to be sterilized because they want to leave open the possibility of having another child in the future. For example, in the event that her husband dies, a woman will likely want to have a child with a future husband to seal and strengthen the marriage bond. Second, some women who have undergone surgical sterilization now suffer from debilitating abdominal pain. This condition sometimes leads to deterioration of the marriage or divorce. Stories of these women's experiences frighten others and effectively eliminate this option for them.

There are Hmong women who have had tubal ligations and do not now suffer any physical discomfort. Some have successful careers in the service, health, or education sectors. It would seem that they would be community models for the success of this family planning method, but some deeply regret having stopped child-bearing after two or three children. This choice was most commonly made by couples who arrived in the first years (1975–80) of the Hmong immigration to the United States. Well-meaning U.S. sponsors counseled Hmong mothers who had two or more children, some as young as in their twenties, to be sterilized because the economic realities of life in the United States would make having more children difficult for them. Now, years later, the women regret having made the decision to be sterilized at such a young age; they long to have more children, know that they could have supported more children, and feel guilt about leaving their children without same-sex siblings. Although these families are successful by U.S. standards, they may not be role models for Hmong families.

## Hormonal Contraceptives

Like the Mouas, some Hmong fear using hormonal contraceptives. Women who have tried the various methods sometimes experience undesirable weight fluctuations or irregular or decreased menses, conditions regarded as detrimental to a woman's health or as symptomatic of disease. Accounts of women who became pregnant while using hormonal contraceptives tell of children being born with mental retardation or other birth defects (Spring, Davis, & Rode, 1997). Other women have experienced infertility or developed cancer after taking hormonal contraceptives. Hormonal contraceptives are available as pills and as injectables. Hmong women are more likely to use oral contraceptive pills than injectables, and many prefer the Chinese-made monthly estrogen-progesterone pill that they purchase in some local Asian pharmacies. Hormonal implants, an option that is no longer available, were the least favored hormonal contraceptive. Women value being able to stop taking the pill and find that it has fewer side-effects and is more likely to regulate menses. Injections and implants frequently eliminate menses. As a result, many who receive an initial injection do not return for another. However, for those who have difficulty remembering to take the pill daily, injections are the preferred form of hormonal contraception. The recently introduced skin patch has become an attractive option and may soon be the most popular form of contraception for women who choose hormonal contraception.

## Barrier Contraceptives

Generally, barrier contraceptives are less acceptable to Hmong and are considered to be less reliable than hormonal methods. Women sometimes experience abdominal pain when a diaphragm or an intrauterine device is in place, and the latter is sometimes thought to cause uterine damage. Condoms are gaining in popularity, but some people object to them because they cause vaginal irritation and injury and they decrease sensitivity. Some women fear that any of the barriers, including condoms, may migrate and become lost inside their bodies.

## Birth Control "the Hmong Way"

Many Hmong Americans, including the Mouas, prefer to use Hmong birth control methods because they find Western contraceptive methods unattractive. Mrs. Moua first employed an herbal contraceptive. It may have been sent to her from Southeast

Asia because plants that Hmong women use to effect sterility in Laos are not grown in the United States (Spring, 1989). The identity and efficacy of these plants are unknown to Western scientists. These methods, as well as Western hormonal contraceptives, are thought by some Hmong to cause permanent dark spots on women's faces, thereby identifying those who use them.

Precisely what behavior the Mouas meant by "natural family planning" was not conveyed in the case story. It is important for clinic staff to ask what the phrase means because it implies different behaviors to different people. The Hmong word *caiv* is often interpreted as "natural family planning." *Caiv* means prohibition or taboo, but in a discussion of sexual relations, there is no consensus about its interpretation or the precise behaviors associated with some interpretations. Other interpretations include "the natural method," "the Hmong way," "abstinence," "periodic abstinence," "abstinence at ovulation time," "rhythm," and "withdrawal." Since people do not talk about details of their sexual practices, many couples, interpreters, and clinicians are not aware of the multiple meanings for *caiv,* and they make assumptions about the behaviors in which couples engage. Making assumptions can lead to faulty communication between patients and physicians as well as unintended outcomes.

Similarly, clinicians cannot assume they know what behaviors are associated with English interpretations of *caiv.* For those who take *caiv* to mean abstinence, the associated behavior is usually infrequent intercourse in order to reduce the risk of pregnancy. Others understand *caiv* as abstaining from sexual intercourse only at ovulation time. However, opinions about when ovulation occurs vary widely. Those who understand fertility based on Hmong concepts of reproductive physiology believe that ovulation occurs during or immediately following menstruation. People who were taught about family planning in the refugee camps in Thailand may understand that this belief is not true, but most are unclear about the exact timing of ovulation. A few have consulted reference books to try to determine when to avoid sexual intercourse. People who have learned about fertility in the United States have a better understanding of the menstrual cycle and the timing of ovulation, but few understand in practical terms how to apply their knowledge to avoid pregnancy.

Hmong also report that *caiv* refers to practicing coitus interruptus or withdrawal. Some report that their elders counseled them to avoid this technique because, according to Hmong concepts, a condition known as *piv ncev* can occur if a man withdraws and does not ejaculate. In *piv ncev,* the unejaculated semen is thought to go into the abdomen, where it forms a hard painful mass that is potentially fatal. Because withdrawal was proscribed in some villages, some Hmong learned of it only after arriving in the United States, and others have never heard of it.

The case story does not specify how the Mouas tried to prevent conception when they were practicing "natural family planning" and withdrawal. Given the dearth of accurate and practical knowledge in the Hmong community about natural family planning strategies, and the desire of both Mr. and Mrs. Moua to avoid pregnancy, it is likely that they failed twice to prevent pregnancy because they lacked adequate knowledge.

## A Long-Term Solution

The case story suggests that the clinic staff did not query or counsel the Mouas about their natural family planning practices. A Western medical bias toward pharmacological, technological, and surgical contraception may have prevented clinic staff from discussing contraception with the Mouas. Instead, staff continued to urge the couple to accept one of several methods that they feared. Eventually Mrs. Moua independently requested a contraceptive injection that would provide her with protection for three months. At the end of the three months, she will again face the questions of how she can avoid another pregnancy and whether she will act contrary to her husband's wishes.

Two important considerations argue for the clinic staff to accept the Mouas' position and work with them to find a mutually acceptable family planning method. First, Mrs. Moua's decision to receive an injectable contraceptive without the knowledge or agreement of her husband could have long-lasting negative consequences for the family. Although she asked clinic staff to keep her confidence, it is likely that Mr. Moua will find out through other means. Hmong people may not talk about or question others about their sexual practices, but they do freely discuss contraception use. In the future, Mrs. Moua may tell relatives or friends about the injections, and it may get back to her husband. He may also become suspicious and question why her menstrual cycle is disrupted. When he learns that she received the injection without his agreement, their marriage could deteriorate because of this breach of trust. Further, should Mrs. Moua become ill or incapacitated in any way in the future, it would confirm Mr. Moua's initial fear that contraceptive medications are unsafe. Rather than being sympathetic to her malady and helping her, Mr. Moua may blame her for bringing the illness on herself. By receiving the contraceptive injection without her husband's knowledge and support, Mrs. Moua faces a variety of possible unpleasant consequences, and she must reconsider these consequences every three months when she decides whether she will return for another contraceptive injection.

A second consideration is that the Mouas want to avoid another pregnancy and have a contraceptive method in mind, which is natural family planning, but they lack the knowledge required to successfully implement it. These methods are often overlooked by clinicians because of bias or the lack of staff time and knowledge to thoroughly instruct patients. Clinic staff could refer the Mouas to Hmong people trained to counsel and teach conception prevention using an ovulation method of natural family planning. Complete, accurate, and practical knowledge about natural family planning methods will give the Mouas a better understanding of the contributions and responsibilities of each in preventing pregnancy, and they will be in a position to make an informed joint assessment of the risks and benefits of using natural methods. They may join a growing number of Hmong couples who have learned from qualified trainers and are successfully using the cervical mucous observation method of natural family planning to prevent or to space pregnancies.

Alternatively, the Mouas may find that they do not want to follow the prescribed periodic abstinence or realize that they want to use a more reliably effective contraceptive at this time in their lives. In this case, the Mouas will be adequately informed about human fertility and better able to formulate questions about and consider the risks and benefits of all contraceptive methods.

Teaching Hmong couples current and practical information about human fertility will help them find acceptable contraceptive methods throughout their lives.

## References

Dunnigan, T., Olney, D. P., McNall, M. A., & Spring, M. A. (1997). Hmong. In D. W. Haines (Ed.), *Case studies in diversity: Refugees in America in the 1990s*. Westport, CT: Praeger, 145–166.

Kunstadter, P., Kunstadter, S. L., Podhisita, C., & Ritnetikul, P. (1989). Hmong demography: An anthropological case study. In *International Population Conference, New Delhi* (Vol. 3). Liege, Belgium: International Union for the Scientific Study of Population, 317–330.

Spring, M. A. (1989). Ethnopharmacologic analysis of medicinal plants used by Laotian Hmong refugees in Minnesota. *Journal of Ethnopharmacology, 26*, 65–91.

Spring, M. A. (2001). *Reproductive health and fertility of Hmong immigrants in Minnesota*. Unpublished doctoral dissertation, University of Minnesota, Minneapolis.

Spring, M. A., Davis, K., & Rode, P. (1997). *Prenatal care among Southeast Asian women in Saint Paul and Minneapolis: A survey of Cambodian, Hmong, Laotian and Vietnamese women in the Twin Cities*. St. Paul: Urban Coalition.

Symonds, P. V. (1991). *Cosmology and the cycle of life: Hmong view of birth, death, and gender in a mountain village in Northern Thailand*. Unpublished doctoral dissertation, Brown University, Providence, RI.

*Commentary*

# Social, Cultural, and Ethical Aspects
# of Controlling Fertility
# in the Hmong Community

*Peter Kunstadter, Ph.D.*

This case raises several issues related to fertility control among Hmong patients in the United States and raises broader questions relating to provision of effective and acceptable health services for Hmong (and other nonmainstream) patients in the U.S. health care system. Among these questions are the following:

- Why do some Hmong patients not comply with advice from health care providers even when they say they understand and accept the reason for doing so?
- Who makes health care decisions in Hmong society, including decisions concerning fertility control, and what processes and criteria are used in reaching these decisions?
- What are the cultural and biomedical explanations for "side-effects" that may vary from the descriptions in medical literature but are used by Hmong patients as rationales for discontinuation or noncompliance with medicines or activities prescribed by U.S. providers?
- What are the patterns of relationships between Hmong and their non-Hmong health care providers? What has determined these patterns? And how do they affect the acceptance and effectiveness of health care?
- What are the implications of applying ethics derived from Western culture to the practice of medicine with people whose values differ markedly from those of Western culture?

In considering these questions, I start with three assertions. First, although reproduction is a biological process, the promotion or inhibition of fertility are behavioral phenomena and must be understood in terms of the cultural and socioeconomic background of the individuals involved. Traditionally, Hmong in Southeast Asia have maintained very high fertility with practices supported by traditional religion and values and closely integrated with traditional household economics and local political systems.

Second, although Western health care services are nominally directed at specific biomedical conditions of individuals, these services involve social relationships modeled on and influenced by other aspects of the patients' and the providers' societies. Health service "problems" that doctors term "lack of compliance" imply that the "doctor knows best." Doctors may not intend to exercise power or be coercive in such relationships and may not recognize that they are doing so. Nonetheless, doctors' manner and practices may be interpreted as prejudicial by Hmong patients.

Third, for Hmong refugees in the United States and for nonrefugee Hmong in Thailand, changing social and economic conditions are affecting the customary supports for high fertility. Comparison of Hmong in these two locations sheds light on some of the practical and ethical issues related to delivery of appropriate health care for Hmong living in the United States. This commentary is based on information gleaned from twenty years of demographic research with Hmong in Thailand and California.

## Factors Affecting Fertility in Traditional Hmong Society

Hmong refugees and nonrefugees generally have had very high fertility rates, but fertility is influenced even in the absence of modern contraception by both biology and culturally sanctioned behaviors. Biological controls on fertility include the age of reproductive maturity and of senescence, which limit the length of men's and women's reproductive life spans, and which can be influenced by nutrition and disease. Biological factors, including the suppression of ovulation by breast-feeding, affect the length of postpartum infertility for women, which in turn affects birth spacing and the total number of possible births over a woman's life span. Biological variables are affected, however, by such factors as social sanctions on intercourse and marriage, desires for children, and attempts to meet fertility goals.

In traditional Hmong society, there are strong pressures for all men and women to marry and strong motives for everyone to reproduce. In a 1987–88 survey of nonrefugee Hmong in Thailand, out of 1,053 men and 1,125 women age thirty and above, only 1.3 percent of the men and 1.0 percent of the women had never married, because of physical deformity, mental handicap, or personal desire. Most women traditionally marry at a young age; half of the women had married by age seventeen, and half of the men by age nineteen. A common Hmong attitude concerning the age of marriage is that marriage partners should be mature enough to fulfill adult economic and social roles, including providing and caring for children. Under traditional conditions, this usually means that boys and girls can marry when they are physically mature.

Almost all Hmong marriages result in reproduction. Hmong women may and traditionally do continue bearing children well into their forties and even beyond age fifty. There does not seem to be any traditional custom or norm that inhibits fertility beyond any specific, biologically determined age. Traditionally, the Hmong try to have as many children as possible, for many reasons. For their parents and each other, children provide affection, social support, economic support in the labor-intensive subsistence agricultural economy, and political support in disputes with other families. Sons are essential both to maintain the patrilineal family line that is an integral part of ancestor worship and to provide economic support for their aging parents. Hmong parents traditionally want to continue to have children, regardless of how many daughters they have, until they are sure they have one or more surviving sons. An equal number of sons and daughters, however, is ideal: in this way, the money needed by sons to pay for bride-prices will be balanced with the money gained from daughters' bride-prices.

Women want children as much as men do. Women depend economically and socially on their husbands and children (especially their sons) rather than on their own biological parents or siblings; thus, for their own well-being, women want sons. Because infertility, low fertility, or failure to have sons is usually blamed on women, women have another strong motive to reproduce. They also wish to avoid the possibilities that their husbands will divorce them or marry a second wife. Some women believe that they are fated to have a certain number of children, and if they do not have them in this life, they will have to have them in the next reincarnation.

The result, on average, is relatively early onset and a prolonged period of child bearing for Hmong women. Total fertility rate (TFR) among nonrefugee Hmong in Thailand was about eight children per woman until the early 1980s. (TFR is the total number of children that an average woman will bear by the time she reaches the end of her childbearing years, if current age-specific rates are maintained throughout that period.) Our surveys of Hmong refugees in California indicate their TFR in Laos was about the same, or slightly higher.

Despite the strong social reasons for high fertility, under some circumstances people may want to prevent pregnancy, delay child-bearing, or increase the interval between births. For example, people may feel they are too old or that they cannot afford the expense of another child. Traditionally, "everyone knows" about abortion, and "everyone knows" there are herbal medicines that render a woman infertile (supposedly for life). However, there does not seem to be any deliberate attempt to teach unmarried children about contraception to delay pregnancy, increase birth intervals, or limit the number of births.

Research shows that Hmong in Thailand have effectively and rapidly reduced their fertility. Fertility began to fall rapidly in the 1980s, from a TFR of eight or more in 1982 to five or more in 1987. Hmong relate their reduction in fertility to several factors. Most important, the Thai government restricted their access to land, forbade them to clear trees, and outlawed opium production. Parents seeing that their children might not have enough land to carry on their traditional land-extensive, labor-intensive form of agriculture, reduced their fertility by increasing their use of modern contraception, rather than by delaying marriage.

## Factors Affecting Fertility among Refugee Hmong in the United States

As some traditional attitudes and behaviors persist while others change, Hmong refugees in the United States have maintained high fertility rates. For Hmong who migrated to the United States, physical maturity comes at a younger age (probably because there is more food and less infection) than for Hmong in Southeast Asia, while social maturity comes at an older age (given the general society's requirements for education and minimum legal age of consent). Nonetheless, age at marriage, especially for women, remains low, and their reproductive span therefore remains long. While some families support education and delaying marriage for boys and girls, many other families do not encourage and support education as much for daughters as for sons, because investment in the education of daughters is not seen as economically beneficial to parents. Thus, daughters may be available for marriage before their education is complete.

Comparisons of birth histories collected among nonrefugee Hmong in Thailand with birth histories of refugee women in California before and after they arrived in the United States show that birth intervals are shorter after arrival in the United States. The reduction in birth intervals and the consequent increase in fertility appear to be related to a decline in breast-feeding, from over 95 percent among Hmong women in Southeast Asia to less than 10 percent in California. In the absence of deliberate contraception, breast-feeding increases birth intervals by delaying postpartum return of ovulation. Refugee women perceive that breast-feeding interferes with their normal school or work routines and that it is discouraged by the practice of separating newborn infants from their mothers after delivery in hospital. Many Hmong also believe that in the United States women do not breast-feed, apparently because they do not see American women breast-feeding. This perception contrasts with behavior in Thailand, where rural Hmong women do not believe breast-feeding interferes with their normal farming activities, where newborns are put on the breast immediately after birth, and where women normally breast-feed their infants semi-publicly for a year or more.

Parents and grandparents in the United States maintain a strong desire for children to contribute to household economics, for sons to perpetuate the lineage, and for daughters to provide emotional support or balance bride-price economics. Although most young adults honor their parents' wishes and continue to believe in the importance of sons to perpetuate the lineage, many also feel that it is neither practical nor important to have many children under U.S. life conditions. Use of modern contraception remains low, though, since many Hmong fear them.

## Similarities between the Case Study and the Experience of the Hmong in Thailand and California

Similarities between the Mouas' attempts to control fertility and the experience of Hmong men and women in Thailand and California suggest persistent cultural influences on determinants of fertility and on responses to modern methods of fertility control. For example, Mrs. Moua was quite young when she married, and she had four or five children in the first eight or nine years of her marriage, indicating high fertility and short birth intervals. Mrs. Moua used traditional medicine to attempt to prevent further pregnancies. Like many other Hmong, Mrs. Moua and her husband believe that tubal ligation will result in chronic abdominal pain and will limit her ability to work. Their dislike of vasectomy is shared by other Hmong who, contrary to medical experience, fear that it will limit sexual function. Also, their unsuccessful use of both natural methods of birth control and condoms echoes other Hmong people's reports of contraceptive failure.

The Mouas' belief that contraceptives that disrupt regular menstrual periods are unhealthy because normal and regular periods are important for cleaning out the uterus is widely shared by other Hmong couples. Hmong fear the side-effects of modern medicine generally because they believe that Western medicine is too powerful and fast for Hmong bodies, and—unlike traditional herbal medicine—likely to lead to poorer health. Long-term consumption of medicine, many Hmong believe, increases the likelihood of side-effects. These similarities in beliefs and fears indicate that there are consistent Hmong cultural patterns with regard to modern methods of contraception. The most commonly mentioned reason for discontinuation of family planning by Hmong in Thailand is the fear or experience of side-effects of Western contraceptive medicine. Hmong (especially those who grew up in Southeast Asia) generally have smaller body size; thus medications that are not adjusted for body mass may result in overdosage. The contraceptive pills given to Hmong women in Laos during the 1960s and 1970s still had a relatively high estrogen dosage. (The dosage has been significantly reduced since then.) This early experience may explain their bad reputation among Hmong. Since no systematic investigation of consistent reports of side-effects of contraceptive medicine among Hmong has been undertaken, real side-effects that may be related to either body size or genetic composition cannot be ruled out.

## Patient-Provider Relationships in the United States

Ineffective use of prescribed contraceptives because of real or feared side-effects suggests poor communication between providers and patients regarding possible side-effects, or systematic problems underlying relationships between Hmong patients and their Western medical providers. Most Hmong age forty and above, especially Hmong women, have limited English-language skills and little or no formal education. The leaders in the Hmong community are generally people of this age category. They are the people most likely to have suffered as a result of poor communication with Western health care providers, and they are the people most likely to be consulted in regard to any important family matter.

Inadequate interpretation can lead to incorrect use of medications and lack of understanding of side-effects and methods to correct them. Few health care facilities have trained interpreters. When medical interpreters are not available, younger, English-speaking family members may be asked to interpret for their elders. The normal pattern of Hmong social relationships is that younger people defer to their elders. When younger family members function as interpreters, the danger of misinterpretation because the person doing the interpretation lacks medical training, knowledge, and vocabulary is compounded by this disturbance in the normal social order. Moreover, since fertility control is an embarrassing topic in Hmong society, older women are unlikely to speak frankly when younger family members interpret.

Even where medical interpreters are available, most health care providers have not been trained in the effective use of interpreters.

Hmong patients are likely to view doctors as authority figures because of their extensive training and use of instruments that can see inside the body. They do not generally like to confront or challenge authority directly. If they experience side-effects, they are more likely either to discontinue the prescribed treatment or to seek advice from another provider, rather than return to their doctor to discuss alternatives.

Doctors may be reluctant to explain side-effects or medication risks for fear that their prescriptions will be rejected. Interpreters who lack the knowledge or do not have good working relationships with the providers may be unable to provide this information. The patient may therefore be unprepared for possible side-effects, such as interruption of the normal menstrual cycle.

Hmong patients' beliefs concerning patient-provider relationships may differ significantly from those held by providers. Research in California shows that most of the 210 household heads surveyed consider the social aspects of relationships to be more important in choosing primary care physicians than are measures of biomedically defined quality of care. They value providers who speak the same language, have interpreters, and respect their culture. In general, they deeply distrust providers who they believe are in the business of making money, will experiment on them, or will provide inferior care to patients on welfare.

For many Hmong refugees, their first contacts with modern medical care occurred in refugee camps in Thailand. In some cases the health services were run by fundamentalist religious organizations whose personnel strongly disapproved of traditional Hmong religious and curing beliefs and practices. Many Hmong came to believe that disapproval of Hmong culture was a characteristic of modern health care. Many Hmong think that health care providers are attacking their culture and identity and coercing them to accept treatment they do not want. These beliefs are exacerbated by widely shared stories of very difficult conflicts between Hmong, health care providers, and police.

## Ethical Implications of Fertility Control
## among Hmong Refugees

Ethical concerns arise when there are real or potential conflicts of interest or values, or where the "best interests" of the patient are in dispute. In the cross-cultural practice of medicine there will always be a basic issue: Whose ethics are paramount, those of the patient, the individual provider, or the dominant society?

The key ethical issue in this case concerns the interests of Mrs. Moua and the interests of her husband. Both husband and wife have expressed the desire to have no more children. The husband says he objects to use of Depo-Provera because he believes it poses a risk to Mrs. Moua's health. The decision of the clinic to give Depo-Provera to Mrs. Moua poses an ethical problem because the decision is to be concealed from the husband.

Because of where U.S. society is at this point in history, the decision is made to honor Mrs. Moua's request for Depo-Provera without her husband's knowledge. I interpret this as follows. The primary care doctor or clinic views Mrs. Moua as a mentally competent individual adult who has the right to make this decision. The doctor or clinic in turn has the right and duty to honor Mrs. Moua's request because it lies within the standard of practice.

In Hmong society, however, Mrs. Moua is seen not just as an individual but also—and primarily—as a member of a kin group. Her body, including her reproductive capacity and her ability to work, was bought and paid for when she married. Mr. Moua is the head of the family, and he has the right and obligation to look after the health of his family members. He views Depo-Provera as risky for Mrs. Moua's health, and it is likely that in a discussion with extended family or clan leaders, his opinion would be upheld.

Did the primary care physician or the clinic consider the social and psychological risks to Mrs. Moua if her husband learns that his wishes have been overruled? Should they consider those risks in their decision? If they agree to administer the drug as Mrs. Moua has requested, the risk that Mrs. Moua will have an unwanted child is reduced. At the same time, the risk of Mr. Moua's distrust (of wife, clinic, Western medicine, and U.S. society in general) is greatly increased.

What does Mr. Moua really want? Does he say he does not want more children because he knows that this is the "proper" answer in the United States? Are Mr. Moua's rejections of various methods of family planning his way of rejecting contraception while avoiding direct confrontation with the clinic or physician? Are his rejections of these methods ways of protecting himself from criticism from his kin-group elders if something goes wrong?

What procedures should a clinic use in evaluating the ethics of this situation? Who should set the criteria? Are Hmong represented on the ethics committee? If so, what should their ages, genders, status be? Should the criteria be exclusively those of the Western medical profession that stress individual rights and minimize the rights of families? Should Hmong social realities, in which wives are viewed more as members of a kin-group than as individuals, be considered in making decisions in cases like this?

Answers to these questions have a bearing on the long-term happiness of both Mr. and Mrs. Moua and their children, as well as for the future operation of the clinic and the relationships between health care workers and Hmong patients.

## Other Works by the Author

Helsel, D., Petitti, D. B., & Kunstadter, P. (1992). Birth weight and other reproductive charac-teristics among the Hmong in California. *American Journal of Public Health, 82*(10), 1361–1364.

Kunstadter, P. (2003). Hmong marriage patterns in relation to social change. In G. Lee, J. Michaud, C. Culas, & N. Tapp (Eds.), *The Hmong in Southeast Asia: Current issues*. Chiang Mai: Silkworm.

Kunstadter, P., & Kunstadter, S. L. (1990). Health transitions in Thailand. In J. C. Caldwell, S.

Findley, P. Caldwell, G. Santow, W. Cosford, J. Braid, & D. Broers-Freeman (Eds.), *What we know about health transition*. Canberra, Australia: Health Transition Centre, Australian National University. 213–250.

Kunstadter, P., Podhisita, C., Leepreeca, P., & Kunstadter, S. L. (1991, November). Rapid changes in fertility among Hmong of Northern Thailand. *Proceedings of the Thai National Symposium on Population Studies*, pp.103–132.

Kunstadter, P., Kunstadter, S. L., Leepreecha, P., Podihisita, C., Laoyang, M., Sae Thao, C., Sae Thao, R., & Sae Yang, W. (1992). Causes and consequences of decline in child death rates: Ethnoepidemiology among Hmong of Thailand. *Human Biology, 64*(6), 821–841.

Kunstadter, P., Leepreecha, P., Kunstadter, S. L., and Sae Thao, R. (1992, November). Cultural determinants of Hmong age at marriage in relation to modernization. *Proceedings of the Thai National Symposium on Population Studies*, 500–525.

Kunstadter, P., Kunstadter, S. L., Podhisita, C., & Leepreecha, P. (1993). Demographic variables in fetal and child mortality: Hmong in Thailand. *Social Science and Medicine, 36*(9), 1109–1120.

Kunstadter, P., Kunstadter, S. L., Leepreecha, P., & Podhisita, C. (1994). Infrastructural, economic and demographic change: Hmong in Thailand. *High Plains Applied Anthropologist, 14*(2), 97–114.

Podhisita, C., Kunstadter, P., & Kunstadter, S. L. (1990). Evidence for early fertility transition among the Hmong in northern Thailand. *Journal of Population and Social Studies, 2*(2), 137–156.

## Acknowledgments

Data referred to in this article, unless otherwise indicated, result from the author's fieldwork, including research among Hmong in Thailand supported by a contract from the Ministry of Public Health of Thailand for research on use of modern health facilities and family planning by Karen and Hmong, by research grants BNS 7914093 and BNS 8040684 from the National Science Foundation, and by grants from the Pacific Rim Research Program of the University of California. Research among Hmong refugees in California has been supported by NICHD Grant RO1HD22686, grants from the Andrew W. Mellon Foundation, the Henry J. Kaiser Family Foundation, the James Irvine Foundation, The California Endowment, and the Pacific Rim Research Program of the University of California. Opinions expressed are those of the author.

# 3

## Woman with Pregnancy Complications

### *A Case Story*

In her fourth month of pregnancy, Mrs. Thor sought prenatal care at the midwifery clinic for the first pregnancy of her second marriage. A twenty-five-year-old woman, Mrs. Thor had lived in a Thai refugee camp for twelve years before coming to the United States with her family when she was fourteen years old. She attended high school for three years but did not graduate. She had a son from her first marriage who now lives with her ex-husband and his new wife. Three years ago she married her present husband, who is the youngest son of a large family, and they live with her husband's parents. She and the family had been concerned about her apparent difficulty with becoming pregnant and they attributed this pregnancy to the successful combination of shaman ceremonies, Hmong herbal medicines, and Western infertility treatment including pills and shots. Mrs. Thor was dedicated to making her marriage a success and was excited about this long awaited pregnancy.

Prior to coming to the midwifery clinic, Mrs. Thor sought prenatal care from an obstetrician. The doctor ordered five tubes of blood for a variety of tests, but Mrs. Thor refused, stating she was too weak and tired to have any blood drawn and she questioned why they needed so much blood. During the prenatal pelvic exam, the doctor wiped her cervix with a wooden spatula for a Pap smear and her cervix began to bleed. Seeing the blood, Mrs. Thor became frightened that the doctor's exam was causing her to miscarry. Despite reassurances that the bleeding was not related to a miscarriage, she left the clinic concerned about the viability of the pregnancy and did not return.

Afterward, on the advice of her sister, she sought prenatal care at the local midwifery clinic. There the midwife and Hmong nurse heard her story, listened to her concerns, and tried to reassure her that the examination had caused no harm to the fetus or to herself. They explained why a blood sample was desired and negotiated to draw a single ten-milliliter syringe of blood. They also recommended prenatal vitamins, but Mrs. Thor declined to take them, stating she did not want a large infant.

A test revealed that Mrs. Thor had an elevated level of alpha-fetoprotein (AFP) and she was called by telephone and asked to come to the clinic for further testing. Hearing the nurse's explanation that a high value may mean that the baby has a birth defect, such as a spina bifida, Mrs. Thor reluctantly agreed to a repeat blood test, the result of which was also high. A fetal ultrasound revealed no evidence of an abnormal spinal formation and the midwives explained the option of seeing a specialist who could test the fluid around the fetus for genetic abnormalities (amniocentesis). Mrs. Thor and her husband were horrified at the thought of using a needle to draw fluid from around the fetus and declined to consult the specialist.

Mrs. Thor did not keep her prenatal appointment at twenty-two weeks. One of the Hmong clinic staff called to schedule a new appointment and to ask whether she had any concerns. Mrs. Thor said she was fine and the baby was moving strongly. At twenty-four weeks, Mrs. Thor experienced labor pains every three minutes and called the clinic. At the clinic the midwife found that Mrs. Thor was in premature labor with regular contractions and her cervix was dilated to two centimeters. She was admitted to a hospital's labor and delivery unit, where obstetricians took over her care, placed her on strict bed rest, and gave her parenteral medication to stop the contractions (tocolytics) and to help the baby's lungs mature more quickly (corticosteriods). The next day she refused to receive any more medications because she was feeling quite ill, her contractions had stopped, and her cervix had stopped dilating. The doctors and midwives were very concerned about the welfare of Mrs. Thor's baby and tried to explain the risks of pre-term delivery to her, her husband, her husband's parents, and her father, who was visiting from out of state.

Mrs. Thor's father was the most vocal family member, explaining to the doctors that taking the medicine was unnecessary because his daughter's contractions had subsided. He explained that he had helped his wife deliver six healthy children without any sort of medical assistance—in some cases, under very difficult circumstances. He and his wife had had three children before they were forced to flee their village in the mountains of northern Laos and five children thereafter. Mrs. Thor and a younger brother were born while the family was living on the run in the jungle. During these two births, the father was on lookout for communist soldiers, and his wife delivered the children by herself. Finally, he assisted with the delivery of each of their last three children, who were born in a Thai refugee camp. His assessment was that his daughter's child was fine and did not need any interventions.

After the long family conference, Mrs. Thor left the hospital, signing a paper stating she was leaving the hospital against medical advice (AMA). A Hmong nurse called Mrs. Thor at home several times, but her family did not wish for her to speak on the telephone.

Two weeks later, at twenty-six weeks, Mrs. Thor came to the hospital with abdominal pains and a fever of 102.5°F. Her membranes had ruptured two days previously, her cervix was dilated to four centimeters, and her fetus was lying in a transverse position. The doctors recommended a cesarean-section, but the family wanted instead to try to have the fetus turned. The family arranged for a traditional Hmong medicine woman to come to the hospital to turn the fetus, but her efforts were unsuccessful.

Several hours of family discussions followed in Mrs. Thor's room, though she never offered an opinion. No medical interpreter was available in person and those family members who spoke English did not understand the medical terminology. A medical interpreter, who was not known to the family, was engaged by telephone. The telephone did not allow three-way conversations, so it was passed between the physician and the family. The physician spoke to the interpreter. The interpreter translated this to a family member who relayed this to the collected relatives. They discussed the matter in Hmong. Their questions and responses were relayed to the interpreter, who translated back to the physician. The family then spoke again with Mrs. Thor's parents in North Carolina. Her father remained opposed to any intervention. Although Mr. Thor and his parents found the physician's behaviors (e.g., anxious pacing, raised voice, impatience, and stares) disrespectful, they reluctantly supported an emergency cesarean-section and Mrs. Thor signed the consent form for the procedure.

Following a general anesthetic with a classical incision, a baby girl was discovered crying between her mother's legs, having delivered vaginally. Shortly thereafter the baby required resuscitation and was brought to the neonatal intensive care unit, where she remained for three months before going home and doing well.

Mrs. Thor stayed in the hospital for six days requiring IV antibiotics to relieve her fever. She was upset about the unnecessary cesarean-section and expressed deep sadness over not having followed her father's wishes. Her dismay increased when the doctors recommended that for her own safety she should postpone her next pregnancy for two years, she should be carefully monitored throughout any pregnancy, and she would have to have cesarean-sections for all future babies. She wished to have a son and so she had planned to get pregnant as soon as possible.

For many months after the cesarean-section Mrs. Thor felt weak and unable to perform her household responsibilities. She was depressed about the events in the hospital and upset about having agreed to sign the consent form allowing the unnecessary operation over her father's objections.

## Questions for Consideration

### Questions about Culture

When in pregnancy do Hmong women tend to seek Western health care services?

What does Mrs. Thor want from a Western prenatal care provider? Why would she be reluctant to accept certain routine aspects of prenatal care, such as blood tests, pelvic exams and prenatal vitamins? Why might she and her husband have refused amniocentesis?

How are genetic abnormalities understood in Hmong culture? How do these understandings compare with those of Western biomedicine?

What role did traditional healing practices play in this case?

When Mrs. Thor was in pre-term labor, why did she and her family consult Western health care? What were they expecting to receive?

What might explain why her family wanted her to sign out AMA and refuse the tocolytics?

What might explain why Mrs. Thor and her family accepted six days of IV antibiotics in the hospital after the delivery, whereas she had left the hospital AMA before?

What cultural values explain the physician's emphatic attempts to persuade the
family to agree to an emergency cesarean-section?

## Questions about Cross-Cultural Health Care Ethics

How might Mrs. Thor's family weigh the risks and benefits of recommended
interventions differently from members of her health care team?
Who tends to make obstetrical decisions in Hmong families? What factors do they
consider in making these decisions?
What role did Mrs. Thor's father play in the decision making?
Who in traditional Hmong families tend to sign consent forms for obstetrical
interventions?
What explains why Mrs. Thor signed the consent form for the cesarean-section?
Why did consenting to the cesarean-section over her father's objections cause her so
much sadness?

## Questions about Culturally Responsive Health Care

What role did negotiation play in this case?
In what ways, and from whose perspective, was the relationship between Mrs. Thor
and her health care providers successful? In what ways could it have been
improved?
What steps can the health care professionals consider if they remain concerned
about Mrs. Thor's well-being?

*Commentary*

# The Cultural Complexity
# of Obstetrical Care

*Helen B. Bruce, R.G.N., S.C.M., M.T.D., C.N.M., and Chue Xiong, R.N.*

> While the process of childbirth is, in some sense, everywhere the same, it is also everywhere different in that each culture has produced a birthing system that is strikingly dissimilar from the others.
>
> Brigitte Jordan, *Birth in Four Cultures*

The belief that childbirth is grounded in cultural and social settings that channel the biological is daily evidenced in obstetrical clinics and hospital units throughout the United States.

Traditional Hmong childbirth and modern Western obstetrics rise from different realities. Mrs. Thor's story acutely portrays how difficulties can arise when two such realities meet. Both worlds have the same basic goals: a safe pregnancy, a birth completed at term with a healthy mother and infant taking their place within a family and community. Yet Mrs. Thor and her U.S. caregivers journey toward these goals along very different pathways with dissimilar philosophies, attitudes, and language.

Consider the expectations of a health care team educated in Western biomedical traditions that seeks to lower maternal and infant mortality and morbidity rates. Aided by the latest medical technology, they question, examine, and test their patients. The information clinicians glean is collated with statistical evidence to guide their recommendations and to enable patients to make informed choices. Obstetrical teams have taken responsibility for the outcomes of pregnancy and the delivery of babies. Only since the 1980s have clinicians attempted a more holistic approach and considered the significance of cultural beliefs on patients' well-being.

## Traditional Cultural Practices and Beliefs

Mrs. Thor belongs to a culture where childbirth is seen as part of a life-death-rebirth cycle shaped by ancestor worship and animism. Her childhood would have flowed with the rhythms of those Hmong traditions. Before marriage, parents and extended family are responsible for a daughter's life; after marriage, husbands and their families become responsible. Daughters-in-law cook for the household members and care for children while their parents work. They shop in Asian stores, socialize with other women at family gatherings, and supplement the family income with their embroidery *(paj ntaub)* and sewing talents. While young wives may respectfully express their opinions within their families, they do not make any major decisions or take any actions without first consulting with their husbands, parents-in-law, or the male heads of the familes.

After three years of U.S. education Mrs. Thor understood and spoke basic English. Her chief contacts with mainstream American life likely were limited to her teachers, social service personnel, clinic and hospital staff when her first son was born, and her child's preschool teachers.

Mrs. Thor's understanding of pregnancy came from watching and listening to the women of her family and her husband's family. Pregnant women practice careful eating habits, do not lift heavy objects, avoid raising their arms above their head, work regularly, and avoid excessive sleep. Lying down for a rest or sleeping in the daytime diminishes strength and is considered counterproductive to labor and childbirth. Pregnant women avoid ponds and lakes for fear of the evil spirits that lurk within their still waters. When minor discomforts arise, pregnant women consult with older women in the community. Wise in the use of herbal remedies *(tshuaj ntsuab)* and adroit in massage *(zaws)*, these elders recognize and treat problems, including moving a baby lying in the wrong position.

Prior to labor, a shaman ceremony *(ua neeb)* prepares women for their well-being in labor and birth. If serious problems arise, the shaman's services are required earlier in the pregnancy. At a family gathering, the shaman *(txiv neeb)* listens carefully to the mother's problems and what she thinks might have caused them. Then the healing ceremony begins. The shaman enters into a trance. Aided by his assistant and helping spirits, his soul departs into the spirit world to recapture the mother's wandering soul. Restoration of the soul is symbolized by tying strings around the mother's wrist. An additional copper bracelet protects against the bad spirits and maintains well-being.

Mrs. Thor expected her mother-in-law and husband to guide her in labor and birth. Before her first pregnancy she would have had little knowledge about labor since she would have been considered too young to be burdened by such information. In labor she would be told to be still, tolerate pain, and not cry out, because noise would scare the baby from wishing to be born. In subsequent births, she would require the presence only of her husband and would receive help from others only if problems arose.

If the birth becomes prolonged and painful, certain rituals can be undertaken. Drinking water with a key in the cup *(tshuaj qhib kev)* may unlock the birth canal. Drinking certain herbal remedies increases the pregnant woman's power to push the baby out. Making two joined paper dolls *(ntawv faib thiab)* and then ritually cutting them apart separates the souls of the mother and her baby. Having an elderly woman, wise in birthing, reposition the baby *(tig menyuam)* helps allow the birth to proceed. The mother may ask forgiveness for disrespect shown toward family elders to ease the labor. She might also ask her husband to stroke her abdomen while calling the baby to descend and be born. Had she or her husband previously done anything to upset the baby's soul, her husband might ask for forgiveness. The mother-in-law might invite the baby to be born by chanting to the infant while lightly touching the mother's abdomen and telling the baby his clothes and his family are ready to receive him. Finally, Christian family members may pray and ask for God's assistance.

Children are a great blessing to Hmong families. In Laos they ensure help in the home and farm. They care for their parents when their parents are ill and old. Sons continue the family's name and traditions and the eldest arranges the parents' funerals *(lub ntees tuag)*. Their daughters and daughters-in-law hand stitch their burial pillows *(loob ncoos)* and burial clothes *(khaub ncaws laus)*. They provide spirit money for their journey into the next world *(dab teb)*. In the United States, they are also an immense help in their parents' transition into American society, for they learn English quickly.

## Prenatal Care

Mrs. Thor certainly expected that her caregivers would ensure her well-being and that of her unborn child. She accepted, without necessarily understanding, the noninvasive routine prenatal examinations, such as weighing, blood pressure tests, abdominal ultrasound, and palpation. However, when advice, medication, or procedures at the prenatal clinic disturbed her feeling of well-being, she refused them. Invasive techniques such as venipunctures, pelvic examinations, and amniocenteses are less familiar and acceptable. Hmong women experience the blood drawn in the first, second, and third trimesters as painful and frightening. Blood draws make them feel weak and they fear that it takes months to replace the blood, if it ever is replaced. Women already feel tired, lacking energy in their first and early second trimesters and blood drawing makes them feel even more vulnerable to the evil spirits. Even worse, the second blood draw for alpha-fetoprotein (AFP) to test for the defect of spina bifida is done in the hospital, a place abounding with the ghosts of patients who have died there, who seek sexual or marriage partners, and who may cause her death (Bliatout, 1988).

Mrs. Thor's decision to have blood drawn was compounded by her need to negotiate for the amount of blood to be taken. U.S. prenatal testing requires five tubes for laboratory testing but Mrs. Thor allowed only one tube of blood to be drawn. The negotiating continued until an agreement was reached that satisfied the patient and the clinicians. The time spent discussing the venipuncture allowed Mrs. Thor to voice her fears, and the staff to respond until she no longer felt threatened by the procedure. This enabled Mrs. Thor to have more control. A single ten-milliliter syringe of blood was sufficient and was distributed to the five tubes for testing.

As an Asian woman, Mrs. Thor was very modest in discussing or revealing her body and was disturbed by the touching that is commonplace in U.S. medicine. She was embarrassed undressing for examinations and ashamed to have her vulva and vagina touched, especially when the exam was performed quickly with no acknowledgment of such feelings.

Undoubtedly, Mrs. Thor heard many women's tales of pelvic examination woe. The recurring themes for Hmong women who refuse pelvic exams are:

- My husband does not want me to be touched there.
- If my husband has never seen that part of my body, why should another man see and touch me there?
- Many different people want to examine me there and I feel shy.
- I feel dirty and ashamed after such touching and do not want to feel that way again.
- Although it may be wrong to feel ashamed, nevertheless, this is how I feel. I hope my U.S.-schooled daughters will feel differently about their bodies.

Also discussed, though less frequently, is amniocentesis. A sharp needle inserted through the abdomen into the uterus to remove abdominal fluid is very invasive and unknown in the collective Hmong experience. Concerned by the absence of a 100 percent guarantee that no harm will come to either the baby or the mother, Hmong parents often decline amniocentesis, believing the procedure does not warrant the risks. Abortion would be an unlikely option to be chosen by Mrs. Thor and her family, even if the baby was abnormal. If the baby is born with such a severe abnormality that it dies immediately after birth, that is its fate *(hmoov)*. If the abnormality is not life-threatening and the infant survives its soul-calling ceremony *(hu plig)* on the third day of life, the family accepts their fate and takes good care of the baby.

## Obstetrical Care

When Mrs. Thor came to the clinic at twenty-four weeks with contractions, she expected to be given medication to stop the labor. She accepted hospitalization because she and her family recognized the dangers of early birth. However, the side effects of the tocolytic agents can be frightening. Palpitations, nausea, feeling hot at all times, and feelings of weakness throughout the body are disturbing to women. Mrs. Thor's family viewed such symptoms as signs of illness and felt it was obvious the drug must be stopped. The drug had, after all, accomplished its goal of halting the contractions. Allowing a vulnerable daughter-in-law to remain in a place containing ghosts of dead people was unthinkable to the family.

Prior to Mrs. Thor's leaving against medical advice, the doctors urged her to remain in bed at home and to increase her fluid intake to six to eight glasses a day. These instructions are quite contrary to Hmong health beliefs and practices. Lying in bed in the daytime encourages muscle weakness and illness during pregnancy. Drinking more fluid was also hard for Mrs. Thor. In childhood she drank only a cup or glass of water with twice daily meals. It was too much to expect her to triple, even quadruple, her liquid intake when she already felt full with the growth of the baby.

Mrs. Thor returned to the hospital, clearly ill, with her family recognizing a need for help. The physician's clinical assessment identified uterine infection and the fetus in transverse lie. The standard of care for such infections is an intravenous antibiotic to prevent septicemia. For the transverse lie, an emergency cesarean-section is required to prevent rupture of the uterus. Both septicemia and uterine rupture are life-threatening to mother and baby. It was difficult for the obstetrical staff to communicate the urgency and danger to Mrs. Thor's family with no language interpreter available. Explanations were repeated several times to the family elders before a final decision was made. The clinicians agreed not to use metal sutures, not to remove any part of the body, not to give a blood transfusion without a family consultation, and to be particularly careful to ensure the mother's future fertility. It is important for clinicians to be aware of the common belief that actions taken in this life directly affect what happens in future lives. One reason Mrs. Thor feared the operation was that on her reincarnation *(thawj thiab)* she might have a deformed uterus. It is helpful at such times for clinicians to remain patient and respectful of the time required to make a final decision.

Two lives were at stake: the mother's and the infant's. In complex situations such as this, male elders of the husband's family and of the wife's family are called for advice and discussion. In this situation both sides of the family decided to postpone a cesarean-section until a Hmong medicine woman could manipulate the baby in the head-down position. When this failed and the baby was still transverse, the husband's elders agreed to consent, but Mrs. Thor's father did not. It was only after much further discussion that Mrs. Thor signed the consent for surgery.

Spontaneous delivery of a live baby girl occurred under general anesthetic while a classical cesarean-section was being performed. The baby required resuscitation and was taken to the neonatal intensive care unit, where she remained for three months before going home.

After her surgery Mrs. Thor felt very vulnerable. She had the discomfort of the wound, the effects of the general anesthesia, and recurrent chills and fevers. Her husband, she knew, was disappointed that she had not presented him with his hoped-for son. She had disrespected her father when she had signed the consent form against his advice. Without his forgiveness she would find it hard to rebuild her strength. After listening to the physician's description of her surgery and the subsequent dangers to her future pregnancies, she knew there was even less chance she would be able to provide a son in the near future. The extended stay meant longer exposure to hospital ghosts and to staff with whom she could not easily communicate.

The physicians clearly were relieved that the baby was alive and responding to supportive care, that the mother's uterus had not ruptured, and the infection was responding to antibiotics. But they were uncomfortable with a vaginal birth during a cesarean surgery. They knew the dangers of a classical cesarean scar to subsequent pregnancies—possible rupture of the uterus with resultant fetal death and further maternal morbidity. In each subsequent pregnancy, Mrs. Thor would have to be evaluated as a high-risk pregnant woman who required extra surveillance and a cesarean-section birth. They would have preferred a vaginal birth for this preterm baby without such dire consequences for future pregnancies, but they accepted the risks of cesarean-section as necessary, given the circumstances.

For Mrs. Thor and her family, the level of success was much less. Their baby girl required intensive medical attention. Mrs. Thor was unable to resume her household role after the traditional month allotted for Hmong mothers to recuperate following childbirth. Indeed, she felt weak for many months with the pain from her abdominal wound. The medically required family spacing would delay the birth of a son so desired to carry the family name. The extra surveillance in subsequent pregnancies would interfere with her role as wife, mother, and provider and make her a burden to her husband.

Could the outcome of this pregnancy have been different? The many variables do not allow simple answers. Where does the responsibility for a pregnancy and birth lie: with the individual woman, the family, the medical team, or a community within the larger society? Would it have made a difference if on Mrs. Thor's first admission the clinicians had spent more time on explanation and mediation and if a medical interpreter had helped convey the seriousness of the pre-term labor? Could a family conference without the pressure of a clinical emergency have altered the course of events? Could that conference have been used to negotiate a common pathway? Would a Hmong-speaking home-visiting nurse have tipped the scales positively by opening more avenues of communication? Would there have been more trust and less frustration on the second admission if medical interpreters had been available twenty-four hours a day and present in labor and delivery? Would it not be practical to have written information and informed consent documents in the patient's first language?

Within the past decade, the idea of cultural competence has emerged within the practice of medicine. "Knowing about cultural differences is a necessity for health care providers. It is no longer an issue of compassion, but a practical means for improving compliance, patient satisfaction, census" (Thiederman, 1997). Explicit to cultural competence is an awareness of the beliefs, values, and behaviors of our own and other cultural backgrounds. Clinicians must ask questions to elicit patients' health beliefs (Kleinman, 1980). Had the clinicians been more aware of cultural values, had they asked about beliefs, and had they kept negotiations open, the Thor family and the medical team might have reached their goals more successfully and with more healing for Mrs. Thor.

Cultural competence is an acceptance of the differences that exist and respect for the strengths inherent in each group. Had the U.S. obstetrical caregivers and the traditional Hmong family had more acceptance of their differences and greater regard for their respective strengths, would the outcome have been better? We believe so.

## References

Bliatout, B. T. (1988). Hmong attitudes towards surgery: How it affects prognosis. *Migration World, 16*(1), 25–28.

Kleinman, A. (1980). *Patients and healers in the context of culture: An exploration of the borderland between anthropology, medicine, and psychiatry.* Berkeley: University of California Press.

Thiederman, S. (1997, September 17). The cultural challenges: Overcoming barriers to patient involvement. *Group Practice Journal,* 42–43.

*Commentary*

# Conflicting Cultural Practices in Deciding about a Cesarean-Section

*Carol A. Tauer, Ph.D.*

Two aspects of this case raise important ethical issues. (1) In the case story, the risks and benefits of possible medical interventions are weighed according to two different conceptual schemes. While the medical providers use scientific methodology to assess risks and benefits, the patient and family rely on cultural beliefs and values, as well as medical advice. The question is, how does one determine which conceptual scheme should take precedence? (2) The practice of informed consent follows a model that is ethically and legally accepted in Western culture. However, this model poses difficulties for traditional Hmong patients and families, since they customarily view important decisions, including medical decisions, as the responsibility of the family rather than of the autonomous individual. Should Western informed-consent practices be modified to accommodate culturally diverse decision-making practices?

## Risks and Benefits

In some respects, similar ethical issues could arise regardless of the cultural background of the pregnant woman. If a Western woman presented in the same situation as Mrs. Thor, there might be disagreement between her and her care providers about the relative risks and benefits of an immediate surgical delivery as compared with an attempt at vaginal birth. While most obstetricians would urge a cesarean in view of the premature rupture of membranes, the transverse presentation, and the presumed infection endangering the fetus (Schwartz, personal communication, November 27, 1998), some would argue that the uncertain viability of a compromised twenty-six-week fetus supports not pressing a cesarean that might turn out to be useless or harmful overall (Anderson & Strong, 1988). Moreover, predictions of caregivers regarding the dire outcomes expected from nonsurgical delivery have often been wrong, and these unavoidable uncertainties support relying on the pregnant woman's assessment of the risks and benefits to herself and to her fetus (Rhoden, 1987; Annas, 1987; Tauer, 1993).

In Mrs. Thor's case, the assessment of risks and benefits includes elements specific to the Hmong culture. She and her family must consider possible harms that express a complex interaction of the physical and spiritual worlds. In the Hmong view, illness may be caused by spirits or by the loss or absence of the soul. General anesthesia resulting in unconsciousness may permit the soul to wander away. The soul might leave the body as a result of a surgical incision, requiring rituals including animal sacrifice to call it back. Moreover, an incision that violates the integrity of the physical body may cause it to remain in a mutilated state in a later life (see Chapter 1; see also Thao, 1984; Center for Cross-Cultural Health, 1997; Fadiman, 1997).

In evaluating the caregivers' recommendations, Mrs. Thor's family also relies on its own experience of pregnancy and childbirth. Family members probably place high value on Mrs. Thor's ability to have future children and to deliver them vaginally. A surgical delivery with classical incision would appear to rule out future vaginal deliveries. Mrs. Thor's father believes he is capable of judging his daughter's situation on the basis of his own experience with the births of his eight children. He and the rest of the family appear to welcome the interventions of Western medicine when they find them effective and appropriate, for example, medications to stop the contractions and antibiotics to eradicate infection. These interventions have fairly immediate and apparent results. The family judges interventions on the basis of observation and experience, using traditional healing methods when it believes such remedies are more effective than Western medicine.

Disagreements between Western patients and health care providers regarding the risks and benefits of particular interventions are ordinarily based either on individual preferences or on differing interpretations of scientific data. A pregnant Western woman may be willing to accept certain risks for the sake of a vaginal delivery to which she personally attaches high value; or she may be aware that certain interventions, such as electronic fetal monitoring, have not been shown to be necessary in most situations (Tauer, 1993).

In the case of Mrs. Thor's family, the assessment of risks and benefits is based on a long cultural tradition in which information about how to have a healthy pregnancy and delivery is culled from experience and communicated orally. New expectant mothers receive advice from female relatives as well as from husbands and boyfriends regarding what to eat and drink, what activities to avoid, and when to seek prenatal care (Spring, Davis, & Rode, 1997). Interviews with fifty Hmong women who had sought prenatal care in the United States suggest that care providers are valued more highly for the characteristics of communicating well and exhibiting cultural sensitivity and a friendly attitude than for medical competence, which these interviewees ranked fourth in importance (Spring et al., 1997).

Care providers can capitalize on the Hmong people's reliance on lived experience and on good communication for guidance in making decisions by ensuring that there are no misunderstandings regarding medical recommendations. For example, Mrs. Thor refuses vitamins because she does not want a large infant. Was enough time taken to explain to her that health, rather than size, was the aim? Did her care providers realize that Hmong community members might also have advised Mrs. Thor to take prenatal vitamins (Spring et al., 1997)? The suggested amniocentesis seems to imply that Mrs. Thor might have an abortion if the test showed abnormalities. Since this choice would be highly unlikely in Mrs. Thor's case, the decision by her and her husband to refuse screening is reasonable in view of the risks of the procedure itself.

While not all differences of opinion regarding risks and benefits can be resolved by good communication, surely some of them can. In the end, however, there may be a residue of unresolvable issues that stem from a difference in worldviews: the Hmong view, which includes spiritual causes of illness and ritualistic remedies for certain problems, and the view of Western medicine, which relies on scientific and empirical evidence. If issues relative to treatment cannot be resolved, the final decision must lie with the Hmong patient and family. They have the same right as any others who consult health care providers to refuse the providers' recommendations.

In the case of Mrs. Thor, the care providers' medical assessment of the need for immediate cesarean-section delivery turned out to be incorrect. Several harms to Mrs. Thor—the general anesthesia, the incision into her body, and the precluding of future vaginal deliveries—were totally unnecessary. The fetus, assumed to be at risk for both mortality and morbidity, survived intact (with the neonatal intensive care required by any infant born prematurely at twenty-six weeks). Care providers could justifiably argue that these outcomes could not have been predicted or anticipated at the time. A question that is left unanswered by the case story, however, is whether the patient had been evaluated for labor or how close to the commencement of the surgery such evaluations were done.

## Consent

The second major ethical issue raised by this case is the role of Western practices of informed consent, particularly the consent for the cesarean-section delivery. It is true that any pregnant woman in Mrs. Thor's situation may be reluctant to consent to a surgical delivery, if she feels it is unnecessary. However, in the absence of mitigating cultural factors, the care providers would regard the pregnant woman as the only person they need to consult for decisions regarding labor and delivery.

In the Hmong culture, however, major decisions are the responsibility of the family, and the larger community may also be involved. Women in particular do not make or express health care decisions publicly. While they ordinarily participate in family discussions and state their views, in the end the decision is asserted by the family or even the clan, represented by the men of the group. In particular the male elders have the responsibility for the decision.

In this case, the care providers respected these cultural practices by engaging the appropriate decision makers—Mrs. Thor's father, father-in-law, and husband—in the discussions. It is apparent that a great deal of time, "several hours," was devoted to the discussion of the surgical delivery. The family's request to have a traditional healer come to the hospital and attempt to turn the fetus was respected, even though obstetricians might have questioned the value and medical propriety of an attempted turning under the circumstances (Schwartz, personal communication, November 27, 1998).

The way this discussion was carried out, however, was not ideal and thus not as conducive to a good outcome as it could have been. The lack of an on-site interpreter was a major problem. With Mrs. Thor's condition as serious as described, accurate communication is essential, and a telephone interpretation creates obstacles to accurate communication. The demeanor of the physician as portrayed is problematic. Any care provider who works with Hmong patients should be aware of the high priority this community attaches to a respectful and friendly manner. Hmong patients decide whether to trust a physician on the basis of their perception of the interaction, not simply on the basis of medical competence (Spring et al., 1997).

By the end of the discussion, key members of the extended family remained divided on the central question: whether to proceed with an emergency cesarean-section. While Mrs. Thor was, according to Hmong practice, considered part of her husband's family, she and her husband's family nevertheless were expected to show deference to the wishes of her father. In this situation Mrs. Thor's husband and father-in-law agreed to the cesarean-section, knowing that her father still opposed it.

Time for exploring other options was clearly limited. Ideally this quandary might be referred to clan leaders or other mediators who could resolve a difference of opinion between two different family authorities. Since a husband and wife ordinarily come from different clans, this negotiation would likely involve leaders of different clans. Because Mrs. Thor's parents live in North Carolina, it is possible that the clan leaders are far-flung geographically, thus making discussion in these emergency circumstances even more difficult.

But no matter how limited the options, the worst possible resolution is for Mrs. Thor to be expected to take the public action of signing the consent form. In Western practice this act indicates that she is responsible for the decision, that it is her independent and autonomous choice. But within Hmong culture, she is not regarded as an autonomous and independent decision maker. As a woman, she is expected to follow the guidance of those who have authority, particularly her husband, father-in-law, and father. While her husband and father-in-law support her consenting to surgery, her father does not. In signing the form, Mrs. Thor is publicly choosing between two authorities in her own culture. She is being forced to take responsibility for a choice that will affect her and her family for the rest of her life and perhaps into the afterlife.

The informed consent process is intended to protect the rights and dignity of the patient. Yet this process may have a very different effect within a culture that expresses respect for persons in a more relational way and that stresses the embeddedness of the individual within community. In Lawrence Gostin's words:

> The formal specifications of informed consent . . . may faithfully advance individual autonomy and human dignity for many patients in dominant Western cultures. But this same formalism may be alienating and dehumanizing to those who view caring and healing not as a bilateral contractual relationship with a physician, but within a mutually supportive, loving environment in the family and community. (Gostin, 1995, p. 844)

Is it necessary that the care providers put Mrs. Thor under such stress by insisting on a Western mode of individual consent? It is apparent that the decision was reached through discussion and that Mrs. Thor was willing to accept her husband's and father-in-law's guidance. Culturally her husband's family is responsible for making decisions about her pregnancy, for taking responsibility for the outcome of the decision, for answering to her birth family's different desires, and for addressing or redressing any potential future charge that a harmful action was taken (K. A. Culhane-Pera, personal communication, May 10, 1999). However, it could easily be inferred that Mrs. Thor would be distressed at publicly going against her father's wishes. In this type of situation, might it be possible to have a multiple signing of the consent form? If Mrs. Thor's husband and father-in-law signed it first, then it would be obvious to the Hmong community that she had agreed in order to follow cultural practice. And in terms of Western ethical and legal requirements, her signature would signify her consent just as adequately as if it stood alone on the form.

What about the aftermath? It is unfortunate that Mrs. Thor was given long-term recommendations at a time of great stress. Since she is anxious to become pregnant again, the health care providers might have shown more sensitivity by telling her that she must wait six months and come in for an evaluation at that time. At the evaluation, the waiting time could be extended if necessary. The discussion of future deliveries could also have been postponed for a while. Care providers may feel that they need to give her all this information to protect themselves in case she does not return for future evaluations. However, it would certainly be kinder and less distressing to her to take things one step at a time.

Regarding her relationship with her father and family of origin, that is a matter for the Hmong communities involved. One can only hope that they will help her to resolve what must be a very troubling and painful situation.

## Summary

In this case the care providers made attempts to recognize Hmong cultural practices, particularly through discussing proposed interventions with the entire family. At times these discussions were quite lengthy. However, the lack of an on-site interpreter, the impatience communicated by nonverbal cues, and the care providers' apparent lack of interest in learning the reasons behind family objections resulted in a process that left family members feeling uncomfortable and disrespected.

The world views of the medical staff and the Hmong family included elements that were incompatible with each other. Better communication might have resolved some of these differences, particularly as they affected assessments of risks and benefits. If the family had felt that their views were understood and respected by care providers, they might have been more willing to trust the recommendations of medical professionals.

The providers followed Hmong practice in seeking consent for the cesarean-section from Mrs. Thor's husband and father-in-law. However, they partially negated the significance of this discussion by requiring Mrs. Thor alone to sign the consent form. Without violating Western ethical and legal norms of informed consent, the providers could have offered the option of a multiple signing of the consent form, a formal act that would have been more consistent with Hmong community practice.

Most important, in this case it could have spared Mrs. Thor the suffering that resulted from her public act of opposition to her father's expressed wishes.

## References

Anderson, G., & Strong, C. (1988). The premature breech: Caesarean section or trial of labour? *Journal of Medical Ethics, 14*, 18–24.

Annas, G. J. (1987). Protecting the liberty of pregnant patients. *New England Journal of Medicine, 316*(19), 1213–1214.

Center for Cross-Cultural Health. (1997). *Culture and health: The Hmong community in Minnesota.* Minneapolis: Center for Cross-Cultural Health.

Fadiman, A. (1997). *The spirit catches you and you fall down: A Hmong child, her American doctors, and the collision of two cultures.* New York: Farrar, Straus, and Giroux.

Gostin, L. (1995). Informed consent, cultural sensitivity, and respect for persons. *Journal of the American Medical Association, 274*(10), 844–845.

Rhoden, N. K. (1987). Cesareans and Samaritans. *Law, Medicine & Health Care, 15*(3), 118–125.

Spring, M., Davis, K., & Rode, P. (1997). The Hmong community. In *Prenatal care among Southeast Asian women in St. Paul and Minneapolis: A survey of Cambodian, Hmong, Laotian, and Vietnamese women in the Twin Cities.* St. Paul: Urban Coalition, 25–43.

Tauer, C. A. (1993). When pregnant patients refuse interventions. *Association of Women's Health, Obstetric, and Neonatal Nursing's Clinical Issues in Perinatal and Women's Health Nursing, 4*(4), 596–605.

Thao, X. (1984). Southeast Asian refugees of Rhode Island: The Hmong perception of illness. *Rhode Island Medical Journal, 67*, 323–330.

# 4

# Woman with Vaginal Bleeding

## *A Case Story*

Mrs. Foua Yang is a forty-two-year-old woman who is the single parent of four children, aged fourteen to twenty-four years old. Four years ago she had an abnormal Pap smear (strong class III) and was advised to undergo a colposcopic exam and possible biopsy of the cervix. She refused, insisting that she was having no pain and no problems. She wondered how she could suddenly have problems with her womb when she had been divorced for ten years.

A year later another Pap smear yielded the same result. A Hmong nurse called Mrs. Yang every few months to ask how she was doing and to encourage her to come in for follow-up. During one of these conversations, Mrs. Yang told the nurse that she was using herbal remedies and had consulted a shaman about her health. She had learned that the reason she had started to have some abnormal bleeding was that the ancestors were angry that her family was not performing the yearly spiritual ceremonies. Several years before Mrs. Yang's oldest son and daughter had converted to Christianity and her son had stopped performing the traditional rites. Her husband's brothers, who lived in California, were not able to perform them for her either.

A colposcopy was scheduled three times and each time Mrs. Yang failed to show up. She said that she was afraid of the biopsy because it could cause infection and death of the tissue and interfere with her reincarnation. Mrs. Yang was persuaded to come to the fourth scheduled appointment. A woman physician spoke very gently and explained that she would simply scrape the lesion. Mrs. Yang agreed to a colposcopy without a biopsy. The colposcopy revealed an ulcerating mass.

After this exam the nurse arranged a family conference with her oldest son and daughter. Mrs. Yang's children pleaded with her to follow the doctor's advice. They told her how much they needed her and wanted her to have a long life. They tried to convince her to give up her fears about surgical interventions and removal of tissue and encouraged her to become Christian. Neither the shaman's intervention nor the herbs were working. Mrs. Yang decided to convert to Christianity and to undergo a biopsy. The biopsy came back positive for invasive cancer. Her physician explained the options gently and clearly and recommended a hysterectomy. Mrs. Yang was very reluctant. She believed and trusted the physician and nurse but still feared the removal of her uterus.

Eventually, with the assistance of her minister, her church community, and her children, she agreed to a vaginal hysterectomy on the condition that her physician be the one to perform it and that the Hmong nurse accompany her. The procedure went well. Her son and daughter were there to support her during her two-day hospitalization. On a follow-up visit, Mrs. Yang was relieved and happy. She expressed her gratitude that her cancer had been removed and that her life had been saved.

## Questions for Consideration

### Questions about Culture

What is the significance of the uterus within traditional Hmong culture? What is its significance for U.S. health care professionals?

What are the signs of uterine health and illness according to traditional Hmong women?

What are the prevailing assumptions about the relationship between sexual activity and gynecological health or disease?

How did beliefs about etiology influence Mrs. Yang's and her providers' beliefs about appropriate care?

What factors were most important to Mrs. Yang's decision to undergo a biopsy and accept a hysterectomy?

How common is it for Hmong patients who hold animist views to become Christian before accepting Western interventions? What is the significance of these religious conversions for patients and their families?

### Questions about Cross-Cultural Health Care Ethics

What factors contributed to Mrs. Yang's trust in her caregivers?

When patients believe they are well, despite biomedical evidence that they are not, is this reason to question their decision-making capacity?

How did Mrs. Yang, her adult children, and her health care practitioners differ in their assessments of risks and benefits?

What criteria did Mrs. Yang's care providers use to define a good cross-cultural health care relationship?

### Questions about Culturally Responsive Health Care

How can U.S. health care practitioners understand and work with patients who choose to prioritize life and spiritual integrity differently than they do?

How can health care practitioners make these types of health care decision easier for patients like Mrs. Yang?

In what ways was the relationship between Mrs. Yang and her health care providers a successful one?

*Commentary*

# Culturally Responsive Care for a Hmong Woman with Vaginal Bleeding

*Deu Yang, L.P.N., and Deborah Mielke, M.D.*

Western medicine has been able to decrease the rate of cervical cancer ten-fold through screening for precancerous changes and treating them. The Pap smear is one of the most valuable screening tools for cancer prevention ever developed. Its effectiveness depends on adequate follow-up and treatment if the Pap smear is abnormal. A colposcopy done with a biopsy is the standard recommendation after any abnormal Pap smear; this procedure allows visualization of abnormal lesions on the cervix and confirms the diagnosis by evaluating the biopsied tissue with a microscope.

## Uterine Health

In Hmong traditional life, the uterus has profound significance for women. It is the home or house for the baby before birth. Without a womb, a Hmong woman is not a "true" woman and cannot fulfill her responsibility to her husband and family. Being a mother—conceiving, bearing, and raising children—is the most important role of a woman in the Hmong community. A husband is allowed to end a marriage if his wife is unable to conceive. At the very least the husband may find a second wife if the first wife cannot bear children. Hence, every attempt needs to be made to preserve the uterus for a Hmong woman.

The primary sign that the uterus is healthy is a woman's ability to become pregnant and deliver a healthy baby. Not menstruating for a long time is considered not good for uterine health. An absence of menses for three or four months is acceptable, but no menses for longer intervals is worrisome. A woman who bleeds too much during one cycle may use herbal medicine or *khawv koob* to treat the excessive blood flow. If the menses is prolonged and heavy every cycle, a shaman is likely to be consulted to identify and to treat a spiritual cause for the bleeding. Cramping during menses is considered normal for young women and is a sign that the woman needs to have a child. In older women, painful menses is not considered healthy. Problems with menstruation and fertility may be caused by evil water spirits if the woman washes bloody clothes near a lake or stream.

Many Hmong have encountered sexually transmitted diseases for the first time after immigrating to Thailand and the United States. Most abnormal Pap smears are caused by an infection of the cervix with human papilloma virus (HPV), which is considered a sexually transmitted disease. Mrs. Yang had a serious diagnosis when she presented with her first abnormal Pap smear. She had a high likelihood of developing cervical cancer if not treated. Mrs. Yang probably had a hard time understanding how she could develop the abnormal Pap smear when she had had no sexual relations since her divorce ten years before. She may have felt some shame, which is common in many women who are diagnosed with cervical HPV or any other sexually transmitted disease.

## Risks and Benefits of Western Interventions

Mrs. Yang was willing to have a colposcopy to look at the cervix and to take pictures, but the idea of "taking a piece of tissue" was frightening to her. In Hmong rural settings, a cut or opening in the skin could lead to infection that would spread to the rest of the body. Whether the damage was caused by evil spirits or bacteria coming into the body, the end result could have been disastrous. Sterile technique and antibiotics were not easily accessible in the mountains of Laos where Mrs. Yang grew up. Some of the fears about removing tissue also come from beliefs about what happens to the body and spirit after death. A biopsy might interfere with the spirit's ability to be at peace after death. And a biopsy might prevent a successful reincarnation in the future. For Mrs. Yang, the description of "scraping the lesion" or white spot was probably reassuring. She was willing to have the colposcopy done when the biopsy was described as a less invasive procedure.

Because of the severity of her cervical disease, the therapy ultimately recommended for Mrs. Yang was a total hysterectomy. The cancer was likely to spread if a less complete procedure was performed. For Mrs. Yang, a hysterectomy meant removing a significant part of her body. She would not be considered a complete woman any more. It also would mean a loss of status and respect within the community. Without her uterus, she could not have any more children and might have believed she would no longer be able to have sexual intercourse and would be a less desirable sexual partner.

Mrs. Yang's physicians clearly had a different view of her best interests than she did. Western physicians are used to having their advice followed. Doctors are trained to feel that their responsibility as clinicians is to do what is in the best interests of the patient. When confronted with a patient who is unwilling to accept their recommendations, it is easy for them to become frustrated. Sometimes, as in the case of Mrs. Yang, a strong sense of compassion is needed. Mainstream Americans are often willing to take much bigger risks with surgery than are Hmong patients. Western patients often have so much confidence in the medical system that they do not pay as much attention to the risks of procedures as do Hmong patients. Even with a clear understanding of the risks and benefits of surgery, Mrs. Yang might not have felt comfortable with the small but real risks of surgery. A 50 percent chance of curing the cancer may be sufficient for some patients, but probably not for Mrs. Yang. Her children agreed that the benefits of surgery justified taking the risks. Their confidence in and understanding of Western medicine probably helped her put the risks and benefits into a new perspective.

## Decision Making

Sometimes patients like Mrs. Yang believe they are well because they have no symptoms, even when doctors provide them with evidence that a disease is severe. In such cases, doctors may question the decision-making capacity of the patient. Mrs. Yang was presented several times with the biomedical evidence that she had a significant illness that could shorten her life if it were not treated in a timely fashion. Yet she apparently had great difficulty believing she could have such a significant disease and not feel sick from it. Deciding to have major surgery, with little direct evidence of the need for it, was not easy.

In general, Hmong patients make excellent health care decisions for themselves if given enough time and information. Sometimes, as in Mrs. Yang's case, the medical recommendation from the Western clinicians needs to be supported by the family and community. The fact that the doctor alone recommends something is usually not enough. When the rest of the clan can be enlisted to help confirm the diagnosis and recommended treatment, then the patient is much more likely to be able to make a wise decision. Rumors and stories of patients within the community who have had bad outcomes with a procedure can strongly influence the patient to shy away from the procedure. If Mrs. Yang goes along with the decision of her family and clan, she is assured of support should adverse outcomes occur. If she makes the decision entirely on her own, she may not get any support if things go badly. The family decision-making process helps to determine what is in the best interest of the patient, especially if symptoms of disease are not present and the risks of a procedure are significant. A greater problem exists if the family structure and clan support are inadequate to help the patient or if the patient is isolated from the community. Also, decisions that need to be made quickly are hard to accomplish when multiple family and clan members need to be consulted. As more Hmong Americans are educated and comfortable with the biomedical aspects of Western medicine, some of these medical decisions may become easier. In the end, Mrs. Yang made a decision with her family's help, knowing that whatever the outcome they would be there to help her. She also had spiritual support from her Christian minister.

Usually, the woman's husband, her family, and his family would make the best decision for her, taking her opinion seriously into account. In Hmong tradition the male head of the household or his male relatives perform animist ceremonies for the household members. Women cannot perform any of the usual ceremonies by themselves. Traditionally the men in the family teach each other how to conduct the rituals. They are taught by their fathers, uncles, or brothers-in-law. The household animist ceremonies are performed, in most cases, before the shaman is consulted. Shaman, however, are not always able to help with problems of the uterus because damage to the uterus is usually not considered to be caused by a spiritual problem. The rituals can help also protect the patient from spiritual problems that may arise when undergoing a major operation. Hmong patients may be more willing to undergo Western medical procedures if they feel they have sufficient spiritual support.

Mrs. Yang could not go to her son for these animist ceremonies because he had converted to Christianity. Her other option was to convert to Christianity to find the spiritual support she needed. Her son could then help her with both the decision to have surgery and Christian ceremonies that would help her spirit survive the surgery. Certainly not all patients need to convert to Christianity to participate in Western medical treatment. Mrs. Yang, however, probably felt that the traditional animist religion had not protected her because she had not been following the standard ceremonies. The change to Christianity offered her new hope.

## Building Trust

Many Hmong immigrants need time to trust Western medical doctors and nurses. This trust may not develop until the patient has been seeing the same provider for several years. The role of the interpreter can be essential in building this trust. Ideally, that person has a respected role within the Hmong community and acts as a cultural as well as a medical interpreter. Medical interpretation training is also beneficial so that procedures and treatments can be described in a way that is both accurate and understandable to Hmong patients. Many words and concepts may not be translatable directly from one language to another. The interpreter's task is both to help the clinician understand the patient's issues and to help the patient understand the risks and benefits of treatment. Using a female interpreter is important when dealing with gynecological or obstetrical issues, since patients may be very shy about their body and sexual functions. Patients also need to have confidence that the exchange is entirely confidential.

Mrs. Yang needed many visits and significant time to make her decision. Her caregivers were successful because they did not give up. They expressed caring and acceptance, regardless of her final decision. She repeatedly delayed treatment until she was comfortable with allowing the colposcopy, the biopsy, and the surgery to be done. They apparently never became angry or impatient with Mrs. Yang. They offered Mrs. Yang evidence that her diagnosis was significant and that surgery would benefit her and were willing to repeat several times the benefits and risks of the interventions.

## Suggestions for Improving Care

American health care providers can best understand and work with patients from the Hmong community by understanding how their patients' spiritual and personal needs may be incorporated into diagnostic and treatment plans. The integration of Western medicine and traditional Hmong healing can help the patient maintain wellness and health. Many Hmong patients use herbal remedies, *khawv koob,* and shaman ceremonies alongside Western medicine. Some of these ceremonies help to protect the spirit when the patient is ill. Providers should ask patients whether they are using any traditional healing methods and support the patient's desire to use both systems. Some traditional ceremonies can be done in the hospital. Many others involve strong smells, sacrificing animals, or burning spirit money, so they have to be done in the patient's home. But the use of traditional Hmong medicine can delay treatment, as in Mrs. Yang's case. Mrs. Yang's emphasis on the spiritual aspects of her health may have helped her survive and recover from surgery as well as she did. Fortunately, the delay in surgery did not seem to have an adverse effect on her long-term health.

The relationship between Mrs. Yang and her health care workers was successful for many reasons. Her providers were supportive of her right to make her own health decisions. They involved the family of the patient in decision making early on, recognizing their important role in the decision. The doctors did not abandon their patient just because she was not following all their advice. They took time to listen and try to understand her concerns about the procedures and therapy. When Mrs. Yang originally refused surgery, the nurse and physician did not take this refusal as her final decision. When she did agree to surgery, arrangements were made to have the Hmong nurse present during surgery as her advocate and support. The patient felt confident that the health care team was going to support her during the surgery and afterward.

A skilled, respected, and compassionate interpreter is an invaluable asset for patients and for Western non-Hmong–speaking providers. Especially in cases of a woman with a sexually transmitted disease, a woman interpreter may be more effective in obtaining an accurate history and communicating sensitive information. Outreach to the family by a nurse or caseworker can help identify the support needed for the patient. The time clinicians spend with the patient is more efficient if family members are included in a family conference where pertinent medical information can be given. Follow-up visits are important to allow the patient an opportunity to reassess her condition and treatment options. Sufficient time needs to be allowed in nonemergent medical decisions so the patient can pursue traditional as well as biomedical healing methods.

The path to Mrs. Yang's decision to have surgery was complicated and long. She eventually made her choice to have life-saving surgery in a way that allowed her to have a successful outcome and to be satisfied with the whole process.

*Commentary*

# Influence of Conversion to Christianity on a Hmong Woman's Decision about Hysterectomy: A Pastor's Perspective

*Lu Vang with Phua Xiong, M.D.*

Mrs. Yang came from Laos, where Western health care was neither available nor familiar. She probably never experienced Western health care before coming to the United States. Western concepts of diseases such as uterine cancer and surgical procedures such as removing cervical tissue were foreign to her. Because Hmong and Western health care beliefs are so different, health care providers should not assume that Mrs. Yang understands that she has uterine cancer and that she is knowingly refusing the most appropriate treatment. Rather, they should assume that Mrs. Yang does not understand Western health beliefs and practices.

Western health care providers need to understand what patients like Mrs. Yang believe and fear so they can help make health care decisions easier for these patients. Mrs. Yang's providers need to understand her spiritual, emotional, and physical beliefs about health and illness first as an animist and then as a converted Christian.

### Mrs. Yang's Spiritual and Religious Beliefs

Hmong men and women in Mrs. Yang's generation came to the United States with rich cultural and religious convictions. As an animist, Mrs. Yang believes that most illnesses have spiritual causes. For example, her soul might be separated from her body by a fall; or it might be sold to, or stolen by, evil spirits. With her soul out of her body, she can become sick and can even die if her soul is not reunited with her body. The soul can sometimes by reunited with the body by performing a soul-calling ceremony *(hu plig)* or a shaman ceremony in which a Hmong spiritual healer *(txiv neeb)* retrieves the soul from the spirit world. If her soul is sold to, or stolen by, evil spirits, a ceremony to appease the evil spirit is performed in order to return the soul to her body—its proper "home."

Mrs. Yang probably also believes that she was born with certain predetermined good and bad fates *(nws tiam ntawv los li ntawd)*. Hmong animists have passed this idea of fate from generation to generation. She likely believes that it is her destiny to have uterine problems and that she can do nothing but accept this condition and its consequences. Furthermore, she is probably frightened by the recommended biopsy because she has never heard of or seen any biopsies before. "Why biopsies, for what?" she must wonder. Taking pieces of tissue out of the body can be scary, especially for animists. Hmong animists believe that people need all of their body parts for reincarnation. If parts are missing, then bodies are born incomplete, which can cause more problems in the next life. Mrs. Yang probably fears that removing tissue from her uterus, and certainly removing her entire uterus, will cause her to face devastating consequences in her next life.

It is difficult for Mrs. Yang to accept that her uterus is diseased because, according to the animist worldview, it is not the uterus but a spiritual component that is the problem. She cannot understand how a biopsy and an operation could produce a cure since the underlying spiritual cause has not been "cured." "Why would the doctors want to operate on me when an operation cannot cure me?" she must wonder. From this perspective, her next consideration might be, "Perhaps they want to take advantage of me, experiment or learn on me, or use me to improve their skills. Or even worse, maybe they want to kill me instead of help me."

## Blending the Old with the New

The integral connections between spirits, souls, ancestral worship, and bodies in health and illness have been ingrained in the minds and lives of the Hmong for thousands of years. Even with conversion to Christianity, it is not easy to set aside or forget beliefs that have been the cornerstone of people's lives for generations. As a Hmong American pastor, I have to be careful not to be too critical of traditional ways and not to offend others who still hold onto the old traditions. When a pastor is in the middle of culture change, it is important to understand and try to balance the old and the new.

Converted Christians take new concepts or ideas and incorporate them into their old ways while doing away with some parts of animist traditions. At Christian funerals, for example, instead of singing *qhuab kev* (the ritual song sung to the dead, leading the soul to its birth place and into the spirit world) or beating the funeral drum, Christian families hold several services of hymns followed by sermons. Similarly, although Hmong Christians no longer pay respect to ancestral spirits, some may continue to think of spiritual causes when family members are sick. They may call a pastor to help instead of calling a shaman or performing a soul-calling ceremony. However, some people continue to use traditional animist therapies, especially if prayer and other healing methods fail. Many Hmong find it difficult to completely give up their traditional ways of doing things and fully adopt American Christian ways.

To illustrate, we just have to look to my own family, which converted to Christianity eighteen years ago. My mother still thinks of spiritual causes as possible explanations of illness. When my son was about four years old, he apparently hurt his leg while playing outside without anyone's noticing. When he woke up the next morning he crawled around the house complaining of leg pain. Despite the fact that I am a pastor and my mother has been a Christian for eighteen years, she thought that perhaps Bryant was sick because our family did not use a cow to welcome him into this world when he was born. She thought perhaps his soul was unhappy and had caused the pain in his leg.

Likewise, when Mrs. Yang converted to Christianity, she probably did not totally give up her animist beliefs about illness. However, her conversion may have allowed her to accept more readily the doctor's recommendations. To understand why she might have changed her mind about the biopsy and operation, we need to understand more about conversion to Christianity and the influence of pastors and church leaders.

## Religious Conversions in the Hmong Community

When discussing matters of health and illness, it is important for health care providers to ascertain whether a person and his or her family is of the "old religion," animism *(coj kev cai qub)*, or of the "new religion," Christianity *(coj kev cai tshiab)*. Providers need not be concerned about offending people when asking about their religious orientation, since Hmong want doctors and nurses to be sensitive to their ways of living and their beliefs.

Some Hmong converted to Christianity in Laos, but the great majority converted in Thailand and the United States. Conversion to Christianity and being a Christian are two separate activities. The Hmong word for religious conversion is *lawb dab*, which literally means "be rid of the spirits." Many Hmong use this term to refer to Christian conversions while others use the term to refer to any religious conversion.

Not everyone who converts to Christianity believes in Jesus or knows what Christianity really is. Some Hmong do away with the spirits but do not believe in God or Jesus *(lawb dab xwb tsis ntseeg)*. When most people throw away the spirits, however, they believe they are hiding their souls away from the spirits that can cause illness.

Many sick Hmong men and women convert to Christianity as a last option or hope for recovery after unsuccessful results with traditional Hmong therapies, such as shaman, soul-calling, or magic healing *(khawv koob)*. If they cannot reunite their souls with their sick bodies or appease the spirits that have brought them harm, they may try to sever their relationship with the spirits as a last chance for survival. Converting to Christianity or other religions may help sick people regain their health because they believe it breaks the bonds between their souls and the spirits. By converting to Christianity, Mrs. Yang may believe that her ancestral spirits can no longer find her and that the spiritual forces that caused her illness are no longer effective. She may believe that she is now under the protection of God.

All Hmong people, but particularly elderly illiterate Hmong, are greatly influenced by the people that surround them. Mrs. Yang is likely to either accept or reject the doctor's recommendation according to who influences her. Pastors and church leaders have a tremendous influence on the members of their congregation, both at home and in the church. When Mrs. Yang converted to Christianity, she may have had a pastor and church leaders who had some understanding of Western medicine and who encouraged her to choose the curative surgery. But if she had been influenced by a pastor and church leaders who did not believe in Western medicine, they might have persuaded her to reject her doctor's recommendation. Hmong pastors and leaders use their position to do what they think is right for the person, though their perspectives, like everyone else's, are limited by their personal and educational experiences.

## Alternative Views of God's Healing Power

Hmong people's perceptions of the Christian God and Jesus, His power, and how He works miracles are found in two distinct views. The first is the belief that God intervenes in matters Himself and works miracles directly with the person in need. In Mrs. Yang's case, if God wills that she be cured from her disease, then He would take away the cancer and make her uterus normal again without any human intervention.

The second view is the belief that God works through people and circumstances. God gives doctors the knowledge and skills to perform curative operations on those who need them. God works through people's hearts so that they do not take advantage of others. According to this view, God works through Mrs. Yang's doctors, nurses, and others involved, giving them skills and kind hearts to help her through her illness. Mrs. Yang's willingness to accept the doctor's recommendations suggests that her circle of influence holds this view of God's healing power.

There are people who believe that God works in both ways, depending on the circumstance and how quickly God answers prayers. God may directly work miracles for people or use others to carry out His work. In the Hmong community, however, older and less literate persons tend to hold the first view while younger and more literate persons hold the second or combined view.

Mrs. Yang may have changed her mind about the biopsy and operation after she converted to Christianity because she now has different spiritual beliefs. She may feel that her soul is able to successfully hide from evil or ancestral spirits and that her soul's destiny is no longer connected to her body's physical integrity. Or she may no longer believe that she was born with a bad fate and has to suffer with cervical cancer but believes that she can change her fate through God's help. The most likely reason she accepted the operation, however, was that she was influenced by her pastor and church leaders who believe that God sends doctors to help people and that a surgical procedure was her best path to a cure.

## Conclusion

Mrs. Yang did not refuse the doctor's recommendations out of stubbornness or ill will. She did not understand her disease in the same way the doctors did. She made decisions supported and encouraged by the people who influence her socially and spiritually. Her conversion to Christianity probably helped her accept the operation because her church community supported the doctor's recommendations. The patience, perseverance, and respect that Mrs. Yang's health care providers displayed probably also enabled her eventually to accept the recommended interventions.

# PART III

# Children's Health

## *Case Stories and Commentaries*

# Children with High Fevers

## *Case Stories*

### Daisy's Story

Daisy Fang was a six-month-old girl who was brought by her young parents to their primary care physician with a fever of 103°F. The chart indicated that the mother had made few prenatal visits and had a normal delivery. Daisy had been to the clinic for three well-child checks but had not received any immunizations, since her parents did not want her to receive them until she was older.

The child had had a fever for three days but had no other symptoms of sickness such as runny nose, sneezing, coughing, difficulty breathing, vomiting, diarrhea, or rash. No one else at home had been sick. Her parents had given her Tylenol, placed a Thai medicine on her temples, wrapped her in a blanket, stopped frying foods, and kept her inside. Still her fever persisted and she became sicker. She was sleeping more and not waking up to drink, cry, or play, so the parents brought her to the clinic.

Concerned about a bacterial meningitis or a bacterial infection in the bloodstream, the doctor recommended—in simple English, since no interpreter was present—hospitalization, blood cultures, urine culture, lumbar puncture, and intravenous antibiotics. The baby's parents were smiling as they listened intently to the doctor. The father asked a few questions about the tests, called his parents, and then agreed to the work-up, stating he was concerned that Daisy was very sick and needed the doctor's help.

The septic evaluation was done quickly. By the time the grandparents arrived, the baby was in the hospital's intensive care unit, receiving intravenous fluids, antibiotics, and oxygen. The test results were consistent with a bacterial meningitis, which required fourteen days of intravenous antibiotics.

Afraid that the child would not get better because there was no rash on her skin, the grandparents told the parents that the child needed the traditional healing rituals of *khawv koob*. The parents asked the nurses whether they could do the healing ceremony in the hospital; the doctor agreed to allow the ritual but refused to let the healer burn incense because of the oxygen Daisy was receiving. The grandparents became angry, but the parents remained quiet and did not challenge the doctor's authority.

Daisy remained feverish, lethargic, and weak for the next two days. Ultimately, she suffered a cardiac arrest. Immediately, the doctors attempted to resuscitate her and her family rushed to the bedside. The nurses told them to wait in the waiting room, but the primary care physician allowed them to stay and tried to explain what was being done to save their daughter. The doctors' efforts were futile. Once they stopped trying to resuscitate Daisy, the family gathered around her, crying and wailing in grief.

After the infant died, the primary doctor heard the nurses and doctors say that if Daisy had had her immunizations, she would have lived. At the Christian funeral, the same doctor heard two elderly people tell the parents that if Daisy had had the *khawv koob,* she would have lived.

## Neng's Story

Neng Song was a three-month-old boy whose young parents brought him along to the mother's prenatal visit and asked the doctors for a medicine to reduce his fever because he had a cold.

The infant was fussy but consolable, with a fever of 103°F., and a normal physical exam. The doctors were concerned about a possible life-threatening bacterial meningitis or bacterial infection in the blood. With a Hmong medical assistant acting as interpreter, the doctors told the parents they needed to draw blood, get a urine specimen with a catheter, and do a lumbar puncture to identify whether he had bacteria in the blood, urine, or spinal fluid.

The parents were shocked at the doctors' evaluation, since the infant had only a cold, and refused the recommended interventions because they feared they would be harmful to their infant. The doctors tried to explain and convince the parents of the need to treat their child aggressively, since the feverish infant without an obvious cause for infection was at risk of dying from meningitis or bacteremia. The parents refused and wanted to take their son home. The doctors called a security guard to take the family to the emergency room while they obtained a police hold and started to get a court order to do their septic work-up and treatment.

The parents telephoned their family members, and by the time the father's parents came, the infant's fever had decreased to 100.8°F. and the boy was alert and playful. The grandfather recommended they take the son home for *khawv koob,* but the doctors refused, wanting to examine the blood and spinal fluid. While the security guard was distracted, the parents escaped out the emergency exit with the infant and drove away in a car. The police went to the child's home to bring the child back, but the boy was never found.

The primary care provider was distraught at the family's departure and worried that the infant was seriously ill and without life-saving medical care. She related that Hmong parents had once taken their sick infant from the hospital and she had worried that the baby had died of meningitis. Feeling responsible, she had vowed that in the future she would always do everything she could to save Hmong infants from their parents, who did not understand the gravity of the illness or the necessity of medical therapies.

Months later, the Hmong interpreter saw the boy in the community. The parents explained that their son had recovered with *khawv koob* at a relative's house and then expressed their anger at the doctors. Why did the doctors want to do such awful things to their son when he was not very sick? Why did the doctors treat them like dogs, without rights and responsibilities toward their beloved son? Did the doctors just want to learn or experiment on their son or just make money, or did they purposefully want to harm him? Had not the doctors lied, saying the baby would die in thirty minutes to scare the parents into allowing the doctors to collect lumbar fluid that could then be used to benefit other babies? And how could the police make them do what the doctor said—was this not a country based on freedom?

## Questions for Consideration

### Questions about Culture

What might explain why these parents had different reactions to the doctors' septic work-up of their sick infants?

On what basis are Hmong parents likely to accept or refuse invasive diagnostic tests in a child with a high fever?

What signs and symptoms do Hmong parents and grandparents evaluate in sick infants? How do these compare with the signs and symptoms that U.S. providers evaluate?

What role did intergenerational conflict play in these cases?

### Questions about Cross-Cultural Health Care Ethics

How do Hmong families and U.S. health care providers differ on the roles they assign to families, healers, institutions, and the state?

Who is responsible for making decisions for seriously ill children in traditional Hmong culture? Who is responsible in U.S. culture?

What are the different ways in which the families and the U.S. health care providers assessed the best interests of Daisy and Neng?

What do these cases suggest about the level of trust Hmong families have for U.S. health care practitioners and what factors support and undermine trust?

### Questions about Culturally Responsive Health Care

What role does the presence or lack of interpreters play in cases like these?

Should hospitals make adjustments to allow families to perform *khawv koob?*

What can hospitals do to accommodate families' desires to perform *khawv koob?*

When is it appropriate to seek a court order to treat children over the parents' objections?

What steps should be considered prior to seeking a court order?

How might institutions and health care practitioners work to repair damaged trust with patients and communities?

*Commentary*

# Hmong Health Beliefs and Practices Concerning Childhood Fevers

*Kathleen A. Culhane-Pera, M.D., M.A., and Va Thao, L.P.N.*

Daisy's and Neng's cases demonstrate the range of situations that can arise when physicians want to evaluate febrile Hmong children. In some, family members agree with everything physicians want to do; in others, family members disagree with everything physicians propose. In some, children die despite receiving what doctors perceived to be necessary life-saving biomedical therapies; in others, children live despite not receiving necessary life-saving biomedical therapies. What is different in these situations? Why do parents and health care workers find common ground in some cases, while in others they get caught in a culture gap and work against each other?

The following commentary relies on in-depth interviews conducted with parents, grandparents, Hmong healers, and doctors concerning nineteen situations in which doctors recommended septic work-ups for Hmong children who had fevers but no identifiable source of infection (Culhane-Pera, 1989). It is also based on our observations of interactions between parents and doctors during years of experience with sick children in Thailand and the United States.

Three aspects of these situations need clarification: biomedical concepts of septic work-ups for children with febrile illnesses; Hmong concepts of childhood febrile illnesses, reactions to biomedical procedures and providers, and familial decision-making practices; and the power issues involved in cases involving young children. Recommendations for how to approach these situations emerge from a clearer understanding of these areas.

## Biomedical Concepts of High Unexplained Fever in Children

When children have fevers without identifiable sources of infection (such as colds, bronchitis, or ear infections) and are lethargic, inconsolable, or unresponsive, doctors are concerned about serious bacterial infections in the brain (meningitis), kidney (pyelonephritis), or blood (septicemia). The standard biomedical approach is to initiate a septic work-up, which includes drawing blood, collecting urine with a catheter, and collecting spinal fluid to test for bacteria. Intravenous antibiotics are started before the completion of test results, which can take up to seventy-two hours.

The antibiotics are continued for three days for kidney infections and two weeks for meningitis; they are stopped if there is no bacterial infection.

For each individual, doctors compare the serious risks of untreated infection (mental retardation, deafness, kidney failure, or death) with the small risks of the interventions (pain and bruises from blood draws, pain from catheters, pain from the lumbar puncture, skin reactions or cellulitis from intravenous fluids, and allergic reactions from antibiotics). They generally decide that it is better to act and deal with any side-effects of interventions than to not act and risk the consequences. Nonetheless, since not all children with fevers need septic work-ups, assessing children's risks for serious infections is an integral part of a doctor's job.

Daisy "looked septic" (feverish, lethargic, and unresponsive) to her doctors, and since there was no identifiable infectious source, they initiated the septic work-up. While Neng was "fussy, but consolable," the high fever in an infant without an identified source of infection alarmed the doctors. Neng's doctors probably were convinced that the parents did not understand the risk of a potential infection, the importance of germs, the accuracy of bacterial cultures, and the effectiveness of antibiotics to treat their child successfully. They discounted Neng's family's evaluation of the child's condition and desire for traditional Hmong treatment. They may have thought that the family's desires for treatment were based on superstition and not worthy of doctors' consideration.

Doctors' decisions to obtain court orders and to render potentially life-saving care to minors against parents' wishes are based on political and legal precedents. States have decreed that physicians must act on behalf of children's medical best interests when their welfare is being jeopardized by parents' decisions. Doctors can feel caught in the middle: between biomedical standards of the appropriate treatment for infections and state requirements that they protect children from harm, on one hand, and a commitment to working in a patient-centered, culturally sensitive manner with parents to effect the best short- and long-term outcomes for the individual, the family, and the community, on the other hand.

The doctor taking care of Neng did not describe a desire to balance culturally sensitive care with life-saving treatment. Rather, she described her concerns about the child's physical well-being and her feeling responsible to "save Hmong infants from their parents, who did not understand the gravity of the illness or the necessity of medical therapies." Her understanding of the importance in medicine of dealing with parents' beliefs and desires seems sorely limited. Because the child later appeared to be "alert and playful," we wonder whether the court-ordered septic work-up was even necessary or whether the doctor's zeal to protect children from their ignorant parents did not result in overuse of her medical authority.

## Hmong Concepts of Childhood Febrile Illness

### Types of Childhood Febrile Illness

Many types of childhood illness can cause fevers: fright or startle *(ceeb)*; a cold *(khaub thuas)*; diarrhea *(thoj plab, zawv plab)*, which can be differentiated by the stool's appearance *(quav dej, quav liab)*; bronchitis *(mob hlab ntsws)*; pneumonia *(mob ntsws)*, which can be differentiated by whether or not it has mucous (dry *mob ntsws qhuav* or wet *mob ntsws ntub)*; impetigo *(kiav txhab)*; bladder infections *(mob zais zis)*; draining ear infections *(pob ntseg muaj paug los)*; and many others. One type of febrile illness, *qoob,* is described in depth below.

As in all translations from one language and one disease categorization system to another, there is not necessarily a one-to-one correspondence of a Hmong disease term to a biomedical disease term. When words are translated, both Hmong parents and U.S. providers may mistakenly think they have similar ideas about a disease.

### Etiologies

We do not know specifically what Daisy's and Neng's parents believed caused their children's fevers. Of the four categories of etiology the Hmong assign—natural, personal, social, and supernatural—children's febrile diseases are most often assigned natural or supernatural causes (see Chapter 1). Natural etiologies of childhood illnesses include germs *(kab mob)*, which can be spread *(sib kis)* by touch or smell; a build-up of wind or air *(cua)* pressure in the body; ingestion of spoiled food or sour milk *(mov zaub tsis huv; mis qaub)*; and diseases that come by themselves *(tuaj ib leeg)*.

Supernatural etiologies include soul loss *(poob plig)* and interactions between spirits *(dab)*, people *(neeg)*, and their souls *(ntsuj plig)*. Children are more vulnerable to soul loss, since their souls are not yet well connected with their bodies. Soul loss occurs when the wandering soul leaves the body after the child is awakened suddenly and the soul stays in the dream world, after the child falls and the soul does not get up, after spirits steal the beautiful child's soul for themselves, and after the child is frightened *(ceeb)* by a loud noise or angry voices. Reincarnation souls can leave the body *(mus thawj thiab lawm)* if they believe that their parents do not care for them or if they are angry with their parents from a previous life. (See Plate 3.)

### Evaluation of Signs and Symptoms

When children are lethargic, not responsive, or not playful or when they have seizures or shaking chills, Hmong parents and Western providers share a similar concern about the child's welfare. Other physical signs may lead to disagreements, however. Parents may look at the pattern of fever in the body (hot body with warm extremities, or hot head with cool body) or look at the pattern of blood flowing through the child's ear to add diagnostic information to their assessment. Parents will be concerned about soul loss or fright by spirits in a child with a hyper-startle reflex. Doctors' words about abnormalities in the blood, urine, and spinal fluid have no direct meanings in Hmong. And while doctors are particularly concerned about fevers in children less than three months old, parents interpret signs and symptoms in an infant in the same manner as they do the symptoms of an older child.

One major difference between Daisy and Neng was each child's presentation. Daisy was "lethargic and weak in her mother's arms," and her father stated "he was concerned that Daisy was very sick and needed the doctor's help." According to Neng's parents, "the infant only had a cold." Families seem more willing to tolerate the risks of invasive biomedical interventions when they judge their child is seriously ill. This was the key difference between Daisy and Neng; Daisy was lethargic and nonresponsive, while Neng was alert and playful.

## Treatments

Treatments for childhood febrile illnesses include wrapping a child in a blanket, rubbing a child's body with a boiled egg *(hau qe kav)* or with a coin, and giving medicines. Medicines include Hmong herbal medicines, U.S. medicines, such as Tylenol, and Thai medicines bought at Asian grocery stores such as antibiotics, paracetamol (which is the same as Tylenol), oral aspirin, and topical aspirin in a tape that is placed on the patient's temple. Also, if there is concurrent fright and startle *(ceeb)*, then ritual healing *(khawv koob)* can calm the baby's soul, or if there is soul loss *(poob plig)*, then soul calling *(hu plig)* is needed. Finally, if a child has had recurrent or persistent symptoms that do not improve, animist parents may pursue a spirit cause and call a shaman. Christians may pursue prayerful healing at any time.

## Qoob

A major type of childhood febrile illness is *qoob* (pronounced "kong"). *Qoob* is a disease entity that must mature and "grow out" of the body for the child to be well. Once *qoob* "grows out" of the body, people can see a rash and then label the illness by the characteristic rash. (For this reason, it may be referred to as a verb *ua qoob* rather than as a noun *qoob.*) If the rash looks like a hemp seed, it is *qhua maj;* when it is filled with water, it is *qhua dej,* and Western doctors may call it chicken pox. If it looks like a millet seed, it is *qhua pias,* and doctors may call it measles. If it looks like a black bean, it is called *qhua taum dub,* and it might be smallpox. If the extremities are covered with a dark blue discoloration, it could be the lethal *ua yeeg,* which doctors might recognize as meningococcemia. Until one is certain what type of *qoob* is present, Hmong people may use the general term *qhua maj qhua pias.*

The power of *qoob* is not to be underestimated. If anything disturbs the disease's growth, it will stay inside of the body and make the child sicker *(phiv mob)*. If *qoob* stays in the lungs, doctors may call it pneumonia, and if it stays in the brain, doctors may call it meningitis. Ultimately, every Hmong parent worries that the illness can cause death. To avoid these complications, parents must adhere to a long list of proscriptions. When any child is sick with a fever, parents must assume that it might be *qoob* and not let the child get chilled, not bring the temperature down quickly, not let the wind enter the child's body, not let the odor of fried foods reach the child, and not give certain foods or medicines to the child. All of these could interfere with *qoob*'s "growing out" of the body. All of these actions could make the child sicker and possibly die. (For more information about *qoob* and the 1990 measles epidemic, see Henry, 1999.)

There are also prescriptive actions that can encourage *qoob* to grow out of the body and thus cure the child. At home, parents may give the same treatments as with all febrile illnesses (see above). In addition, ritual healing *(khawv koob)* is the most effective, because the healer connects with the illness and helps it grow out of the body. The healer *(tus ua khawv koob)*, trained in apprenticeship with other healers, calls his helping spirits *(dab khawv koob)* with incense and chanting, and directs them with water, silver, and words to entice *qoob* to grow out of the body. The power of *khawv koob* healers to communicate with *qoob* and to prevent death is legendary.

Probably both Daisy's and Neng's families were concerned that their children had *qoob*. This would explain why Neng's family wanted to perform *khawv koob* before consenting to the invasive and potentially harmful medical approaches. It would also explain why Daisy's extended family members stated that she would have been cured had she been treated with *khawv koob*.

## Families' Reactions to U.S. Medicine and Providers

While Hmong people may look to the U.S. health care system for assistance with childhood sickness, they also have concerns about U.S. practitioners, and their preventive, diagnostic, and therapeutic practices.

Hmong families may accept vaccinations to protect their children from American diseases, but they weigh the benefits against the risks of injecting dead or weakened germs into children. People have witnessed and heard stories about children who developed high fevers, sicknesses, and paralysis, as well as children who died after receiving vaccinations. Parents are most protective of the children they perceive as most vulnerable: infants *(mos mos liab)*; skinny *(yuag yuag)* rather than chubby *(pham pham)* children; and heavy-boned *(pob txha hnyav)* rather than light-boned *(pob txha sib)* children. Hence, parents may decide to delay getting vaccinations for their most vulnerable children out of their desire to love *(hlub)* and take care of their children (Xiong & Culhane-Pera, 1995). Risk assessment—weighing the risks and benefits—of vaccines for children is a key process for family members. Daisy's family may have decided to wait to have her vaccinated until she was older in order to reduce the risks of the vaccination.

Parents are concerned that U.S. responses to their children's fevers could make their children worse. While giving Tylenol and slowly reducing the fever makes sense, parents may refuse to unwrap or sponge-bathe their children, because the wind or the cold may make *qoob* worse. While giving intravenous fluids and antibiotics are often desired, some parents fear that the cold fluid and the medicine going directly into the child's veins could make the child sicker *(phiv mob)*. Performing lumbar punctures has been associated with death and paralysis in Thailand refugee camps, as well as in the United States. Placing a catheter into the bladder can harm a child's ability to urinate. Taking blood from children can result in weakness, interfere with blood flow on one side of the body, or increase susceptibility to diseases. Blood has traditionally been evaluated by examining a drop of blood from the finger, so the amount of blood Western providers draw seems out of proportion to what is necessary.

Finally, parents have many concerns about health care workers' motivations in treating their children. Do doctors and nurses really want to care for them? Or do they use Hmong people to learn or experiment on or to make money? Such concerns are sharpest during times of conflict between doctors and parents and when doctors get angry and raise their voices or predict the child will die if parents do not do what the doctor says.

## Familial Decision Making

Several value commitments are evident in Daisy's and Neng's parents' decision-making processes. First, family members believe they, not healers or doctors, are responsible for taking care of sick children and for all the consequences of their decisions. If parents make wrong decisions, they are the ones who have to live with the painful consequences of those mistakes. But if doctors make decisions about sick children, and children die or suffer side effects, the doctors can never make it up to the parents. Clearly, Neng's family believed that family members have the right and responsibility to make decisions about Neng.

Second, although parents (and paternal grandparents, especially when parents are young) are responsible to raise their children, they are not alone responsible to make decisions. When a child is seriously ill or doctors recommend potentially harmful procedures, family members are asked to help make decisions. The father's side of the family *(kwv tij)* has more responsibility than the mother's side of the family *(neej tsa)*. And although the evaluations of respected and responsible people carry a lot of weight, no one person makes the decision for the parents and grandparents to follow. Rather, the process is a consensus model, in which opinions are heard, evaluated, and discussed, until the group reaches an agreement. In this way, everyone shares responsibility for the consequences of the decision, whether good or bad. If parents make a decision about an invasive procedure without or against the group's opinion and dire consequences occur, the parents are alone in bearing the responsibility. In Daisy's case, the extended family members disagreed with her parents' decision and blamed them for her death.

Third, there is a general orientation that it is better to not act and to accept the consequences of not interfering than to act and be responsible for the negative consequences of the intervention. This evaluation of risks and benefits is in direct conflict with Western biomedicine's belief that it is better to act and deal with the consequences of interfering than to not act and deal with the consequences of inaction.

Young parents are caught between the old and the new ways. They are told to obey and honor their parents, and they are told to learn U.S. ways in order to survive and thrive in U.S. society. Wanting to do what is best for their children's health, they wonder whether to leave the feverish child wrapped up or to unwrap the child. They want to fry foods for their family to eat but wonder whether they should avoid frying foods when their children have fevers. They want to allow their sick children to have ice cream or cold soda pop but wonder if they could be bothering *qoob*.

Daisy's parents were caught in between. They allowed the doctors to proceed with the septic work-up and treatment but then were criticized by family members for choosing the harmful U.S. ways rather than the traditional Hmong healing ritual. They may have been guided to delay vaccinating Daisy by their grandparents' concerns about vaccinations, and then they were criticized by health care workers for not getting the protection. Trying to provide the best care for their child, they succeeded in angering both communities.

## The Doctor's Power

Doctors and families may disagree about who should have the right to decide. Neng's parents believe that, as the parents, they have the right to decide. Neng's doctors believe that, as the doctors, they have the right to decide.

This tug-of-war escalates until the doctors decide whether they will get a court order or not. If they decide that the child's life is in serious immediate danger, then they contact the hospital attorney, who contacts the judge, who invariably agrees with the doctor's assessment. The judge issues an order allowing the doctors to act without parental consent. Once the police arrive to enforce the court order, the family has no recourse and the septic work-up and treatment ensue unless they successfully flee with their child—out the emergency exits, back staircases, or side doors; in waiting cars, vans, or planes; to relatives' homes, or to other states. The consequences of court-ordered treatments are felt throughout the community and contribute to suspicion and distrust of the health care system and health care professionals. All parents have heard the stories and the accompanying advice: don't go to those providers because they will call the police and force your child to be tortured; don't go to that clinic because the providers will use your child to study or learn on.

Through these conflicts, Hmong families are being socialized into U.S. society. They are learning about the capacity of medicine to heal. They are learning how to interact with professionals of higher social status, when to answer questions and when to ask questions, when to accept what is said and when to challenge, when to refuse and when to comply. They are learning the limits: when they can make decisions for their children and when the doctors, through their connections with the state, will force them to conform.

The consequences of these conflicts are painful for health care professionals as well. U.S. doctors relate stories about their pain and anguish in not being able to provide a sick Hmong child with the best modern medical care, their frustration in spending inordinate amounts of time and still not arriving at an acceptable resolution, their anger at being treated disrespectfully by families, and their ambivalent feelings of relief and sorrow about forcing families with court orders. The pain of Neng's doctor was evident; her previous difficult experience seems to have galvanized her to enforce her medical perspective with a court order, rather than work with family members and jeopardize what she considered to be in Neng's best interest. But in her fear, she may have acted in a paternalistic and ethnocentric manner and she may have overstepped the bounds of her authority.

Some U.S. providers are changing. Exposed to patients' different ideas, desires, and demands, they are experiencing cross-cultural health care. Some providers are learning to ask questions and listen to answers, including answers that reveal parents' understanding of childhood illnesses, their experiences with suffering, and their struggles to find healing. And some health care workers have made a greater effort to communicate with extended family members and negotiate other options.

## Recommendations

Health care workers need first to be aware of their own experiences of working with patients from different cultural backgrounds. This awareness involves being reflective about their own cultural beliefs and values and being willing to learn about cultural beliefs and values from other people.

Health care workers also must consider how to communicate with Hmong families. What languages are needed—White or Green Hmong? What language assistance is accessible—family members, untrained interpreters, or trained interpreters in person or by a telephone service? Who is available to discuss the situation, and who needs to be present (parents, grandparents, family leaders, and community leaders)? Given the urgency of responding to a child's febrile illness, the best approach is to arrange for a family conference with the family's decision makers and a trained interpreter in a timely manner.

It is crucial that professionals avoid verbal and nonverbal expressions of anger or impatience with family's concerns, resistances, or desires; these can raise families' suspicions about providers' motivations to help their child. Saying that the child "will die" can be insulting ("hurt parents' hearts"), can be interpreted as a curse ("If you don't do as I say, your child will die"), and can be inaccurate. It makes more sense to express concern in other ways, for example, by saying, "Your child is very sick" or "I am concerned about your child's future" or "I am concerned your child will not get well without medicines, but I am hopeful because I have seen other children with the same problem get better with medicines."

Health care workers should follow the LEARN model: Listen, Explain, Acknowledge, Recommend, and Negotiate (Berlin & Fowkes, 1983; see Chapter 16). Before presenting the clinical information and viewpoint, it is helpful to ask the family members about their assessment of the child. Listening to the family's beliefs, fears, and desires for the child demonstrates respect, interest, and willingness to work together. Eliciting parents' concepts of disease (including *ua qoob* and *phiv mob*), evaluations of their child's illness (mild, moderate, or serious, and specific concerns) and desired treatments (herbs, Western medicines, or *khawv koob*) provides important information.

Then it is appropriate for health care providers to explain the biomedical viewpoint, using patient education skills to empower parents and referring back to their ideas, fears, or concerns. Providers need to share evidence from the physical exam with family members, draw diagrams, and explain lab results to them. Generally, Hmong families want information and they feel respected and empowered when they understand the biomedical information. They should also acknowledge similarities (such as physical findings, severity of illness, and role for medications) and differences (such as diagnostic tests or therapeutic options) in order to find common goals (such as decrease fever, give medicines, keep the child healthy).

Following the explanations, providers should recommend diagnostic and therapeutic procedures. They may need to explore the family's reactions to the recommendations (medicines, sponge baths, IV fluids, blood tests, lumbar punctures, and so on) and gently provide information to counter families' fears and concerns. They should consider building on the trust they have with specific people (primary care doctors, clinic nurses, interpreters, and so on) and emphasizing clinicians' ages and expertise in performing procedures (for example, "This nurse is our best in starting IVs").

For situations like Neng's, in which families refuse to allow septic work-ups, providers should be willing to negotiate and compromise. Consider obtaining a second opinion quickly from other clinicians, clinics, or hospitals; admitting the child for observation; allowing the parents to take the child home and return the next day; warming up IV fluids; using warm water for sponge baths; allowing families to be present during procedures; allowing traditional therapies such as *khawv koob* in the hospital (some intensive care units allow incense to be burned in the presence of oxygen as long as there is no open flame); and treating with antibiotics without complete medical data. While each of these options presents health care providers with less than optimal conditions, the risks may be worth the benefits.

Following these avenues is likely to increase trust between providers and families, improve relations between clinics and communities, and provide excellent care to sick children.

## References

Berlin, E. A., & Fowkes, W. S. (1983). A teaching framework for cross-cultural health care. *Western Journal of Medicine, 139,* 934–938.

Culhane-Pera, K. A. (1989). *Analysis of cultural beliefs and power dynamics in disagreements about health care of Hmong children.* Unpublished master's thesis, University of Minnesota, Minneapolis.

Henry, R. R. (1999). Measles, Hmong, and metaphor: Culture change and illness management under conditions of immigration. *Medical Anthropology Quarterly (new series), 13*(1), 32–50.

Xiong, P., & Culhane-Pera, K. (1995, April 7). *Hmong perceptions and attitudes about immunizations.* Paper presented at the Hmong National Education Conference, St. Paul, MN.

## Commentary

# State-Ordered Medical Care
# for Our Son: Parents' Perspective

*Parents (Anonymous)*

Neng was three months old when my husband and I took him with us to my prenatal visit. We thought since Neng had a fever and we were at the clinic, we could ask for medication to reduce his fever.

Although Neng had a fever of 103°F., he was playful and happy and was not fussing at all. Through a Hmong interpreter, our physician told us that our baby had bacterial meningitis and would not make it through the night; he probably would die within twenty-four hours at most. My husband and I were very shocked. We could not believe that our baby was going to die, and we refused to have his spinal fluid and blood drawn with a needle and syringe.

We told our physician that we would go home first, talk with my husband's parents, and have our uncle do traditional healing *(khawv koob)*. If Neng was not better, we said we would bring him back to the hospital, and then they could do all the necessary tests and treatments. We gave our promise to the doctor, but no matter what my husband and I said, our physician just would not listen to us as parents. She preferred seeing our child in her medical way and ruling us, our child's birth parents, out of the health care decision-making process. It was at this point that things got so out of hand that we began speaking to each other in loud voices.

Our physician said that if we refused the interventions, we would be arrested by a police officer. She told us we did not have any right to stop the treatment of our baby, since he was too young to make his own decisions even though we gave birth to our child. She stated she had the right to get a court order, have our child removed from us, and have us arrested if we continued to refuse the treatments.

Her remarks really offended both of us. I was trembling and frightened while holding onto my baby, with questions running through my mind: "What have we gotten into with this physician? What did we do wrong as parents to encounter such a mess with this physician? Is she mad, wanting to do experiments on our child, as though our baby is not a human being?" But my husband was strong and argued against her intervention. If she wanted to have us arrested we would not stop her, but we would not allow her to perform such tests and treatments, since we as parents knew that our child was only having a nonserious cold with fever. She then told us that if we held back for too long or ran away with our child, and our baby died because of delayed treatment, we would be held responsible for our child's death. And worst of all, both of us would be put in jail for the death of our child. This really angered my husband.

My husband called his parents and they also disagreed with the physician's intervention. They knew for sure that Neng did not have meningitis and knew that the spinal needle would only make the illness worse and damage our child's well-being. They wanted us to bring our child home for traditional healing. They were sure we would lose our child if we allowed the doctors to do such testing and treatment. Our father told my husband that they were on their way to the clinic and to tell the physician to hold their testing and treatments until they got there.

Neng was very alert and when the nurse took his temperature again, his temperature was down. Both of us were really relieved, but still they did not allow us to go home with Neng.

We repeatedly told the doctor to wait for our parents. The security guard pushed my husband to the door and said he would be cuffed and arrested if he did not cooperate. I was very frightened and thought that no matter what we say or do now, we just cannot convince them to wait for our parents. A police officer arrived and told us with a very rude gesture that the doctors had obtained a court order for us to bring Neng to the hospital and if we refused, he could arrest us. We asked for the interpreter to return, but she had left for the evening.

We were escorted to the Emergency Room. People came to examine Neng. A male doctor said our child was very sick. We did not respond because it was no use to speak, the officer was in the room, and it would just be a waste of our words. Two nurses held Neng down so the man could look into Neng's ear with the otoscope. Neng's cry was very sharp and I knew my baby was in pain from the otoscope being forced into his ear and that he was frightened by the many different people surrounding him. I forced myself between them and said to the man that he is hurting my baby. He responded that Neng is fine, that he needs to see whether Neng has any ear infection. I picked him up crying. The man said our child does seem to have an ear infection, and a blood test would be drawn. After they left, my husband and I were able to calm Neng down. We were afraid that his fever might come back, and the physicians would do whatever they wanted to do. My husband felt Neng's forehead and there was no fever; he was fine and his cheeks were not cherry pink any more.

Our parents and brother arrived shortly and informed us that the security guard was still guarding the door. Nurses came to draw Neng's blood. Our father asked them how much blood they were taking and the type of test they would be doing, but he did not get any response. They just told my mother-in-law to hold Neng for them. Neng cried while they drew his blood.

Then another male physician whom we had never seen or known before came in with the officer and informed us that he would be doing a spinal fluid test and said if there was an infection in the spinal fluid, a surgery may be required to save him. He said that Neng's blood was normal, but they still needed to do the spinal fluid test to make sure he did not have meningitis. Without doing the spinal fluid test, they would not give or prescribe any medication and would not let us go home. My heart was beating as fast as ever and my tears rolled down my cheeks because of all the commotion and disagreement going on in the room. We demanded to speak with our primary physician but were only told that she had left for the evening. We never saw our physician again.

The physician told us that our child was going to die within thirty minutes if we refused testing and treatment, and that the intervention was necessary to save our child's life. We decided that we would not allow them to do such testing and that we would have to protect our child. We knew that once they took the spinal fluid, they would only tell us that our child did have meningitis, and more tests and treatments would be needed. And we knew that Neng was not that sick, since he had no symptom other than fever, and if we went along with them, we would lose our child.

We made a plan to run off with our child. If we were caught, my in-laws would take our child away from the hospital and care for him. My husband went out with Neng tucked in his jacket, and I followed after him along with our brother. We were able to reach the emergency exit when the security guard noticed that we were leaving with our baby. He shouted, and we all started running out. Since our brother was holding onto Neng's blanket, the security guard caught up to him and stopped him, thinking that he was holding Neng. My husband and I headed toward our parents' car with the security guard, nurse, and physician chasing after us. When we reached the vehicle, the officer was close behind, but we were able to drive away quickly.

We drove to our uncle's home and asked him to perform *khawv koob* for Neng. Our parents called us at midnight and told us two officers and a Hmong interpreter had come to our home, questioned where we went with our child, and laid out the consequences if our child died. But our parents said they did not know where we were. That night Neng's fever never returned (no medication was ever given for Neng's fever that evening at the clinic and hospital), and in the morning he was well and playful, sitting and clapping hands with our cousins.

What my husband and I experienced with our physician was something so traumatic that we never want to go through the same thing again. This experience has really affected our lives, our trust with health care services, and the way we use clinic and hospital services. We think our physician never realized what this experience did to us psychologically. We changed clinics and delivered my second child at a different hospital. Whenever our children come down with a fever or are sick we are always afraid of what could happen if we take them to see a physician. We prefer to use our own traditional healing, home remedies, and over-the-counter medications first, as well as have our child's fever come down before using the clinic. We now think twice before seeking medical advice.

When it comes to health care for a young or old non-Caucasian patient, before proceeding to do anything, physicians ought first to give their perspectives and discuss the risks and benefits of the test procedures, medications, and type of surgery necessary with the patient's family members who make health care decisions within the family. The physicians must be open-minded and sensitive to the family's need to use traditional healings. They must realize that Hmong families have been practicing traditional healing such as *khawv koob*, herbs, and other forms of treatments for generations. They should allow these fundamental forms of healing within the clinic and hospital.

Physicians should not use force with a court order or use threats to make family members comply with their recommendations. Using threats and force is unethical medical practice. Experiences like the one we encountered will only trigger more Asian families to think that physicians are opportunistic, doing things only for their own benefit.

The doctors—who indicated to us that our child would die within thirty minutes to twenty-four hours, threatened us with a court order to use our child for their treatments, threatened to arrest us if we took our child away from their care, and stated vindictively that we would be held responsible for our child's death—should have their medical licenses revoked for their missed diagnoses and wrongful accusations. Doctors must respect parents' rights, responsibilities, and love for their children and never act so unethically and disrespectfully.

*Commentary*

# Family-Centered Cultural Collaboration in Pediatric Care

*Donald Brunnquell, Ph.D., and Stephen Kurachek, M.D.*

Daisy's and Neng's parents face a crisis of cultural faith: Whom should we believe? Should we trust our parents and extended family, who are telling us that if we want our child to live, we must take our child home to receive a gentle, well-known, and trusted treatment? Or should we trust the doctors and nurses, strangers vested with all the trappings of power and authority in this new homeland, who are saying we must not only stay and reject our own parents' way of life but also subject our child to painful and invasive treatments with no guarantee of success?

The ironic outcomes of these two cases reinforce both sets of cultural beliefs and perpetuate misunderstanding between two communities who share a deep love and respect for children. These cases demonstrate that health care decisions have meaning only in the context of the culture from which each party understands the world. A fact becomes a fact only in a particular cultural context, and successful pediatric care, in our view, requires attention to the cultural assumptions of both the practitioners and the families.

## The Fallacy of Medicine as "Culture Free"

Western medicine views itself as a scientific endeavor based on principles of physics, chemistry, and biology, and it often presumes that its assessments and interventions are "objective." This view raises two fallacies, one epistemological and the other practical.

The epistemological fallacy is the Western scientific notion that what can be seen, or at least measured, is all that is real, and that one understands something best by breaking it down to simpler and simpler processes and units. This approach has proven to be powerful in improving the lives of people all over the world, but it provides neither a complete nor universally accepted explanation of the universe. Rather, it reflects cultural assumptions about the world.

The practical fallacy is that medicine can be pursued without reference to the values and goals of the individual person or the group to which that person belongs— that is, their culture. In fact, the decision to pursue each medical treatment reflects a decision that the anticipated outcome has value. Value is culturally influenced, and every decision to pursue a medical treatment is in practice a culturally based decision. The value element is often invisible because of practitioners' and patients' culturally shared values. When assumptions are challenged, as in Daisy's and Neng's cases, the cultural dimension of medical decisions emerges sharply.

One constructive response to this practical fallacy is to attempt to identify the "cultural lens" each person brings to his or her work as provider and as parent—a way of seeing that helps shape both external reality and the meaning of that reality. Each practitioner must acknowledge this lens and also avoid the fallacy that only the practitioner has a "cultural lens." Each party brings one to the dialogue. In the end, the outcome for the child is in part determined by the encounter between cultures. Understanding such encounters is an important element of improving patient care.

## Family-centered Cultural Collaboration

Family-centered care should lie at the core of every pediatric health care encounter (Shelton & Stepanek, 1994). This philosophy of care begins with recognition that the family is the constant in a child's life, while the service systems and support personnel within those systems change. Collaboration is difficult enough with families whose basic beliefs about causality and illness derive from a tradition the practitioner shares with the family. The ethics literature is replete with stories of failed collaboration between providers and patients or families within the Western tradition. The cases of Neng and Daisy demonstrate the magnitude of the challenges all parties face in achieving true collaboration. What follows is an exploration of the problems and struggles Western practitioners experience when applying a family-centered collaboration model to cases such as Daisy's and Neng's.

The family-centered care model calls for practitioners and families to explicitly name and pay particular attention to the differences that may arise as they interpret events and their causes and meanings. Explicitly recognized, such differences offer an opportunity to collaborate in establishing their meaning and relevance; ignored, they become obstacles to action. Although recognition of differences does not in and of itself guarantee eventual agreement, it does recast the relationship between the family and practitioners in a way more likely to achieve agreement.

Consider Neng's case. How might it have been different if, at the point of initial explanation of bacteremia, the physician and team had acknowledged that there might be differences in how they and the family understood Neng's outwardly minor illness, and that their goal was to work together to achieve what was best for Neng? If this theme had been the touchstone of the interaction, especially when the practitioners and family disagreed, the parents' shock and the ensuing polarization would have been reduced if not eliminated.

Even when two parties share linguistic and cultural meanings, they often spend time developing shared definitions of terms. When the two parties have divergent linguistic and cultural backgrounds, such as the Western health care practitioner and the Hmong family, the meanings of key concepts diverge: health, get better, good outcome, painful, cure, choice, soul, spirit. Each concept has a different—sometimes very different—meaning from culture to culture, from family to family, and from individual to individual. To achieve a shared understanding, it becomes necessary to ask and to explain what each party means and understands by these terms.

## Steps in Achieving Family-centered Cultural Collaboration

It is not enough to identify the barriers to collaboration between practitioners of Western health care and Hmong families. The next essential step is to identify actions that can remove or cross those barriers. In this process the interpreter plays an essential role in articulating the data on which our recommendations are based and the reasons for our recommendations. Timely and accurate interpretation signals both that we respect the traditional language of the family and that we are committed to achieving understanding.

Family-centered cultural collaboration includes taking the following steps:

1.  Recognizing the specific cultural lens and assumptions that we as U.S. providers bring to our work; this involves acknowledging potential differences with families. In Daisy's and Neng's cases, both parties would openly recognize that their disagreement is about means to achieve a shared goal.
2.  Achieving a broad understanding of the cultural traditions of the populations with whom we work; this means having some general knowledge of health care beliefs and knowing at least what questions to ask. When encountering an unfamiliar culture, asking directly about families' beliefs is essential.
3.  Acknowledging with each family (not only ethnically identified families) that it is important to discuss the basic beliefs about health and illness that lead them to their conclusions and us to our conclusions. This kind of communication equalizes the power differential that exists and tells a family that we wish to respect their core values and beliefs.
4.  Asking the family to describe their understanding of what might have caused the illness and what might be done about it in their traditional culture, as well as their understanding about the typical approach in the United States. This signals to the family that we are concerned about more than the physical procedures the practitioner believes are needed for the child. In Neng's case this might have opened the door to discussing an integration of Western and Hmong approaches and avoided the life-long distrust of the health care system engendered by involving the police.
5.  Acknowledging differences that are identified and then seeking third parties or other forums to resolve them. This step again may balance the power differential in the health care system and it encourages collaboration.
6.  Asking about decision-making traditions and the degree to which the family adheres to those traditions. Doing so makes it clear not only that the beliefs about health and illness are important to the practitioner but also that beliefs about respect and human relationships will inform our actions.
7.  Pursuing whenever possible a dual approach of Western and traditional treat-

ment. In Neng's case it may have been possible to pursue *khawv koob* in the hospital, as it was with Daisy.

8. Acknowledging at the outset that the parents are the decision makers for the child, that they have the right to include others in that process, and that we will work with them according to their wishes about who should be involved in the decision. But we must also inform patients that when practitioners seriously disagree with the family, and the child's life is in danger, they are required to seek authorization from the court or child welfare services to abrogate the parents' decision-making power. While it is difficult to discuss involving other authorities, such discussions are a respectful way of approaching a situation that becomes even more difficult if, as in Neng's case, police are involved without a chance for the practitioners to explain their reasons and obligations.

9. Describing any questions or concerns we have about the information we receive or our interaction with the family. By focusing on the need to clarify different understandings, we avoid direct confrontations that may be based on assumptions about the superiority of one set of beliefs or culture. In Daisy's case, this approach might have facilitated discussion between the Christian immediate family and other extended family members who held other beliefs.

10. When difficulties arise, refocusing on the shared goal of improving the health of the child and allowing that goal to guide our interpretation of the "facts" and the motivations of others.

The essence of this approach is mutual respect and communication about potential differences rather than making assumptions about any general cultural approach. By implementing family-centered care, we can attempt to achieve a balance of cultures which serves the best interest of the child in the context of the family.

## Challenges to Family-centered Cultural Collaboration

### Collaboration with Extended Family

In Daisy's and Neng's cases, family-centered care leads to collaboration not merely with the parents of the child but with an extended group of decision makers. In each case, the grandparents have significant influence on how the parents frame reality and decisions during and after the medical encounters. Instead of the Western legal assumption that the parents are the agents of the child, staff working with the Hmong family discover that the extended family is the child's agent, with a patriarch as an influential decision maker. Who is really speaking for the child? Do the parents agree with their parents, or are they acquiescing to a tradition that conflicts with their beliefs about what is best for the child? Most pediatric practitioners are used to fathers' acquiescence with the mother in matters regarding young children, or even fathers' total absence. Working with Hmong families, Western providers may observe instead that mothers may not even be consulted.

Who is the legitimate moral decision maker for the child? On this issue no single cultural tradition is correct. In many cases, reliance on the extended family may actually reduce any conflict of interest between a child's individual interests and the interests of the parents as caregivers. With every family, providers should ask how decisions are usually made and work within the cultural and family structure to meet the child's interests while recognizing the U.S. legal realities of parental consent.

## Embracing Only Parts of Treatment Plans

In Daisy's case, the parents indicated that they intended to immunize but wished to delay the process. They had attended well-child visits and complied with some but not all aspects of the recommended best practice of scheduled immunization. Hmong families who do not trust the Western medical system frequently "pick and choose" treatment. Picking and choosing, while grounded in the notion of patient autonomy to choose or refuse treatment, also raises questions about collaboration in making decisions.

Ideally, the physician's recommendation concerns not a single, isolated treatment but rather a plan of care that in this case includes immunizations. If portions of the treatment plan are omitted, the entire plan may be invalidated or rendered less effective. When families object to certain portions of the treatment plan, providers can ask about what is acceptable and why, in keeping with the notion of identifying differences. Providers should also outline their view of the risks associated with partial treatment. When the deleted part of the plan truly invalidates the treatment, providers should articulate that point and withdraw the offer of treatment. When partial treatment renders the plan partially effective, the practitioner must assess the value of the partial treatment compared with the cost of alienating the family and other members of their community.

In Neng's case, some of the staff may have wondered why the family brought Neng to the hospital at all if they were not going to accept what the providers believed was best. While this reaction often occurs when any family questions recommended treatments, it occurs more frequently with immigrant families. The stereotypical question, "Why did they come if they weren't going to listen?" must be reframed to ask what understanding of the health care system and the world has led the family to bring the child to the providers at this time.

Why did Neng's family seek help from the doctors at all? This is a question, reflecting the "caught-in-the-middle" status of many Hmong families, that has as much to do with sociology, psychology, and cultural power as it does with health care. Providers should not be surprised that Hmong have as much ambivalence about seeking Western treatment as they would about engaging with any Western institution. The health care system sends messages of cultural power and sanction to all: enormous, well-appointed buildings; state-sanctioned, licensed providers with honorific titles; the power to impose seventy-two-hour "holds" and to access the police and courts for assistance; and access to techniques only vaguely understood by outsiders that require a long, ritualistic period of training. Most people working within the system take this cultural sanction for granted and presume it will be accepted by anyone seeking treatment. Those unacquainted or only marginally acquainted with the traditions of the culture often respond with deep mistrust.

The actual benefits of Western treatment certainly influence the decision to seek care. Other important elements include beliefs about what causes illness, fears of experimentation disguised as treatment, community stories of court-mandated treatment, family histories of mistrust and miscommunication, and histories of exploitation.

Just as Euro-American families seek "alternative" medicine when "Western" medicine seems inadequate, a Hmong family is likely to explore "alternative" medicine, which to them may mean "Western" medicine. Loving parents may explore all options for their children, even if they eventually choose not to use one of them. The principle of respect for patient autonomy in health care ought not to be translated by practitioners as, "You can exercise your autonomy when you choose to seek care, but once you're here, your choice must agree with mine."

## Mandated Reporting, Medical Neglect, and Religious Exemption

The question of reporting the parents' choice not to pursue Western health care as medical neglect is important to both the Western provider culture and the Hmong culture. Medical neglect is understood here as not providing needed treatment. Such neglect is generally considered a "mandated report," meaning that the health care provider is legally obligated to notify the police or child welfare agency of the parental action (or inaction) that is harming the child. In Neng's case, the Western providers felt that neglect was occurring and thought law enforcement officials should be involved.

Providers who are mandated by law to report medical neglect often struggle with the definition of neglect and particularly with the question whether a particular treatment is truly needed or simply preferred. The degree of concern about sepsis or meningitis cannot be assessed without seeing a child. In some cases the clinical impression of meningitis or sepsis is so strong that to not pursue diagnosis and treatment is clearly medical neglect—but not in all cases. Based on the case material, it is impossible to evaluate the validity of the judgment made here.

Neng's case must be examined in the light of specific exemptions most states have written into many child abuse and neglect statutes for "religious or spiritual treatment." Such an exemption holds that a family's choice to pursue spiritual treatment instead of medical treatment should not be construed as criminal neglect. Many Western providers believe this "religious exemption" introduced into maltreatment laws largely by the Christian Science Church is wrong, since it does not meet a justice standard of equal access to life-saving treatment for all children. Nonetheless, there is no reason it should apply less to Hmong beliefs than to Christian Science beliefs.

Many providers believe that if their treatment choices must be legally enforced, collaboration with families has already gone by the boards. In many cases, however, physician relationships with the family continue after legal involvement. Perhaps the family has no choice, or perhaps the family recognizes the physician's good-faith attempt to achieve what the physician feels is best for the child. Providers who communicate with the family about the decision to involve the legal authorities—stating clearly what they plan to do, why they will do it, and why they believe it is best for the child—

have a better chance of maintaining a relationship with the family and encouraging future use of the health care system.

### Interests of Child, Interests of Culture, and the Question of Justice

Some providers who treat children like Daisy and Neng express concern that the interests of the Hmong culture in maintaining itself seem to take precedence over the interests of the child in receiving appropriate care. The Hmong family seems to be saying, "We choose not to pursue Western health care because it is not consistent with our beliefs, and our beliefs are more important than the welfare of this individual child. If we are not true to our ways, we will all lose our way, and what will happen to all our children if we lose our way?"

In a culture in which individual interests are considered paramount, this argument may make little sense. Should a child's chance for life be allowed to be compromised by parental decisions made to consider larger cultural implications? An important justice question also arises: Does a Hmong child not deserve the same standard of treatment as a European American child, an African American child, a Latino child, or a Somali child in the United States? The definition of justice an immigrant community brings with it will be challenged as the community experiences enculturation and assimilation. The life-and-death crisis of a critically ill child accelerates such a value crisis. There is a strong tendency in precisely such a life-threatening crisis to view what is occurring and to decide what to do in the most familiar and culturally traditional terms; those cultural norms help to guide behavior in life crises such as a critical illness.

Pediatric health care providers often ask themselves about the long-term outcome for the surviving family. For families in the midst of the rapid change entailed in immigration, acts that seem valid in the traditional culture may no longer seem valid as the new blended culture begins to shape the family's worldview. In Daisy's and Neng's cases, providers may advocate Western treatment in part because they believe—somewhat paternalistically, perhaps—that within a generation, the family will view that treatment as the better choice. Perhaps a better strategy would be to talk openly with the family about the concern about how the choice will be viewed in the future—a discussion that should occur with every family facing the crisis of critical illness.

When a good biological outcome can be predicted with high probability, there may be greater justification for insisting on Western treatment. When a good outcome cannot be predicted with high probability, greater parental autonomy to choose something else is reasonable. This does not completely answer the justice question, since similarly situated children will be treated differently: a surgery with a 50 percent mortality may be chosen for one child, but not another, even though their clinical conditions are almost identical. However, not all majority culture children are treated similarly either. Allowing greater family autonomy as we become less certain about outcomes is a reasonable stance that reflects both our sense of duty to protect children and our desire to respect other cultures.

When the question of justice pits the child against the culture, it wrongly separates the outcome of a particular treatment for the child from the child's overall life outcome within their culture. A treatment that saves the child's physical life but could cause a child or family to be ostracized may win the battle but lose the war. Providers must be careful not to overestimate the likelihood of ostracism but must also consider potential stigma that may follow the child or family within their cultural group.

In Daisy's case, her family risks the anger of their extended family and their clan by acquiescing to Western treatment. They take the risk that all their future decision making and actions may be called into question, and they risk their status as accepted members of their family and social group. In the Hmong American culture, in which the primary social contacts are still within the Hmong community, the stakes are considerably higher than for someone with alternative networks of support and friendship through other institutions (e.g., church, educational organizations, fraternal organizations). A decision that jeopardizes all of one's social support in a new environment goes beyond the issues of loss and grief surrounding the particular child. Family-centered cultural collaboration acknowledges these issues and allows the providers and parents to collaborate on how to value them in the decision-making process.

Ultimately, several ethical issues remain: the questions of justice, the duty of the practitioner (to provide access to the resources of Western health care that offer the best chance of ongoing life and future possibilities), the duty of parents (to offer what they believe is best for this child and their other children), and the value of what is offered. The answers to these questions are key to achieving what is best for the child. With Hmong families or with families of other recent immigrant groups, these questions are especially challenging. Providers who discuss with the family the meaning of cultural traditions and values gain the best chance of achieving answers that the practitioners, the family, and the child can live with.

In Daisy's case and in Neng's case, there is no indication that this open discussion ever occurred. Identifying possible disagreement about how to achieve the shared goal of what is best for the child is an important first step. This discussion provides the best means of collaborating across cultures and across individual beliefs about what is best for the child.

## Reference

Shelton, T. I., & Stepanek, J. S. (1994). *Family-centered care for children needing specialized health and developmental services*. Bethesda, MD: Association for the Care of Children's Health.

# Bottle-Fed Toddler with Anemia

## *A Case Story*

Xong Mary Hang was a one-year-old girl whose mother brought her to the community clinic for a well-child check. She lived with her sixteen-year-old mother, who attended high school; her eighteen-year-old father, who worked; and her paternal grandparents, who took care of her during the day. Her mother's primary concern was that Xong's skin was yellow. In response to Dr. Anderson's questions, she reported that Xong was drinking up to eight fluid ounces of whole milk six or seven times a day, as well as once or twice during the night. She was a picky eater, preferring to drink milk rather than eat rice, meat, or vegetables.

On examination, Xong was overweight for her small height, pale but not jaundiced, and had a 9.2 hemoglobin (normal range is 12–14). Dr. Anderson diagnosed iron deficiency anemia, which she felt was related to too much milk consumption. She recommended that the mother give less milk, offer a cup instead of the bottle, and encourage balanced table foods. She also gave iron supplements for the child.

Xong was also receiving services from WIC (Special Supplemental Nutrition Program for Women, Infants, and Children, a federally funded program that provides nutritional support for low-income pregnant women, infants, and children). WIC sent Dr. Anderson a note stating that Xong had low hemoglobin. There was no further communication between the WIC program and the physician.

Xong missed a one-month follow-up visit but was rescheduled and returned two months later. To Dr. Anderson's surprise Xong was clutching a bottle of milk. When Dr. Anderson asked Xong's mother about this, she replied that she had tried to implement the physician's suggestions, but Xong threw a tantrum each time they took the bottle away and still ate very little. Xong's grandparents were concerned that she would starve without the milk. On examination, the child's weight had increased disproportionately to her height, her skin was paler, and her hemoglobin was 8.2.

Dr. Anderson and Xong's mother discussed the child's condition and the mother seemed to understand the adverse effects of the anemia. She said she would try again to implement Dr. Anderson's recommendations to decrease Xong's dependence on milk and give the iron supplement with orange juice. Xong returned one month later, again clutching a bottle, and was clinically worse with pale skin, notched front teeth, a flow murmur, a palpable spleen, and a hemoglobin of 5.8. Dr. Anderson pointed out to the mother where Xong was on the growth curve, her paleness, her heart murmur, and her enlarged spleen.

The mother explained that they simply could not get the child to change her behaviors toward milk, food, and the bad-tasting iron supplement. The mother agreed to injections of iron and agreed to let a public health nurse visit their home. Shoua Moua, the public health nurse, made weekly home visits for a month, evaluated the situation, provided education, and supported behavior change. She reported that the grandparents watched the child every day and that they had trouble insisting that the child give up the bottle and eat solid foods. They felt the child would starve without the bottle, and they could not bear to hear her cry when they withheld it. Two of the grandparents' children had starved to death in Laos, including one infant who had died during the war and refugee flight from an insufficient supply of breast milk. The grandparents told the nurse they only wanted to love and care for *(hlub)* Xong.

Also, Ms. Moua explained that she felt there was tension between the parents and the grandparents. It seemed to her that the parents wanted to be more "American" in raising their children—setting limits about food and behaviors, following a feeding schedule, having a routine nap time, and having the child sleep in her own crib. The grandparents did not believe it was right to force a child to do things she did not want to do; they were against these measures. Furthermore, the grandparents felt insulted that the parents were telling them how to take care of the grandchildren, as though the grandparents knew nothing. Ms. Moua sensed that both grandparents were depressed but especially the grandfather. The grandfather cried while he explained that he had been a leader in Laos and an influential man in the war, but now his role in life had changed and his stature had diminished. Now, he said, he was only good enough to watch children, and even in this endeavor, his son's wife had criticized him and blamed him for Xong's "low blood." The real problem, he believed, was that the child had a frightened soul, which could be returned if only his son would arrange for a soul-calling ceremony *(hu plig)*.

Xong's parents brought her to the clinic two weeks after the iron injections. The parents pointed out that her skin was rosier and she was livelier. Dr. Anderson found that Xong's murmur and enlarged spleen had resolved, and her hemoglobin was 9.2, closer to the desired 12. When Dr. Anderson asked whether Xong's eating had improved, the mother said that Xong now drinks less milk, but she was unable to quantify any significant change. Dr. Anderson congratulated the parents on the improvement but was concerned that the improvement was due to the iron injections alone and not to any substantial behavior changes that would be required to prevent developmental delays caused by nutritional deficiencies.

## Questions for Consideration

### *Questions about Culture*

What cultural beliefs and practices as well as refugee experiences are contributing to Xong's iron deficiency anemia?

What are the prevalent attitudes and assumptions about bottle-feeding in mainstream Anglo-American culture? How do they differ from those in Hmong culture?

What does it mean to have a frightened soul? How can Xong's grandfather tell that this is Xong's problem? How might a soul-calling ceremony help?

Why might Xong's father not have arranged for a soul-calling ceremony?

### *Questions about Cross-Cultural Health Care Ethics*

How did the grandparents, parents, and physician differ in their assessment of what was in Xong's best interests?

In what ways was the relationship between the physician and the family mutually respectful? In what ways was it disrespectful?

How closely must Xong's treatment resemble the U.S. standard of care for children with anemia?

How might the family's and the physician's understandings differ concerning who has responsibility for health care decision making?

What ethical conflicts exist for the health care professionals in this case?

### *Questions about Culturally Responsive Health Care*

How can health care practitioners help refugees whose experience with trauma and deprivation provide barriers to their accepting health care recommendations?

How can the WIC program better assist children at risk for iron deficiency anemia?

How could the health care professionals have provided Xong with more culturally responsive health care?

When if ever might health care professionals be justified to intervene with a court order in a case like Xong's? What steps should be tried first?

*Commentary*

# Iron-Deficiency Anemia
# in Bottle-Fed Toddlers

*Cher Vang, M.P.A., and Christopher L. Moertel, M.D.*

In the late 1980s, while many professionals were trumpeting the success of WIC in reducing nutritional anemia among low-income children (Yip, Binkin, Fleshood, & Trowbridge, 1987), another study clearly described the emergence of childhood iron-deficiency anemia in a population with very high levels of WIC participation—the Hmong of St. Paul, Minnesota (Brown et al., 1986). Later, in a major review in the *New England Journal of Medicine,* the late Frank Oski (1993), a scion of pediatric hematology, stated, "In the past decade severe iron-deficiency anemia has been virtually eradicated in the United States." Doctors in St. Paul, Minnesota (Moertel & Watterson, 1993) and Fresno, California, were slack-jawed: iron-deficiency anemia was virtually epidemic among Hmong children like Xong. Patients like her were commonplace in area clinics and on the hospital wards, and physicians like Dr. Anderson were ill-prepared to deal with this previously uncommon diagnosis. Compounding the problem was providers' poor understanding of cultural issues and a language barrier.

The root of the problem is amazingly simple—bottle-feeding. In Laos, bottle-feeding was not an option for the majority of Hmong mothers. Infant formula and cow's milk, available only to the urban rich, were scarce commodities for the Hmong mountain dwellers. As a result, all infants were breast-fed. Since there was no way for mothers to pump their breast milk and store it for later use, every feeding was fresh. For the first years of life, mothers had their infants with them wherever they went. Children were weaned when the next baby was born, when the mother felt her milk was inadequate, or when the children were between two and five years of age. Parents did not push their infants to eat solid foods. Hmong parents felt that eating solid food was a natural process for children and therefore waited for children to show interest in food. When children were ready, they would reach out or ask for food. Infants were fed rice gruel instead of rice; otherwise, infants generally ate the same foods adults ate, except in smaller amounts.

In the United States today, the majority of Hmong mothers, like Xong's mother, prefer to bottle-feed their infants with infant formula for two reasons. The bottle makes it more convenient for caregivers, such as Xong's grandparents, to care for infants while the mother is out of the home. And formula is readily available; low-income families like Xong's qualify to receive vouchers from the WIC program to obtain infant formula or milk without cost.

Most Hmong people are unfamiliar with the difference between infant formula and cow's milk. Beyond one year of age, families continue to give cow's milk to the child with the same frequency as they did infant formula, without encouraging the child to eat more solid food. Xong's family perceives the bottle as a source of comfort and nutrition, not knowing that too much cow's milk may cause harm.

Pasteurized cow's milk is essentially void of available nutritional iron. Therefore, as Xong continues to grow, her body's iron stores cannot keep up with her increasing mass and ongoing physiologic iron losses, which results in iron-deficiency. As the condition worsens, effective production of hemoglobin, an iron-containing protein, is impaired, and Xong becomes anemic. The pallor and decreased activity we associate with anemia is the most visible manifestation of total-body iron deficiency; the brain, muscles, and vital organs all may suffer from a lack of iron. As a result of her anemia, Xong is very likely to exhibit a learning difficulty when she reaches school age (Lozoff, Jimenez, & Wolf, 1991; Lozoff et al., 1998).

In Laos, if a child had developed symptoms of anemia such as irritability, low energy, and paleness, Xong's grandparents and their community would most likely have perceived the etiology as due to an evil force or Xong's soul wandering from her body, rather than a diet-related chemical deficiency. Since health care in Laotian Hmong communities was provided by shaman, herbalists, magic healers, and local purveyors of over-the-counter medicines, Xong's family might have invited a shaman to come to their house and perform a ritual to diagnose and treat her. By the end of the ritual, the shaman would have described a number of spiritual reasons for the illness and presented his recommendations to solve the problem spiritually. Among his recommendations might have been calling Xong's soul, tying strings to her wrists, or sacrificing an animal to a troublesome spirit. If Xong's family followed the shaman's recommendations and the problem still existed, they could call a different shaman with different healing spirits; if one shaman's spiritual healing power did not work, another healer's might. Western diagnoses and treatments were not options.

Xong's family may have a hard time understanding how Dr. Anderson could make the diagnosis of iron-deficiency anemia. They may feel, like many other Hmong families, that all the laboratory tests are incorrect or fabricated. Such skepticism and lack of trust are widespread in the U.S. Hmong community. It is likely that Xong's grandparents heard rumors in the refugee camps and in the United States that Western providers use Hmong patients for horrifying experiments.

Against this background, health care facilities that provide care to Hmong patients must have dialect-appropriate trained interpreters, bilingual-bicultural workers, and health care providers who are knowledgeable about Hmong culture. The first and most important requirement for non-Hmong providers is to have an interpreter present to serve as a cultural broker and to bridge the language gap. At present, this requirement is just as important in cases where the patient, parents, or family members are or appear to be fluent in the English language.

Second, providers must pursue the diagnosis with care. The key to diagnosis depends upon the amount of cow's milk or formula consumed. Quantifying milk intake can be problematic for those employing Western time idioms. When asked, "How much milk does your child drink each day?" the family usually assumes "day" events are from sunup to sundown. Their response may reflect as little as 30 percent of the child's total intake, especially during long, dark winters. Consuming milk in excess of sixteen ounces per twenty-four hours may prevent adequate iron absorption, but we have seen children consuming up to forty ounces per twenty-four hours, leaving no room for a normal diet. Laboratory testing need not be overly rigorous; a history of high cow's milk intake and a fingerstick or venipuncture blood sample to investigate unusual causes of anemia are generally all that is required.

Third, providers must set aside adequate time for discussions with family members about the diagnosis and significance of the problem. Because Xong's grandparents have significant caregiver roles, they must be included in this discussion. Explaining iron-deficiency anemia to Xong's family is difficult because there is no Hmong word for iron and no traditional concept that blood *(ntshav)* contains components, such as hemoglobin, red cells, white cells, platelets, and so forth. Most Hmong families do not understand why this new U.S. malady afflicts their child. Providers must explain the basic physiology of blood, hemoglobin, and iron; the pathophysiological relationship between cow's milk, diet, and iron-deficiency anemia; and the consequences of untreated anemia on childhood development, in concrete terms with diagrams. Keep in mind that Hmong parents, like other parents, are protective of their children and they want to understand everything before they give permission for the health care staff to work on their children.

Fourth, all caregivers should be encouraged to take ownership in the treatment plan. The cornerstones of therapy for Xong include reduction of milk, introduction of solid foods, and consumption of iron supplements. Families must be assured that reducing milk will not cause children to starve, since children will eat food once they realize there is not enough milk to drink. Palatable foods, especially those that are part of the family's regular diet, must be readily available and encouraged. A tough love philosophy may help families withstand children's tantrums for milk and build upon the Hmong concept of good parenting. Reminding parents that as toddlers they probably were firmly weaned from the breast when their younger siblings arrived also may provide parents with a cultural context that can help them through the tantrums. Several techniques to reduce milk bottles include: giving milk in cups with spouts; using bottles without nipples; giving bottles with water instead of milk; and using pacifiers rather than bottles full of milk for emotional comfort. However, eliminating bottles altogether may be more successful than slowly reducing the use of the bottle. And providers can encourage the family to practice their spiritual healing concurrently at home.

Ferrous sulfate, an excellent vehicle for delivering supplemental iron, does not taste good and so infants and toddlers frequently cough and sputter the first time they receive it. Putting concentrated infant ferrous sulfate drops into a nipple with fruit juice or infant formula (but not cow's milk) frequently helps, since the total volume is small and the dose is not divided so that the rigors of medication delivery need only be suffered once a day. Also, fruit juices contain ascorbic acid, which improves iron absorption. Blood transfusions are rarely necessary for children with hemoglobin values greater than 3. If parents can observe some improvement with Western medicine, they will be more likely to work collaboratively with providers.

Throughout the treatment process, frustrated health care providers must avoid two temptations. They must avoid intra-muscular injections of iron; while they are a quick fix, they do not solve the basis of the condition. However, one-time injections in dire situations may prove useful in convincing parents about the significance of their child's condition and the importance of treatment. Also, they must avoid replacing cow's milk with other liquids such as infant formula or dietary supplements, because doing so continues a dependence on the bottle and does not reinforce appropriate weaning. In addition, continued bottle-use predisposes Hmong children to two additional public health problems: dental caries and obesity.

Employing this multiple-phased approach, we have successfully treated many Hmong children with iron-deficiency anemia. In addition to our recommendations for clinics and clinicians, we believe that the following policy and community education recommendations are required to conquer iron-deficiency in Hmong children:

1. Public policies at the city, state, and federal levels must meet the specific needs of new immigrant groups, such as the Hmong. Because the major Hmong population centers are around Fresno, California, and St. Paul, Minnesota, support of public health programs addressing Hmong health care issues in these communities will have a significant impact across the Hmong population in the United States.
2. WIC clinics must lengthen the time of initial WIC intake and recertification visits with Hmong clients specifically to address bottle-use, appropriate age of weaning, and the differences among cow's milk, mother's milk, and formula. Initiatives that reward breast-feeding and encourage appropriate weaning can be coordinated through WIC clinics serving Hmong clients.
3. Community education staffed by Hmong community members must occur at community events, such as soccer tournaments, Hmong New Year, and other large community gatherings.
4. Federal and state agencies overseeing the WIC program must require education of market vendors who take WIC vouchers and must enforce appropriate voucher use so that nonmilk vouchers cannot be used to purchase milk.

Millions of dollars have been spent to educate the U.S. public about the dangers of dietary cholesterol; a commensurate effort is required to educate the Hmong community about the benefits of breast-feeding, the dangers of cow's milk, and the need to eat healthy solid foods. To effectively deal with the problem of iron-deficiency anemia among Hmong children, a concerned and coordinated effort will be required by public health departments, federal and state nutritional agencies, food vendors, health care providers, and Hmong community leaders. This is a tall order, but achievable.

## References

Brown, J. E., Serdula, M., Cairns, K., Godes, J. R., Jacobs, D. R., Elmer, P., & Trowbridge, F. L. (1986). Ethnic group differences in nutritional status of young children from low-income areas of an urban county. *American Journal of Clinical Nutrition, 44,* 938–944.

Lozoff, B., Jimenez, E., & Wolf, A. W. (1991). Long-term development outcomes of infants with iron deficiency. *New England Journal of Medicine, 325,* 687–694.

Lozoff, B., Klein, N. K., Nelson, E. C., McClish, D. K., Manuel, M., & Chacon, M. E. (1998). Behavior of infants with iron-deficiency anemia. *Child Development, 69*(1), 24–36.

Moertel, C. L., & Watterson, J. (1993, October 22). *Severe iron deficiency anemia secondary to high cow's milk intake among Hmong children in St. Paul, Minnesota.* Paper presented at the Northwestern Pediatric Society Annual Meeting, Rochester, MN.

Oski, F. A. (1993). Iron deficiency in infancy and childhood. *New England Journal of Medicine, 329*(3), 190–193.

Yip, R., Binkin, N. J., Fleshood, L., & Trowbridge, F. L. (1987). Declining prevalence of anemia among low-income children in the United States. *Journal of the American Medical Association, 258*(12), 1619–1623.

# A Culturally Informed Public Health Response to Pediatric Anemia in the Hmong Community

*Elanah Dalyah Naftali, Dr.P.H., R.D., and Mao Heu Thao, L.P.N., B.A.*

In this commentary we focus on nonclinical, cultural aspects of the Xong case that go unaddressed by the medical and public health professionals. We feel strongly that the reason for Xong's deteriorating condition is precisely because these concerns go unattended. In our opinion, the core problem—one that may be relevant to many Hmong American families—is that too little is done by the health professionals to accommodate the realities of the Hang household. The challenge is to understand and appreciate the cultural disparities that the elder generation is experiencing as they reconcile conflicts or seek to balance old beliefs and traditions with new practices and values. Given the grandparents' role as primary caregivers for baby Xong and their once dominant role as respected decision makers for the family, a successful clinical care plan must involve the grandparents.

## Family Dynamics in Historical Context

Xong's grandparents' personal experiences and memories of life during the Secret War in Laos, the refugee flight in the jungles of Southeast Asia, and the Thai refugee camps (1970–97) are important in understanding their child-care practices. During these years, suffering was commonplace: prolonged hunger, thirst, and starvation; injuries and infections; separations, grief, and loss; and daily deaths of infants, children, and adults. The grandparents' extended grief and disillusionment, which the public health nurse discovers, are caused by these traumatic life experiences and are common in many Hmong refugees of their generation (Westermeyer, 1986).

Resettling in the United States adds a layer of economic hardship and malaise for the grandparents. Language difficulties, transportation barriers, and lack of employment skills contribute to their inability to integrate into Western culture and limit their chances to work, which was the cultural norm for healthy Hmong elders. Certainly, Xong's grandparents are experiencing culture shock and are unable to adopt an incomprehensible U.S. lifestyle.

In contrast, Xong's parents seem to be adapting to the demands of life in the United States: her mother is attending school and her father is working. Given their ages, we can assume they were born in the United States. While they undoubtedly live with frequent reminders of the grandparents' hardships in Laos and the refugee camps, Xong's parents appear to be well-adjusted, pursuing work and school obligations that require daily separations from their baby. The intergenerational tension in the Hang household seems to be intensified by Xong's parents' desire to emulate American childrearing values.

## Childrearing in the United States

Xong's caregiving arrangement is contrary to what was traditionally practiced in Laos or Thailand. Breast-feeding was the only viable feeding option in traditional village life where mothers and their infants were rarely parted before a child was weaned from the breast. Short-term separations that were due to illness or travel had to be accommodated by other lactating women, as bottle-feeding was unknown. In the United States, where separations of mothers and infants are often necessitated by obligations outside of the home, breast-feeding is difficult to sustain. Also, the virtual absence of breast-feeding in public places contributes to many Hmong women's conclusion that bottle-feeding is the norm in the United States.

Among older adults, there are strong cultural beliefs about breast-milk that younger people experience as making breast-feeding difficult. Breast-milk must not contact anything or anyone other than the baby or lightening will strike *(xub tua)*, bringing potentially fatal harm to people in the household. Consequently, people are fearful of pumping, storing, or giving breast-milk in a bottle; any spillage or consumption by others could result in disaster. Tradition dictates which foods are to be avoided by nursing mothers in the first postpartum month and when their babies are sick, for fear that their children will be harmed. If long intervals occur between feedings, the foremilk can become "sour" *(qaub)* which could make the infant sick; hence, there are prescribed practices for expressing the foremilk. Also, mothers should refrain from nursing when they are ill, so as to avoid passing the illness to their infants.

It is no wonder that young women in the United States find it difficult to follow the prescriptions and avoid the taboos and so prefer the less encumbered alternative of bottle-feeding formula to infants rather than breast-feeding (Romero-Gwynn, 1989; Tuttle & Dewey, 1994; Dewey, Heinig, Nommsen, Peeson, & Lonnerdal, 1993). Indeed, the convenience of bottle-feeding, the freedom it affords mothers, and its wide availability in the United States makes it the feeding method of choice for the majority of U.S. women, especially minority women (National Academy of Science, 1991). The fact that it is subsidized for low-income families by the Special Supplemental Nutrition Program for Women, Infants, and Children (WIC) makes it nearly ubiquitous in Southeast Asian homes (Brown et al., 1986; Fishman, Evans, & Jenks, 1988; Romero-Gwynn & Carias, 1989; Tuttle & Dewey, 1996). The large size of many Hmong households is another motivating factor for preferring bottle-feeding to breast-feeding, since bottles allow many people to care for infants and allow toddlers to feed themselves.

The abundant supply of infant formula—once unavailable and now a food subsidized by the government—and the commercial endorsement of milk as "healthy" for growing children and adults alike enables others to care for Xong while her mother attends school. Surely, too, as a high school student, Xong's mother is probably modest about her body and eager to fit in with her non-breast-feeding peers. Lacking young adult role models and information about breast-feeding, she probably did not even consider breast-feeding when the baby was born.

Why, however, is milk the only food offered to Xong when she should be eating solid foods that would ensure her adequate nutrition, including vitamins and minerals such as iron? Are the grandparents so pressed for time they cannot prepare the rice gruel *(kua dlis)* traditionally offered to infants? *Kua dlis* is the first semi-solid food typically offered to babies around five to six months (although the recommended age for introducing *kua dlis* varies across and within families) and is followed by a progression of vegetable and meat additions to a staple dish of rice (Culhane-Pera, Naftali, Jacobson, & Xiong, 2002; Toporoff & Xiong, 1998). Or do the grandparents have additional children to care for, and thus cannot give Xong the extra attention she needs?

In traditional practices, infants may be older than five- to six-months before other foods are offered. Infants must show their developmental readiness to eat solid foods by reaching out for table foods, spoon-feeding without spitting up, and being able to feed themselves. This child-paced approach can be acceptable for breast-fed infants who can thrive exclusively on breast milk for the first year of life (Dewey et al., 1993). However, the same approach is harmful for formula-fed infants, who must begin supplementary feedings by six-months of age to avoid nutritional deficiencies such as iron-deficiency anemia. Perhaps some of the difficulty of shifting Xong to solid foods is related to the relatively late introduction of solid foods (in comparison with the U.S. convention); perhaps her grandparents had judged that she was neither ready for nor tolerant of solid foods before a year of age.

An important factor reinforcing Xong's dependence on the bottle is the fussiness she displayed when not given her bottle or when given solid foods instead. This was a common behavioral response reported by parents participating in focus groups sponsored by the Minnesota WIC Program (Culhane-Pera et al., 2002; Toporoff & Xiong, 1998). These parents described their anemic children as picky eaters *(ncauj xim)* content to go all day and night with a bottle as their sole source of nutrition. These children were easily satiated on their liquid diets and because their appetite and interest in solid foods were curtailed, they acquired poor eating habits. Ingesting more than the recommended allowance of twenty-four ounces of milk a day (Pipes & Trahms, 1993; Satter, 1989), young children do in fact gain weight. While this may give the impression that they are thriving, more often their longitudinal growth (height-for-age) is compromised or stunted (Hamill et al., 1979).

### *Hlub:* A Central Hmong Value

A traditional Hmong value that reinforces the picky-eater phenomenon is known as *hlub*. Translated as "love," *hlub* embraces a deep-seated regard for kinfolk and is expressed by actions that fulfill loved ones' wishes. In the realm of family relationships, *hlub* denotes an obligation of parents to take good care of their children. Parents show their love by lavishing special attention on their children, indulging children's desires, and minimizing their crying spells. A crying child could indicate an unhappy soul that if neglected, might leave the body. These practices may be related to the high infant mortality rates in Southeast Asia, where parents and grandparents may have been motivated to please their children and thus appease the children's souls in order to keep their children with them. (See Plate 3.)

In addition to the child-centered focus of *hlub,* there are tremendous social pressures and expectations around being good parents and producing healthy and happy, well-behaved children. Popular phrases that capture this intention are *mivnyuas yog koob moov* (children are precious gifts) and *mivnyuas yog koj txuj sav, xaav rua tej mivnyuas, dlai sav nyob hlub pub* (think about your children in hard times and preserve your life to love and care for them). Model parents are patient *(sab ntev)* and kind-hearted *(sab zoo)* so that their children will grow up to be respectful and responsible, with compassion for all people *(sab dlawb).* In public, a malcontent child can bring shame to the family, since parents are charged with creating model citizens. Also, since public displays of affection are minimized, a bottle can become an easy way to appease an unhappy child in public. From this framework, it is easy to understand how a pattern of milk drinking, attachment to bottles, and iron-deficiency anemia can occur.

*Hlub* appears to be a guiding belief for the Hang grandparents, who are unable to replace Xong's bottle with solid foods, as reported by Ms. Moua, the public health nurse. They essentially give in to her desires rather than endure her crying. The ardor of changing Xong's eating habits appears more distasteful than indulging her seemingly harmless desire to seek comfort in a bottle. Key informant interviews of Hmong parents revealed that parents were inclined to tolerate bottles as poor proxies for missed affection and bonding between nursing mothers and infants (Culhane-Pera et al., 2000). Recall, too, the grandparents' vivid memories of their time spent in the refugee camps; a crying child meant a hungry or a starving child. Their depression is likely fueled by the bitter reminder of their two children who died in Laos, and this affirms their choice of indulging Xong.

In contrast with the grandparents, Xong's parents have a different interpretation of *hlub* and are more intent on enforcing what they understand as U.S. values of setting limits around food and creating rules to guide Xong's behaviors (for example, structured feeding and napping schedules, sleeping in her crib). They are trying to break with tradition but they do not have the power to enforce their desires on the paternal grandparents. Given the new life circumstances they share, the Hang household blends traditional customs with new practices. Ultimately, the parents' dependence on the grandparents as Xong's primary caregivers during the day may be limiting their efforts to enforce rules and change her feeding behaviors. The combined desires of Xong's grandparents and parents create a mixture of childrearing practices that seek to bridge aspects of the new life in the United States while retaining some values from Laos (Rossiter, 1992).

## Interpretation of Physical Signs of Anemia

Dr. Anderson's interpretation of Xong's physical signs of anemia are inconsistent with the family's interpretation. Xong's weight gain between the first and second clinic visits may support the family's illusion that she is thriving. The fact that bottle-fed infants are typically heavier and bigger than exclusively breast-fed infants may contribute to the family's perception that Xong is doing well. Chubby babies *(mivnyuas phaam phaam)* are viewed as growing, healthy babies—a status marker of economic prosperity. Moreover, Xong's pale complexion may not register concern that she is in any imminent danger, because the traditional interpretation of light skin *(nqaj tawv dlawb)* is a sign of beauty.

Following the third clinic visit, when Dr. Anderson discusses tangible evidence of the baby's poor health with the mother, the family seems to comprehend Xong's worsening condition. While it is not clear precisely what they understand about the heart murmur and the enlarged spleen, the grandparents' perceptions of Xong change to accommodate the notion that a once healthy, growing child now needs a formal soul-calling ceremony *(hu plig)* to restore her health. (See Plates 27–29.)

Someone might divine Xong's lost soul *(poob plig)* in several ways: by examining her ears; interpreting patterns in egg yolks; communicating with spirits using goat, cow, or buffalo horns; or considering a previous frightful experience that may have caused a soul to leave. Whether Xong has a lost soul or a startled soul, Xong's grandparents want to shore up her spiritual health and subsequently improve her physical health with a soul-calling ceremony.

The parents' decision to not perform a soul-calling ceremony may be due to one or more of several considerations: the expense; their desire to break with tradition; their struggle with the grandparents; and the influence of Christianity. Refusing to arrange for a soul-calling ceremony, they are being disrespectful to the traditions and the honored role of the grandfather as an influential person in family decision-making processes. Traditionally, the parents' unwillingness to comply with the request for a *hu plig* would trigger the grandparents' authority to act in their stead. Why Xong's grandparents fail to take the initiative in this case remains puzzling; perhaps they do not have the money, they do not want to go against the parents, or they want to hold the parents accountable for consequences that will ensue for Xong.

## The Health Care Providers' Responsibilities

Dr. Anderson is trained in the science of Western medicine that does not consider social relations or spirituality as primary elements in disease and healing processes. Dr. Anderson unintentionally may contribute to the worsening of Xong's condition by discounting the traditional hierarchy for decision making in Hmong families and the spiritual significance of Xong's condition. Efforts to build trust with the family would be aided by inviting all of Xong's caregivers to the clinic. Dr. Anderson is wise to use Xong's physical signs—enlarged spleen and heart murmur—as teaching tools, but she seems to be ineffective in communicating their significance. She should involve a Hmong nutritionist specifically trained in the prevention of iron-deficiency anemia among young children to aid the family's understanding of the clinical picture and the seriousness of Xong's condition. And she should work with a Hmong interpreter, even if the mother's English is good.

The public health nurse reports critical information about the family (the intergenerational tensions and the grandparents' depression), but how much of this is heeded by the health care providers is unclear. Perhaps Ms. Moua should elicit a stronger response from Dr. Anderson and request that a social worker or public health nutritionist work in the home. It is also unclear how well the nurse tailors her care plan (based on the doctor's recommendations) to be sensitive to the cultural and interpersonal dynamics of the Hang household.

Poorly coordinated care may also contribute to Xong's worsening health. The lack of communication between WIC and the primary care clinic, for example, suggests a lapse in timely follow-up. The prolonged deterioration of Xong's condition testifies to the failure of our current health care system. We need a system that coordinates care among all relevant health professionals, balances best-practice clinical judgments with culturally sensitive prescriptions, communicates with all people in their primary language, and tailors educational efforts to patients' and families' specific needs.

## Conclusion

A montage of factors explains the family's tolerance of Xong's attachment to bottles and of her deteriorating health, among them adapting to a U.S. lifestyle while preserving aspects of traditional cultural beliefs. The mixture of old and new childrearing customs adds layers of complexity that are likely inaccessible to clinicians unless they engage in an extensive cross-cultural dialogue with their patients or community spokespersons or both. Health care providers must be cognizant that the relationship they build with the family caring for a loved one will probably determine their success in clinical medicine. It is essential that providers take the time to nurture this relationship and build the trust necessary to ensure optimal health outcomes for the community. Public health nurses can be instrumental in fostering a trusting relationship by getting to know the families' values, beliefs, and customs about sickness and health through repeated visits to families' homes. Trained interpreters should be involved and cultural mediators or community spokespersons should be engaged to advocate on behalf of the family. Finally, working with family members and all decision makers is extremely important. Only by following these measures will health care practitioners create an effective cross-cultural bridge for delivery of health care to Hmong individuals and their families.

# References

Brown, J. E., Serdula, M., Cairns, K., Godes, J. R., Jacobs, D. R., Elmer, P., & Trowbridge, F. L. (1986). Ethnic group differences in nutritional status of young children from low-income areas of an urban county. *American Journal of Clinical Nutrition, 44,* 938–944.

Culhane-Pera, K. A., Naftali, E. D., Jacobson, C., & Xiong, Z. B. (2002). Cultural feeding practices and child-raising philosophy contribute to iron-deficiency anemia in refugee Hmong children. *Ethnicity and Disease, 12*(2), 199–205.

Dewey, K. G., Heinig, M. J., Nommsen, L. A., Peeson, J. M., & Lonnerdal, B. (1993). Breast-fed infants are leaner than formula-fed infants at 1 year of age: The Darling study. *American Journal of Clinical Nutrition, 57,* 140–145.

Fishman, C., Evans, R., & Jenks, E. (1988). Warm bodies, cool milk: Conflicts in post partum food choice for Indochinese women in California. *Social Science and Medicine, 26,* 1125–1132.

Hamill, P. V. V., Drizd, T. A., Johnson, C. L., Reed, R. B., Roche, A. F., & Moore, W. M. (1979). Physical growth: National Center for Health Statistics percentiles. *American Journal of Clinical Nutrition, 32,* 607–629.

National Academy of Science. (1991). Who breastfeeds in the United States? In *Nutrition during lactation.* Washington, DC: National Academy Press. 28–49.

Pipes, L. P., & Trahms, C. M. (1993). *Nutrition in infancy and childhood.* St. Louis, MO: Mosby.

Romero-Gwynn, E. (1989). Breast-feeding pattern among Indochinese immigrants in Northern California. *American Journal of Disabled Children, 143,* 804–808.

Romero-Gwynn, E., & Carias, L. (1989). Breast-feeding intentions and practices among Hispanic mothers in southern California. *Pediatrics, 84,* 626–632.

Rossiter, J. C. (1992). Attitudes of Vietnamese women to baby feeding practices before and after immigration to Sydney, Australia. *Midwifery, 8,* 103–112.

Satter, E. (1989). *Child of mine: Feeding with love and good sense.* Palo Alto, CA: Bull.

Toporoff, E., & Xiong, B. (1998). *Final report of Hmong parent focus group findings.* Unpublished report, Minnesota Department of Health, WIC Program, Anemia Prevention Project.

Tuttle, C. R., & Dewey, K. G. (1994). Determinants of infant feeding choices among Southeast Asian immigrants in northern California. *Journal of the American Dietetic Association, 94,* 282–286.

Tuttle, C. R., & Dewey, K. G. (1996). Potential cost savings for Medi-Cal, AFDC, food stamps, and WIC programs associated with increasing breast-feeding among low-income Hmong women in California. *Journal of the American Dietetic Association, 96,* 885–899.

Westermeyer, J. (1986). Indochinese refugees in community and clinic: A report from Asia and the United States. In C. Williams & J. Westermeyer (Eds.), *Refugee mental health in resettlement countries.* Washington, DC: Hemisphere, 113–130.

# 7

# Infant with Down Syndrome
## and a Heart Defect

## *A Case Story*

Pam Yang, a ten-month-old girl, was brought by her parents for a routine well-child check. Since the physician who had been caring for Pam was no longer with the clinic, this was her family's first visit with her new pediatrician. Through the interpreter, they indicated that she was happy, healthy, and growing without difficulties in eating, sleeping, or activities of daily living and that they had no other concerns. They appeared to be very caring and concerned about her well-being.

Pam demonstrated classic signs of Down syndrome (trisomy 21). Her height, weight, and neurologic development were delayed but within normal limits for a child with Down syndrome. Her cardiac exam revealed a loud and harsh murmur consistent with a large hole in her heart, a ventricular septal defect. With every beat of her heart, blood flowed in the wrong direction and overloaded a normally low pressure system. The pediatrician explained that Pam had a hole in her heart that should be surgically repaired before she was a year old. He cited the overwhelming scientific evidence that children with her condition suffer irreversible physiologic changes to their lungs (pulmonary hypertension) and premature death by age six.

Her parents confirmed that they had been informed of her heart murmur at the time of her birth, when an ultrasound had been performed. The pediatrician read Pam's chart and learned that the parents had kept her up-to-date with immunizations but had failed to come to any scheduled cardiac appointments. The parents said that their daughter had no problem, that they did not want any heart surgery, and that they would not go to any cardiology appointments.

Recognizing the difficulty in communicating the gravity of the situation across cultures, the pediatrician had the parents listen to their own hearts and then listen to their daughter's heart and, with the help of an interpreter, describe what they heard. He drew a picture of the heart with normal and abnormal flow and used the metaphor of a river to explain the difference in sounds and the desirability of smooth flow in the right direction. They responded by acknowledging these differences and restating their fervent opposition to any further cardiac work-up.

They agreed to return for an extended conference with an interpreter. At this two-hour meeting, the parents reported their opposition to further cardiac evaluation.

First, they stated that although their daughter might have a hole in her heart, she was clearly doing well and did not have a problem. They said that they recognized she was "a crooked cucumber" but said they loved her "as much as every cucumber in their patch." Second, they said they were adamantly opposed to surgery because of the accompanying risks of soul loss and bad spirits entering her body. They rejected the physician's assertion that not correcting the hole in her heart would result in serious problems. If she developed problems, they said, they would bring her back to the clinic and consider treatment at that time. They did not accept the physician's assertion that if problems developed, it would be too late to intervene.

When the pediatrician asked the parents why he should treat their daughter any differently from any other child with the same condition, they became frustrated and angry, and they concluded the meeting. Despite several additional meetings and attempts to convince the parents of the necessity for further evaluation and probable surgery, they refused to take any steps in that direction. The parents also refused to grant the pediatrician permission to consult with other members of the Hmong community, including other family members and their clan leader.

When Pam returned to the clinic at one year of age, she looked sick; her respiratory rate and heart rate were markedly accelerated. She was started on Digoxin and Lasix to help her heart work more effectively and was scheduled for an echocardiogram. When her parents failed to keep her appointment for the echocardiogram, the pediatrician obtained a court order to perform a full cardiac work-up. The ensuing evaluation indicated that it was too late to perform corrective surgery. Pam's parents agreed to try an experimental medication, which was later stopped when it failed to work.

## Questions for Consideration

### Questions about Culture

How did the parents understand Pam's condition? How is Down syndrome viewed and treated in traditional Hmong culture? How does this view differ from the cultural perspective prevalent among pediatricians trained in the United States?

What health beliefs might have influenced Pam's parents to accept immunizations and well-child checks, but to refuse life-preserving cardiac surgery?

### Questions about Cross-Cultural Health Care Ethics

How did the parents' assessment of risks and benefits differ from the physician's?

How did the parents view their role and the role of the physician in this case? How does this perspective on roles differ from the pediatrician's?

Is there any reason to question the parents' decision-making capacity given their health beliefs?

How does this case differ from cases in which parents, because they are Jehovah's Witnesses or Christian Scientists, refuse life-saving interventions for their children?

Under what circumstances, if ever, might it be justifiable to permit this child's care to deviate from the standard of care for children with this condition in the United States?

What is the pediatrician's view of good cross-cultural health care relationships?

## Questions about Culturally Responsive Health Care

What beliefs might the family have to give up or change in order to accept the physician's recommendations?

Are there any steps that might be taken to protect against soul loss during surgery?

What other steps could the physician have tried to convince the parents to take action and follow his recommendations? Should the physician have contacted community leaders over the parents' objection?

Is this case an example of the appropriate use of a court order? Why?

From whose perspective is this case an example of a good cross-cultural health care relationship?

## Commentary

# Defining Best Interest for a Hmong Infant: A Physician's Challenge

*Gregory A. Plotnikoff, M.D., M.T.S.*

> The wish to impose order upon confusion, to bring harmony out of dissonance and unity out of multiplicity is a kind of intellectual instinct, a primary and fundamental urge of the mind. . . . The theoretical reduction of unmanageable multiplicity to comprehensible unity becomes the practical reduction of human diversity to subhuman uniformity, of freedom to servitude.
>
> Aldous Huxley, *Brave New World Revisited*

This case raises a series of formidable challenges, among them how to define the "best interest" of a Hmong infant? Should the criteria be biomedical? Legal? Familial? Religious? Cultural? In clinical encounters with recent immigrants, who should define harm? The physician? The family? The courts? A religious leader? A cultural leader? When both options—surgery or no surgery—are considered harmful, how should one define patient advocacy?

This case challenges us to define the meaning and purpose of health care. It challenges us to define parental responsibility as well as parental neglect, child protection as well as child endangerment, and child abuse in cross-cultural contexts. It challenges us to clarify fundamental U.S. legal principles, including equal protection and the separation of church and state. Furthermore, this case challenges us to understand the diversity of religious expression and religion's inseparability from culture.

As a new pediatrician, I lost much sleep over this case. Years later, I still wrestle over what is the "right" answer. Now, however, I believe that this case contains the key to envisioning a more responsible and humane health care system.

### The Biomedical Perspective

From a strictly biomedical perspective, there is no question about what would have been the right action to pursue. "Best interests" of children are determined by the best physiologic outcome. As declared by the American Academy of Pediatrics' Committee on Bioethics (1997, p. 280):

Physicians who believe that parental religious convictions interfere with appropriate medical care that is likely to prevent substantial harm or suffering or death should request court authorization to override parental authority or, under circumstances involving an imminent threat to a child's life, intervene over parental objections.

In this case, the scientific data clearly demonstrate that a corrective cardiac operation by twelve months of age is the standard of care for infants with trisomy 21 and a large ventricular septal defect. Repairing the hole in the heart offers these children a full life expectancy. Without the operation, death will ensue within a few years from irreversible pulmonary hypertension and congestive heart failure. Focusing on physiologic data clearly simplifies the challenges in this case. From this point of view, there is no conflict among medicine, ethics, and the law. The child has the operation and the case is resolved.

Because of the cross-cultural context, I disagreed with the seductive simplicity of this answer. Is surgical intervention against the will of competent and caring non-American parents the best or most appropriate response? Should we define these parents as incompetent, as incapable of giving informed consent? Is their refusing the operation a case of willful harm or extreme neglect? Is this a case where parental rights should be overridden?

The answers to these questions cannot be found in the scientific data regarding surgical treatment of ventricular septal defects. These questions, in my mind, demand review of the ethics of the biomedically sanctioned response. Clearly, limiting one's perspective to the biomedical facts or limiting one's perspective to the biomedical judgment of right action is pure paternalism. Because our society and our laws are grounded on the Enlightenment's explicit rejection of such tyranny, I turned to the law for guidance.

## The Legal Perspective

The American Academy of Pediatrics' support for defining a child's "best interest" by biomedical criteria is well supported by several important legal rulings. In *People v. Pierson* (68 NE 243 [NY 1903]), the New York Supreme Court stated:

> The law of nature, as well as the common law, devolves upon parents the duty of caring for their young in sickness and in health, and of doing whatever may be necessary for their care, maintenance and preservation, including medical attendance, if necessary: and an omission to do this is a public wrong, which the state, under its police powers, may prevent. (Quoted in Swan, 1997, p. 501)

This statement affirmed that medical necessity is defined by physicians and justified by the state's interests in preserving the lives of children. Four decades later, the U.S. Supreme Court ruled in a 1944 case that "parents may be free to become martyrs themselves. But it does not follow that they are free, in identical circumstances, to make martyrs of their children" (*Prince v. Massachusetts,* 321 U.S. 158 [1944]; quoted in Swan, 1997, p. 503). This statement affirmed that in the case of children, religious exemptions to laws do not hold.

These rulings mean that parents must provide life-saving treatment for their children, even if the treatment violates deeply held religious beliefs. Failure to comply with a pediatrician's legitimate medical orders constitutes child endangerment, a form of child abuse. As a pediatrician, my failure to report child endangerment constitutes a prosecutable offense in the state of Minnesota. And the existence of immunity clauses protect me from civil or criminal charges if any of my suspicions are found later to be wrong.

The legally and medically sanctioned response is not as clear, however, as stated above. In 1974, the U.S. Department of Health, Education, and Welfare mandated that "a parent or guardian legitimately practicing his religious beliefs who thereby does not provide specified medical treatment for a child, for that reason alone shall not be considered a negligent parent or guardian" (National Archives and Records Administration, 1975). This mandate was revoked in 1983 during the Baby Doe controversies. However, in 1996, Congress passed a new religious exemption in the Child Abuse Prevention and Treatment Act (P.L. 104–235; cited in Swan, 1997, p. 513). In this act, Congress clarified that it did not create a "federal requirement that a parent or legal guardian provide a child any medical service or treatment against the religious beliefs of the parent or legal guardian." So, federal law, U.S. Supreme Court rulings, and professional society statements appear to be inconsistent.

This approach certainly applies in Minnesota. State law allows for a religious defense to child endangerment, criminal abuse, or neglect charges. Hence, in the most celebrated case in recent state history, the Christian Scientist mother and stepfather of an eleven-year-old boy who died of untreated diabetes were absolved of any criminal liability. However, following this, they were held financially liable for a wrongful death in a civil suit. The U.S. Supreme Court allowed the trial court's judgment to stand as well as a Minnesota Court of Appeals ruling against the mother and stepfather. In declining to review the case, the U.S. Supreme Court affirmed the assertion of the Minnesota Court of Appeals that "protecting a child's life transcends any interest a parent may have in exercising religious beliefs" and that "the parent is not the ultimate decisionmaking authority" (*Lundman v. McKown*, 1995).

In Minnesota, parents are not criminally liable for religious exceptions to life-saving health care, but health professionals are responsible for contacting Child Protection Services and going to the courts for orders mandating life-saving medical interventions over parental objections. However, neither the law nor shared professional experience have addressed the concept of "fair notice" when working with non-English-speaking immigrants who have just entered the technologically and legally complicated United States. Given this twist, a dilemma emerges. Does declining to push for an operation represent a form of discrimination against this child? Or does forcing the operation against the parents' wills represent a form of discrimination?

## Familial, Religious, and Cultural Perspectives

Neither the biomedical nor the legal perspective enabled me to understand this patient's, her family's, or her community's goals and expectations. For the Hmong, the material and spiritual worlds are not separate and cannot be separated. Failure of Western health care professionals to recognize the spiritual nature of illness means failure to address the underlying cause (Fadiman, 1997; Meyers, 1992). Surgery has particular importance for some Hmong people because of fear of loss of soul, fear of bad spirits entering the body, fear of disrupting the spirit's preferred form for a body, and fear of disappointing the spirits (Nuttall & Flores, 1997; Rairdan & Higgs, 1992; McInnis, Petracchi, & Morgenbesser, 1990; Thao, 1984). Spiritual responses to the fear of soul loss include shamanic bargaining with the spirit world, which includes rituals for soul calling, soul retrieval, and prevention of soul loss.

## Seeking a Court Order

I tried to avoid the courts at all costs and diligently sought understanding and compromise. First seeking to understand, then and only then seeking to be understood required me to explore Hmong values, beliefs, and ways of knowing. After much deliberation, and several hours of dialogue over several weeks with the parents through interpreters, I sought a court-ordered cardiac work-up. My reasoning for doing so took the following factors into account:

1. the parents could not or would not articulate why I could not contact their clan leader for his participation in the decision;
2. the twelve-month deadline and the appearance of visible signs of declining cardiac function were approaching; and
3. the parents had repeatedly broken their promises to take the child for a scheduled noninvasive echocardiagram.

I believed that the parents' behaviors were not necessarily "Hmong" behaviors but could easily represent family-specific behaviors. I believed that I needed more input and a broader perspective than what the parents or the interpreters could provide. Throughout the case, I sought to understand their refusal of surgical intervention and tried to understand their reasoning. I believe in my heart that I had tried everything possible to avoid going to court. My biggest regret was that I did not meet this family until the child was ten months old.

## Conclusion

I do not see a day when biomedically focused providers will believe in the Hmong animist perspective. We share with the rest of U.S. society a clear preference for all things technological. However, I do see a day when the corporatization of health care will result in standardized, "objective" clinical practice and a significant narrowing of what the health care management leadership has termed the "appalling" degree of variation that is current health care practice. Although "one size fits all" health care may be efficient, my experience suggests that this approach risks the loss of effectiveness and humanity, as well as medicine's soul. As Frances W. Peabody (1927, p. 814), the eminent Harvard physician, noted, "The treatment of a disease may be entirely impersonal, the care of a patient must be completely personal." Peabody emphasized the importance of what he termed the "intimate personal relationship between doctor and patient." "For in an extraordinarily large number of cases both diagnosis and treatment are directly dependent upon it, and the failure of the young physician to establish this relationship accounts for much of his ineffectiveness." If we cannot accommodate the time-honored and deeply held beliefs of newly arrived refugees, then we certainly will be less capable as a society of honoring and respecting the deeply held beliefs of our fellow citizens.

To answer the questions of best interests, harm, and advocacy raised by this case, one must go beyond the limitations of biomedical and legal knowledge. This case forces us to reflect on what is the goal of health care and goal of technological intervention in people's lives. What if it is what the patient and family define it to be? It might follow then that health care professionals are obliged to seek to understand clearly the beliefs and the viewpoints of each patient, especially when conflicting worldviews undermine effective partnership. This venturing into the cultural and spiritual—that is, into the realm of human values—requires humility as well as interviewing skills not routinely taught or valued in professional health care.

So, we in the mainstream culture are challenged to justify our overriding of a Hmong parent's wishes. This might be daunting if it were not so easy to label the Hmong perspective as an assault on Western rationality. However, might the Hmong, for their part, see legally enforced medical orders as an assault on Hmong rationality, identity, and way of life? As an assault on a Hmong person's very soul and life? We are left with an even more daunting task: can we develop a consensus around the meaning and purpose of health care?

In the future, those who can see beyond narrow biomedical and legal perspectives to articulate the value of deeply held religious and spiritual beliefs will be the prophets of a more responsible health care system. The Hmong community's challenges may be their gift to us. An examination of best interest, harm, and advocacy in such cases may result in a deeper recognition of and renewed appreciation for our own culture's soul. Going beyond the biomedical and legal aspects of clinical care for a Hmong child might humanize health care for all people.

## References

American Academy of Pediatrics Committee on Bioethics. (1997). Religious objections to medical care. *Pediatrics, 99*(2), 279–281.

Fadiman, A. (1997). *The spirit catches you and you fall down: A Hmong child, her American doctors, and the collision of two cultures.* New York: Farrar, Straus, and Giroux.

Lundman v. McKown, 503 N. W. 2d 807 (1995) cert. denied.

McInnis, K. M., Petracchi, H. E., & Morgenbesser, M. (1990). *The Hmong in America: Providing ethnic-sensitive health, education, and human services.* Dubuque, IA: Kendal/Hunt.

Meyers, C. (1992). Hmong children and their families: Consideration of cultural influences in assessment. *American Journal of Occupational Therapy, 46,* 737–744.

National Archives and Records Administration. (1975). 45 Code of Federal Regulations 1340. 1–2 (b)(1).

Nuttall, P., & Flores, F. (1997). Hmong healing practices used for common childhood illnesses. *Pediatric Nursing, 23,* 247–250.

Peabody, F. W. (1927). The care of the patient. *Journal of the American Medical Association, 254*(6), 813–820.

Rairdan, B., & Higgs, Z. (1992). When your patient is a Hmong refugee. *American Journal of Nursing, 92,* 52–55.

Swan, R. (1997). Children, medicine, religion, and the law. *Advances in Pediatrics, 44,* 491–543.

Thao, X. (1984). Southeast Asian refugees of Rhode Island: The Hmong perception of illness. *Rhode Island Medical Journal, 67,* 323–330.

*Commentary*

# "Why Do They Want to Hurt My Child?": The Mother's Perspective

*Phua Xiong, M.D.*

When Pam was six years old, I was fortunate to have the opportunity to interview her parents in their home about their feelings, understanding, and perception of what happened to Pam shortly after birth, as well as the reasons for their decisions about Pam's medical care.

In this commentary, I also discuss the value Hmong people place on children born with disabilities and issues of trust and distrust of U.S. medical and legal systems.

## The Parents' Understanding of Pam's Condition

At the time of delivery Pam's parents did not notice anything unusual about her physically. When she was brought back after several hours with the nurses, however, they asked about a blue bump on her left forehead. The nurses explained that the bump resulted from scraping through a small birth canal. Pam's mother thought, "If my bone scraped her, it would be a streak, not a bump."

Pam's parents worried more when she was taken away again. They wondered what the doctors and nurses were doing to their baby and became suspicious when, after a whole night, they finally saw Pam's little head under a hood and her little body covered with wires. "What have they done to our little girl?" they wondered.

They were unfamiliar with Down syndrome and could not fathom how a hole in her heart could occur. In Laos children were born with deformities and learning disabilities, but no one had ever heard of a child born with a hole in the heart. Looking at their child they could see no signs of trouble. Her breathing was fine. She ate well and had a strong suck. She was no different than other newborns. How could she have a hole in her heart and still be able to do all these things?

The parents wondered how the doctors came up with the story about the hole in their daughter's heart. Why would they want to take advantage of such a little helpless person so early in her life? Perhaps they dropped her and this caused the blue bump on her head and the hole in her heart. Perhaps the doctors created the story because they wanted to operate on her. Pam's doctor was moving to another job and perhaps she wanted to use their little girl for a final learning opportunity. Through word in the community, Pam's parents knew that U.S. providers treat Hmong people unfairly. Americans do not like the Hmong. They see Hmong people as expendable and provide them with poor care.

## Loving Pam

Pam's parents were told that without heart surgery Pam would likely live only to one year of age. With an operation, she might live two years. Pam's parents weighed the risks and benefits of the options offered to them and decided against surgery because her chances for life were slim. Even with surgery, she would live only one additional year. What was the benefit of putting her through the trauma of an operation—cutting up her tiny body—just to give her one additional year of life? And what kind of life would she have in that additional year if she must suffer the pain of surgery? Besides, if she does not make it through surgery, then they would have denied her any chance of life at all.

Love for Pam led the parents to refuse a procedure that would cut open her body, put her in danger of dying on the operating table, and only give her one extra year to live. In their minds, following the doctor's recommendation would mean they did not love Pam enough. They could not allow the doctors, strangers who cared little about Pam, to make cuts and scars that would remain forever with Pam, in this life and the next. They loved her too much. They did not want anything to pierce her, such as a needle or a thorn. In her mother's words, "Americans, they say they love the child that is why they let the doctors do surgery on her, but Hmong, we say we love the child that is why we will not let the doctors do surgery on her."

For her parents, loving Pam means providing for and protecting her from harm. It means allowing her to live as long as she can, postponing surgery until her life energy *(txoj sia)* is stronger. Loving Pam means protecting her from U.S. doctors who might want to use Pam for their own gains.

## My Child: A Public Child?

The parents received a letter telling them they must give their child over for testing and surgery in accordance with the doctors' wishes. The letter included two courses of action after the surgery: the doctors may give the child back or the child may become a "public" child, belonging to the government. In anguish and outrage, Pam's mother exclaimed,

> Did I not give birth to this child? Was I not the one who gave her life? How can Americans claim Pam as theirs, making her a "public child," a property or possession of the government? How can they do with her what they like, including taking her life away on the operating table? Why, just because we are on public assistance can they do this? It's not like this money is free. They came to our country and destroyed it. Our people have died and sacrificed their lives for Americans. We died in the war saving American lives. We lost

our country because of the Americans. That's why we have come to live here and depend on them to help us. We did not come here because we desired to come freely. We are not asking a lot. We are not asking for American lives in return. We are only asking for minimal survival resources, such as medical care and financial assistance for food and shelter. Yet, the Americans do not stop taking advantage of us. They continue to claim anything as theirs, including human life. They say that our child is their child, belonging to them. How many more lives are they going to take?

Pam's mother was outraged at how the U.S. system works, taking away parents' rights without giving them a chance to speak for themselves. She felt powerless because she was on public assistance, could not speak English, and was dependent on government programs for health care. We have suffered more than enough for the sake of Americans.

She felt that as Pam's biological parents, they had no rights whatsoever. As veterans of the Vietnam War, they received no recognition. And as refugees of war, they had no power.

## Pam's Life Energy

The smaller and younger a person is, the less life energy *(txoj sia)* she possesses and the more vulnerable she is to illness and death. To put a newborn on an operating table is almost like placing her on her deathbed. For these reasons, Pam's parents refused heart surgery when she was two and six months old. At such a young age, Pam's life energy was too frail and fragile. They questioned Pam's ability at even one year old to withstand the procedure.

Despite their anguish, Pam's parents could not fight the legal system and had to let the doctors take her. She underwent several angiograms (invasive tests that look inside the heart), ultrasounds, and many other tests. After the work-up, they were told Pam had a 1 percent chance of survival and a 99 percent chance of not making it were she to undergo surgery. The specialist, or *thaj maum loj* (big doctor), could not fix Pam's heart because they could not protect Pam's life energy during surgery to ensure she would live. Even now when she is older and her life energy is greater, Pam's mother reasoned, they cannot ensure her viability. How, then, could they have thought Pam had a chance when she was younger with a smaller and more vulnerable life energy?

## A Crooked Cucumber Will Do Just Fine

Hmong people often speak in analogies or metaphors. Referring to a cucumber allows Pam's mother to talk about sensitive and personal things indirectly. She explains, "All children are not born beautiful physically. Just like a patch of cucumbers or squash, not all will be long, slender and straight. Some will be crooked, short, or be uneven. But, if you take care of the not so perfect ones well, cover them with a leaf to protect them, they will turn out alright, not so crooked in the end."

The doctors had said Pam would live only six months, one year at the longest. But now, her parents say she is six years old and doing just fine. She is not so crooked after all. And she would not still be alive had she had the surgery.

## Trust

Pam's parents distrusted the health care providers for several reasons. They did not accept the "scraping of the head" through the pelvis as a plausible explanation for the bump on Pam's head because the bump was not visible right at birth. It appeared only after the nurses had taken the baby away to a different part of the hospital. Then the doctors' stories were inconsistent. First, Pam had one hole in her heart. Then she had two holes in her heart. Pam was predicted to die at six months without surgery, but she lived. The doctors' motives and the incredible pressure they placed on the parents to consent to surgery seemed related to secondary gain for the doctors. It was not love for Pam that motivated the doctors but rather their own interests.

The court order deepened the parents' distrust of doctors, the legal system, and the U.S. government. Though Pam never had surgery, her parents say they will never trust U.S. doctors and the health care system again. They will not go back to the clinic where Pam's original doctors worked, and now they see a Korean doctor who supports their views and decisions.

Pam's parents believe U.S. doctors have a superior attitude and think they know more than others. If people do not do what they say, U.S. doctors force them to by resorting to the legal system, a system that is unjust to people who are less fortunate, non-English-speaking, powerless, or of lower socioeconomic status.

Their experience showed them that Americans can and will interfere with people's lives, take their rights away, and do with them what they will. Pam's parents felt discriminated against, and powerless to do anything about it.

## Children Are Blessings

Hmong people value children. Children are gifts, blessings; each child is unique, born with his or her own fortune. Having more children is favorable because children raise a family's social, economic, and political prestige in traditional Hmong society.

Although everyone wants to have children that are normal and healthy, children born with deformities, special needs, or handicaps are also valued, in their own way. The Hmong have spiritual, physical, and social explanations for a child's physical features or handicaps. Spiritually, children with physical deformities may be living out fates from their previous lives. Their parents may be living out their own fates by having to care for a handicapped child. Socially, children with deformities may result from a curse (*foom*) or mockery of those who are handicapped or look unusual. Sometimes, the curse may be carried from one generation to the next. For example, if a curse is believed to result in a child born with the inability to speak, or mental retardation, future generations of the same familial lineage may suffer from this curse and will have children born with similar disabilities. Many people do not want to marry into families who have been cursed, or given an unfortunate fate, for fear of having to carry that fate or curse forward to the next generation. This attitude indicates an awareness of hereditary or familial disorders; however, the cause of the disorder is perceived to be a social phenomenon rather than a genetic one. Hmong families choose their prospective in-laws very carefully for this reason.

Physically, children with handicaps may be the product of mischievous or reckless behavior. Certain herbs can cause miscarriages. If an intended miscarriage is not successful, the herbs might affect the development of the baby in the uterus, causing physical deformities. Alcohol and opium have been attributed to fetal problems.

Furthermore, children with certain features may be regarded to have been gifted with certain powers from birth. Historically, children born with certain head shapes (elongated or bald) are regarded by many Hmong as superior human beings, capable of seeing the future. Some of these children have been called *mes nyuam* Saub (children of Saub who is a god or superior being who is omniscient).

Hmong families care for special-needs children well. There are few cases of children with handicaps who are neglected or seen as a burden on the family. Special-needs children or adults usually do not have the same responsibilities as the rest of the family, whether at home or at the farm. They contribute to the family if they want to or can but are not obligated to.

In the United States, Hmong parents provide for special-needs children in much the same way they did in Laos, taking care of their personal, physical, and nutritional needs. However, Hmong parents feel very inept at dealing with the psychological and educational needs of these children. In Laos, few people had opportunities to go to school; therefore, formal education needs did not exist, especially for mentally challenged children. In this country, there are schools for all children—those with and without disabilities. Hmong parents are thankful for these opportunities. They also are worried because they do not know how to help their children at home, especially children with disabilities. Parents feel the obligation and desire to help their children. Yet, many are not equipped with the knowledge or experience to help children who are caught between cultures.

The economic demands on parents to work and provide for the family also put strains on the care of children. Parents no longer can farm and baby-sit at the same time the way they did in Laos. They cannot afford day-care expenses when their income provides for only the basic necessities such as food, clothing, and shelter. Parents no longer have time for children, especially those with handicaps, because the lifestyle and demands of survival in the United States often require multiple jobs and multiple shifts.

Hmong parents feel torn between working for family survival and caring for their children. Survival concerns often overpower other concerns in the stressful lives of Hmong families in the United States and special-needs children may lack appropriate attention and care.

# PART IV

# Chronic Disease

*Case Stories and Commentaries*

8

# Man with Diabetes and Hypertension

## *A Case Story*

Blia Vang was a fifty-two-year-old man who had lived in the United States with his wife and ten children for about fifteen years. He and his wife lived with three of their children and he helped care for his grandchildren while his married children worked and attended school. Concerned about his increasing fatigue, weakness, and weight loss over a period of about eight months, his wife and son brought him to the clinic for a routine fifteen-minute appointment. They implored the doctor to find the cause of his problems and cure him. While they had taken him to see several doctors and Hmong healers, he was still losing strength every day and was losing his ability to work.

After a complete physical exam, the doctor diagnosed diabetes mellitus, prescribed a diabetic diet and exercise, and scheduled him to see the diabetes educator. Over several sessions, a Hmong diabetes educator taught Mr. Vang, his wife, and his son about the physiology of glucose, the pathophysiology of diabetes, the technique of monitoring blood glucose, and the dietary restrictions and exercise regimens.

Weeks later, when he returned to see the doctor, Mr. Vang explained problems he was having with the recommended diet and exercise. He was having difficulty following the diet, which included only a cup of rice at each meal. He felt as though he were starving, just as he had for the two years when he and his family lived off the food they could gather in the forest as they fled from the communist soldiers in Laos.

He was having trouble exercising, too; even walking aggravated an old back injury. Years ago, while running from the soldiers, he had fallen while carrying his two-year-old daughter and a heavy backpack. Later his daughter had died. Also, he was afraid to go outside his apartment because of the gangs in the public housing project. Finally, his family thought he was already too skinny and losing weight would make him even sicker. They asked the doctor whether there was a medicine he could take to improve his diabetes, make him gain weight, and increase his strength. The doctor prescribed an oral diabetes medicine, referred him back to the diabetes educator, and made a referral to a psychologist to evaluate him for possible depression and posttraumatic stress disorder.

Over the ensuing months, Mr. Vang's blood sugars remained high and he was started on insulin. The diabetes educator reported that while Mr. Vang seemed capable of taking care of himself, one of his married sons was going to his house twice a day to

173

give him the insulin and monitor his blood sugar. A month later, neither his blood sugars nor his fatigue had improved, so a public health nurse started making daily visits to monitor compliance with the regimen. In the ensuing month, his blood sugar levels did improve and the patient and his son reported that they liked checking his blood sugar and knowing when his blood sugar was high or low.

When a diabetes support group was started at the clinic, the Hmong nurse educator asked him to join and help others adjust to the demanding regimen. At the first meeting, as people shared their miseries regarding diabetes and their frustration with a lack of cure, one man reported that Thai people had a medicine to cure diabetes. By the end of the meeting, another man stated he would go to Thailand and bring back the cure for everyone. Mr. Vang listened intently. He knew that he could not afford to go to Thailand to obtain the cure but was interested in learning more about the medicine.

Despite improvement in his blood sugars, Mr. Vang continued to feel "not right." The doctor diagnosed hypertension, reiterated the importance of diet and exercise, and prescribed an oral medicine. Mr. Vang was perplexed at the diagnosis, wondering how his blood pressure could be high when his blood sugars were low. Besides, only sometimes did he feel as though his body were under increased pressure. After he attended the funeral of an elderly man who had died from a cerebral hemorrhage brought on by uncontrolled hypertension, he found that whenever his head felt heavy he would feel better after he took the blood pressure medicine. So he started a pattern of taking the medicine when either his blood sugar was high or his head felt heavy.

Still, he continued to feel tired, and so his family pursued other treatment options. He took a Hmong herbal medicine and a tropical fruit juice called "noni" for diabetes; both decreased his blood sugars, so he and his family decreased the amount of insulin he was taking. Since they were Christians, they also prayed to God. But when Mr. Vang's weakness persisted, and the doctor could not offer further explanations, they began to wonder about spiritual causes and sought the assistance of a shaman.

After several sessions, the shaman told Mr. Vang that he was being chosen by the helping spirits to become a shaman. He was startled and worried at first, but over several weeks he and his family accepted the diagnosis. Mr. Vang gave up Christianity and started his apprenticeship with the shaman; as he learned to shake and to enter the shaman's trance, he became stronger and stronger. He reported to the doctor that for the first time, with the assistance of the insulin and becoming a shaman, he felt like himself again.

## Questions for Consideration

### *Questions about Culture*

How were chronic illnesses like diabetes and hypertension understood and treated by the Hmong in Laos?

What body weights are considered ideal? What weights are considered unhealthy?

How might being a war refugee have affected Mr. Vang and his family's health care decisions?

What role did Mr. Vang's spiritual beliefs and practices play in his healing?

How common is it for Hmong persons to shift between animist and Christian belief systems? What are the likely causes of such shifts?

### *Questions about Cross-Cultural Health Care Ethics*

How did Mr. Vang's assessment of his best interests differ from that of his health care practitioners?

How should U.S. health care practitioners assess comprehension and decision-making capacity in families such as the Vangs?

### *Questions about Culturally Responsive Health Care*

In what sense is Mr. Vang's case an example of a successful relationship with U.S. health care practitioners?

From whose perspective does this case have a good outcome?

What diabetes and hypertension management strategies are culturally responsive to the needs of traditional Hmong families?

What can providers learn from this case about integrating traditional and U.S. health care practices?

*Commentary*

# Type 2 Diabetes Mellitus
# in the Hmong Community

*Kevin A. Peterson, M.D., M.P.H.,*
*May Lee Vang, A.A., and Yer Moua Xiong, M.P.H.*

In the United States diabetes mellitus is the seventh leading cause of death and afflicts approximately sixteen million people, or 5.9 percent of the population (Centers for Disease Control and Prevention, 1997). For the Hmong community living in the United States, however, diabetes is still a new disease. The Hmong originally migrated from an area of mainland China that had one of the lowest frequencies of diabetes mellitus in the world, occurring in less than 1 percent of the population (King & Rewers, 1993). However, Hmong migration to the United States has been associated with many changes, especially increased incidence of chronic diseases such as diabetes and high blood pressure (Henry, 1996; Story & Harris, 1989).

Challenges arise for both the Hmong and the health care communities as the Hmong face unfamiliar diseases and must learn how to deal with them. Reviewing Mr. Vang's treatment plan highlights specific cultural barriers that influenced the outcome of this case. Cross-cultural differences in education, dietary practices, family structure, treatment goals, and religion are focal areas for misunderstandings between Mr. Vang and his health care providers.

## Education

When people are unfamiliar with a disease, basic concepts that health care providers sometimes take for granted need to be explained carefully. Questions like these are among the first to arise in chronic diseases such as diabetes:

> The doctor told me that I have *tus mob hu ua ntshav qab zib*\* [sweet blood]. I never eat or drink sweet things. Why and how do I have the disease? Did I catch this disease by using public bathrooms or sharing utensils with other people who have diabetes?

---

\*Hmong terms are in the Green Hmong dialect.

It is important for providers to clarify the noninfectious nature of a chronic illness like diabetes and to stress that the condition can be controlled successfully with attentive care. Providers unaware of cultural beliefs and practices about health and disease sometimes make mistakes unwittingly. For example, it is common for providers to stress the seriousness of a disease by emphasizing the potential for disability or death if appropriate care is not given to the condition. Particularly when explaining the potential for future injury, it is important for health care providers to explain the seriousness of a disease without saying, "This will happen to you if—," since this can be interpreted as a prediction or even a curse.

Mr. Vang was fortunate to receive information from a Hmong diabetes educator, who explained the physiology of diabetes to him. A basic understanding of the disease can help patients understand why diet and exercise are important in controlling their condition. Pictures depicting the pancreas and its function can be particularly helpful in providing information about diabetes. However, even with careful diabetes training, when Mr. Vang was diagnosed with high blood pressure, he understandably became confused.

The Hmong language does not have terms for diabetes and high blood pressure. Interpreters commonly use the words *ntshav qab zib,* or "sweet blood," for diabetes. High blood sugar is often translated as *ntshav qab zib siab* ("high sweet blood"). High blood pressure is translated as *ntshav siab* ("high blood"). The potential for confusion is considerable. Mr. Vang correctly recognized that his headaches from the high blood pressure improved with blood pressure medicine. It is understandable that he thought that the medicine that successfully treated "high blood" *(ntshav siab)* would also treat "high sweet blood" *(ntshav qab zib siab)*. Even with good diabetes training, problems with translation and understanding the difference between diabetes and high blood pressure led to Mr. Vang's confusion about his medications.

Successful patient education begins with an open-ended assessment of a person's understanding, followed by an explanation of a disease that is tailored to that understanding. The concept that a chronic illness has no cure can sound ominous. In diabetes focus groups conducted by the Minnesota Department of Health, one Hmong participant explained,

> The doctor told me that such a disease had no cure. You can cope with it by caring for yourself, but if you don't do that, your hands and feet could become paralyzed. I realized I could die, so I said to the doctor, "If there is no cure, please give me some kind of medication so that I can die. I don't want to live like this." (Minnesota Diabetes Control Program, 1998)

For the health care provider unfamiliar with the Hmong language, assessing comprehension is difficult. Part of a thorough assessment of comprehension includes having the patient and family explain back to the provider their understanding of the disease process and the therapeutic approach. The family should be assured that when questions arise, they can ask the providers about their concerns. For many Hmong people and for those who provide care to them, the lack of experienced interpreters and appropriate educational material impedes educational efforts.

Focusing on anatomical descriptions of disease and providing background information about how the body works can lessen these misunderstandings. Detailed explanations and patience are essential. When introducing techniques such as glucose meters or blood pressure measurements, demonstrating what is normal and then demonstrating the abnormal finding can clarify the relevance of a particular therapy. When explaining a disease, it is often helpful to relate the disease to a concept that is familiar to Hmong patients. For example, a practitioner can use the process of making tofu to provide a conceptual explanation of the role of insulin and its importance:

> *Ntshav qab zib zoo ib yam li tov taum paj. Cov kua qaub muab piv txwv tau rau cov insulin uas tawm hauv lub* pancreas *los. Yog yus muab kua qaub tsis txaus ces cov kua taum yuav tsis ntshiab thiab koj yuav teev tsis tau cov taum paj. Ib yam li ntawd, thaum yus tus* pancreas *tsis muaj peejxwm tso tau cov kua* insulin *los tov cov kua qab zib los ntawm tej zaub mov uas koj noj los yog cov kua* insulin *ua haujlwm tsis zoo, ces cov kua qab zib ntawd yuav nyob nraim hauv koj cov ntshav. Yog li ntawd koj cov ntshav qab zib yuav dhia siab. Cov tshuaj noj thiab txhaj tshuaj* insulin *yuav pab kom cov kua* insulin *ua hauj lwm zoo.*

Diabetes can be compared to the process of making tofu. The lemon juice used to congeal the tofu can be likened to the insulin that comes out of the pancreas. If you do not use enough lemon juice, then the liquid will not become clear as the tofu precipitates. In a similar fashion, if the pancreas cannot produce enough insulin to mix with the sugars from the foods that you eat or if the insulin does not work properly, then the sugar will remain in your bloodstream. As a result, your blood sugar will be high.

Because the explanations require an individual assessment of understanding, it is most effective to provide diabetes and high blood pressure education in one-to-one sessions. The practitioner has time to explain information thoroughly, and the patient has the opportunity to respond and ask questions. However, it is also important to explore other methods, such as group education and community-based efforts. Hmong people value the community's opinion on many issues.

Challenges accompany these educational strategies. When it comes to the Western health care system, many Hmong prefer to wait until their conditions require emergency intervention before they seek help. Especially with silent diseases such as diabetes and hypertension, it is often easy to ignore the symptoms. By the time serious complications arise, it may be too late to effectively decrease the risk of further problems. Early identification of these diseases, followed by effective intervention, is essential. Helping the community to understand the detrimental effects of these chronic silent diseases is a key step in helping people in the Hmong community.

## Dietary Practices

Hmong focus group participants commonly perceive that they were healthier before being introduced to modern U.S. lifestyles and diets. Their very active lifestyles as farmers in Laos have been replaced by more sedentary lifestyles in the United States. A decline in physical activity and an increase in high-carbohydrate, high-fat, low-fiber diets change the risk patterns for disease. Under these circumstances, diabetes, high blood pressure, heart disease, and obesity form a deadly quartet of diseases that appear together; they have been called the "New World Syndrome," "Metabolic Syndrome," or "Syndrome X." Exceptionally high rates of this disease quartet are found in several other populations that have migrated or changed quickly from a traditional rural to a modern urban lifestyle, including Native Americans, Hispanics, East Asian Indians, and Pacific Islanders. Prevalence rates of diabetes in these adult populations sometimes exceed 35 percent.

Altering eating patterns and engaging in physical exercise comprise an effective initial therapy for most people with diabetes. A prescribed food plan can satisfactorily treat diabetes in some cases and can make subsequent therapy more effective. However, inadequate knowledge about the Hmong diet by health care providers can compromise the success of treatment based on altering eating habits. Few health care facilities have a nutritionist who can describe dietary interventions in Hmong, and fewer still understand how to tailor a Hmong diet for an individual with diabetes. Generally, a person with diabetes needs a balanced diet low in saturated fats and processed carbohydrates. Refined sugar plays only a small role in the traditional Hmong diet, and substantial restriction of sugar has little benefit on overall glucose control.

Mr. Vang tried to follow the prescribed diet given to him by his dietician, but that diet raised some particularly difficult issues. For Mr. Vang, the dietician limited rice intake as a way to reduce carbohydrates. Although a reasonable strategy for someone on a Western diet, this requirement was difficult for Mr. Vang, since rice is a staple food, that is, a food eaten at every meal in large amounts. Two cups of cooked rice per meal is common in a traditional Hmong diet and can provide up to half of normal daily calories. Restricted to only one cup of cooked long grain rice at each meal, Mr. Vang quickly began to lose weight.

Weight loss itself can often result in marked improvement in diabetes and sometimes eliminates the need for medicines. Weight reduction using a balanced diet can be a reasonable first step in the treatment of diabetes. For many Hmong, however, weight loss has particularly negative associations. On one hand, the Hmong people have endured a history of flight and starvation, and loss of weight is naturally associated with illness. On the other hand, obesity, uncommon in Laos, has a positive social connotation. In this case, Mr. Vang and his family interpreted his loss of weight as a negative outcome. Reminded of when he nearly starved to death in the jungle, Mr. Vang lost confidence in the treatment. The family became alarmed and sought other solutions.

Although dietary preferences are unique to individuals, a few generalizations about the traditional Hmong diet may help providers avoid misunderstandings. Rice is the preferred staple of many Hmong families. It is cheaper to buy and lasts longer than other foods. Different kinds of rice can have different effects on blood glucose. Short-grain rice (including sticky rice) tends to be sweeter than long-grain rice and should be replaced or at least rotated with long-grain rice for meals. In Laos, a traditional Hmong diet would also include boiled vegetables, limited meat, and little salt. In the

United States, diets are often very high in fats, particularly diets that include fried vegetables, fried meat, and lard. A return to a more traditional diet, including a reduction in frying and an increase in boiled vegetables can substantially alter saturated fat and caloric intake without affecting the use of staple foods. The use of sugar-free fruit juices can also be valuable in caloric reduction. For individuals with high blood pressure, salt reduction can be achieved by avoiding soy sauce and fish sauces. Mr. Vang needed a food plan he could accept and then an appropriate adjustment of medications to accommodate his lifestyle.

Diabetic medicines often affect body weight. Insulin and sulfonylureas often result in weight gain, while metformin is usually associated with weight loss. It is, therefore, important to explain these side-effects carefully. It is also important for the patient to understand that not too much weight will be lost and that losing weight does not imply a worsening of the disease. The provider needs to recognize the traditional belief that a large body size is considered a positive attribute and carefully explain the reasons why weight loss is important. Moderate weight reduction could help control the patient's diabetes and reduce or even eliminate the need for additional medicines to control his blood sugar. The patient and family should be aware of these benefits and, with the provider, identify an ideal or target weight.

## Family Structure

For diabetes, as for many chronic diseases, the most important providers of care are the patients and the patients' families. Most important decisions about day-to-day care are made by patients' families in the community setting, not in doctors' offices. Since they have an important role in care-taking and decision-making activities, the families of most Hmong patients should be involved in educational support and empowerment.

The move to the United States resulted in a reversal of roles for many Hmong families. Younger family members used to rely on the elderly for wisdom regarding health and healing. The elderly must now rely on their younger family members to understand English in order to provide a link to the Western health care system. Mr. Vang's family brought him to the doctor, and it was only with his family's support that he was able to begin insulin therapy. Once he began this therapy, he continued to rely on his son to help him with the insulin injections. His family encouraged seeking other therapies when they became concerned about Mr. Vang's weight loss.

Food preparation is a family responsibility. Even young teenagers frequently have significant responsibilities in preparing meals. Since the timing of meals, as well as their frequency and balance, are very important for a person with diabetes, the entire family should be aware of dietary recommendations to avoid family discord and promote support. Focus group data support this assessment. Elderly participants with diabetes expressed feelings of despair and depression with respect to misunderstandings between themselves and their children. One man shared his hurt feelings: "My daughter-in-law is impatient. When I get up so often to eat, she scolds me and says, 'Why do you old people have to get up so often to eat? You can't even do anything. Why do you eat so much?' It's better to die . . . [than to live this way]."

The Hmong community is family-centered. Family-centered education recognizes this relationship, empowers the patient, and promotes increased support for lifestyle changes.

## Treatment Goals

People with chronic disease often have different treatment goals than their physicians. Mr. Vang's health care providers sought to control his blood sugar and his high blood pressure to prevent the eventual onset of debilitating complications. Achieving this control required Mr. Vang to alter his diet and lifestyle. The goal of a person with a chronic disease, however, is generally to live a normal life with as few changes in diet and lifestyle as possible. Mr. Vang sought a therapy that had the least impact on his life. The family's decisions were consistent with Mr. Vang's best interests as the family understood them.

Patients often continue to seek help from a variety of sources. Health providers need to be responsible in their recommendation of traditional remedies in order to protect their patients from people who prey on vulnerable individuals. Providers must be sensitive to traditional therapies, which provide emotional or spiritual support, but they do not have to recommend unapproved medicines. It is important for physicians to provide an environment that encourages patients to disclose and discuss the full range of therapies they are using. Therapies like noni can affect the blood sugar but also may interfere with medicines offered by the provider.

Struggling to promote openness between providers and patients and stressing the importance of understanding both disease processes and therapies will go a long way in promoting the health of Hmong patients. Communication and a better understanding of each other's treatment goals are cornerstones in improving the partnership between people with a chronic disease and their health care providers.

## Religious Issues

Mr. Vang sought the help of a shaman because he recognized that his disease was affecting both his physical body and his soul. Having tried all possible remedies to treat his physical symptoms, he wanted further explanation for why he was still not feeling right. His doctor referred him to a psychiatrist, but Mr. Vang and his family turned to animism for possible answers.

Many shaman share the view that their healing expertise involves illnesses of a spiritual nature and that diseases that affect the physical body, such as diabetes, are not appropriately treated by their techniques. While some animist Hmong with diabetes do not attribute their illnesses to spiritual causes, those who believe their condition is associated with spiritual causes, as Mr. Vang and his family did, seek advice from a shaman.

Although Mr. Vang is a Christian, he was raised in an animist culture. When his symptoms worsened, he sought assistance in his animist roots. He believed that his soul was not in its right place, making him feel as if he was "not himself." Spirits will often cause people to become ill as a way of communicating to them that the spirits have a specific need. A shaman can assess and determine the specific need. In Mr. Vang's case, the shaman spirits had chosen him to be a shaman; they needed him to heed the call. In order for Mr. Vang to accept their call and regain his health he needed to convert back to animism and become a shaman. Health care practitioners should become familiar with spiritual beliefs and initial assessments should include conversation about the patient's spiritual orientation and how it may contribute to the healing process.

## Conclusion

As the Hmong community replaces a traditional rural lifestyle with a modern urban one, the incidence of "New World Syndrome" can be expected to rise rapidly. Diabetes, hypertension, and their complications may emerge with increasing frequency within the Hmong community, accompanied by significant social and economic costs. People with these chronic diseases and health care providers need to work together to ensure that Hmong people have the tools to prevent and manage them.

## References

Centers for Disease Control and Prevention. (1997). *National diabetes fact sheet: National estimates and general information on diabetes in the United States.* Atlanta, GA: Centers for Disease Control and Prevention, U.S. Department of Health and Human Services.

Henry, R. R. (1996). *Sweet blood, dry liver: Diabetes and Hmong embodiment in a foreign land.* Unpublished doctoral dissertation, University of North Carolina, Chapel Hill, NC.

King, H., & Rewers, M. (1993). WHO ad hoc diabetes reporting group: Global estimates for prevalence of diabetes mellitus and impaired glucose tolerance in adults. *Diabetes Care, 16,* 157–177.

Minnesota Diabetes Control Program. (1998). *Voices from the community: Focus groups with African American, American Indian, Hispanic and Hmong people with diabetes.* St. Paul: Center for Health Promotion, Minnesota Department of Health.

Story, M., & Harris, L. J. (1989). Food habits and dietary change of Southeast Asian refugee families living in the United States. *Journal of the American Dietetic Association, 89*(6), 800–803.

# "I Tell You This Story of Healing":
# A Shaman's Perspective

*Yer Moua Xiong, M.P.H. as told by Nkaj Zeb Yaj*

Daughter, I tell you this story as a lesson in believing and healing. Listen carefully. Do you hear the echo of lost souls yearning for healing? The soul is the life source for the body. When the soul wanders or is lost, the body becomes ill. Do you hear the calls of ancestors sharing their needs? Ancestors communicate with their living family members by bringing illness upon them. Mr. Vang's doctors said that he had diabetes *(ntshav qab zib)* and hypertension *(ntshav siab)*. I believe his illness was related to problems between his soul *(plig)* and the spirits *(dab)*. As a shaman, it was his soul that I knew; it was his soul that I healed.

Each time I heal, I travel to the land of the spirits, and it is like a journey into a foreign land. In the spirit world, I must know a foreign language that I learned from my shaman helping spirits *(cov qhua neeb)*. I summon my *qhua neeb* by burning incense and sending smoke through the wind and the clouds. These spirits are my allies. They speak through me and we heal together. In the spirit world, we fight spiritual battles. In the spirit world, I advocate for my patient, much like a defense lawyer advocates for his client. In that place, we fight spiritual battles. This is how we heal.

The act of healing by a shaman is called *ua neeb*. The first time that I perform a healing ceremony, I must *ua neeb saib,* to search for the cause of illness. I have to *ua neeb saib* first before I can actually heal an ill person. If I do not search for the cause of the person's illness before I heal, then I will not know how to retrieve the person's soul from the place to which it has wandered. The actual healing ceremony is called *ua neeb kho,* which often requires an animal sacrifice. When the wandering soul has been found, the soul of a sacrificial animal takes the place of the ill person's soul, preventing that person from dying and entering into reincarnation. If I perform the healing ceremony prematurely, I will be bringing the animal's soul into the spirit world without first knowing how to lead the person's soul back home. When I performed *ua neeb saib* for Mr. Vang, the spirits revealed three aspects of his life that needed to be corrected before he could get well.

First, when he was frightened *(ceeb)* at the funeral home, he experienced soul loss *(poob plig)*. I asked my shaman spirits to journey to the place where he had lost his soul and bring it back in order to save his body. This alone would have healed him if soul loss had been his only cause of illness. But it was not.

My second diagnosis involved the fact that he was living with his daughter and son-in-law. Hmong culture and tradition do not allow this kind of living arrangement. A married daughter is part of her husband's family and therefore she reveres the household spirits and ancestors of her husband's family. Her parents cannot reside in her husband's home because the husband's spirits would be unwilling to share their house with other spirits. Her parents are considered guests, so her husband's spirits will not protect them. To remedy this problem, I told him that they must move from his daughter's home to his son's home. Still, there was another problem and another sacrifice Mr. Vang had to make.

The spirits also revealed that Mr. Vang and his wife had their deceased grandfather's shaman tools. One of them had to use the tools in the manner that they were intended. It was as though the dead grandfather said, "You have something of mine, so now I want you." The grandfather chose him to become a shaman and expressed this choice by making him sick. You might ask, "Why didn't the grandfather choose his wife?" When the grandfather weighed the strength of their souls, he determined that only Mr. Vang's soul was able to become a shaman. Almost all shaman have experienced a near-death illness, which is a sign that they have been chosen to heal humankind. Chosen people will continue to be deathly ill until they accept their duty. The third remedy involved setting up an altar for Mr. Vang so that he could answer his call of becoming a shaman.

After we pleaded with my shaman helping spirits to heal him and completed the three prescribed remedies, he was better for one month. He then experienced much fatigue and his illness worsened. His doctors could not cure him at this point. He also sought the help of many other shaman, but they were unable to help him. He believed he would die. One day Mr. Vang summoned his son to his bedside and told him of his fears of death. The thought of losing his father brought tears to the son's eyes, so the son came to me and pleaded for me to help his father. He knew that his father did not fully believe in me and apologized on his behalf. You see, Mr. Vang did not accept his call to become a shaman wholeheartedly. He did not fully believe in shamanism, since he had converted to Christianity years before his illness. As a result, his illness continued, and so once again, I journeyed with the aid of my shaman helping spirits into the spirit world in defense of Mr. Vang.

This is how we healed Mr. Vang. In a three-hour healing ceremony, we asked permission for Mr. Vang to be given a new gift of life. We asked for his life to be renewed and requested that his tears and sorrows be taken away. We did not want his children to cry anymore. We did not want his soul to enter into reincarnation. We asked for his name to be taken off of the list of souls to be reincarnated. We offered him as a shaman and said that this time he was ready to welcome his shaman helping spirits into his home and into his life. He was ready to be a shaman with full commitment to fighting spiritual battles on behalf of lost souls.

As I performed the shaman's *ua neeb saib* ritual, I promised my shaman helping spirits that if Mr. Vang became well in fifteen days then I would return with pigs, chicken, or cattle to complete the healing process with the *ua neeb kho* healing ceremony. It only took eight days for Mr. Vang to feel better. We knew he was well because his body felt lighter, he could sleep, and he wanted to eat. As promised, I returned to complete the healing process with the shaman ritual *ua neeb kho.* With renewed breath, strength, and life as a shaman, Mr. Vang experienced two years of restored health.

Then during a ceremony to welcome the New Year, after smelling and consuming the food there, he became very ill again. He became unconscious at one point and needed me to help him again. He could neither eat nor speak, and his family had to take him to the hospital. I asked for and was granted permission to perform the healing ritual of *khawv koob* in the hospital. *Khawv koob* requires a series of chants that can be learned by an apprentice willing to shadow a healer. Soon after the *khawv koob* healing ritual, Mr. Vang felt as though a fist had been taken out of his throat and he could breathe again. He told his family and me that while he was unconscious, he saw me standing in front of a gate to the spirit world, blocking the entrance so that he could not pass through to the other side. He returned to life and has been well ever since.

Several factors contributed to Mr. Vang's recovery. I am convinced that if a person does not have any kind of belief system, he will not heal. Doctors must find out about their patients' beliefs. What helped this patient was his belief in the doctor's medicine and ultimately in the healing powers of the shaman. They were both able to help him. It is also true that his children loved him so much that his soul wanted his body to live on to return their love. In Hmong families, one of the deepest forms of love is through giving of oneself. This act of giving may come in the form of an actual gift, kind words, or time spent helping others. Once a person has given love, the one who receives it is obligated to return that gesture. Mr. Vang wanted to show his love for his family by continuing to care for his grandchildren so that his own children could work to support their families.

I cannot tell you about his diabetes or hypertension. I am a shaman. I only know about *plig* and *dab*, about *ua neeb* and *khawv koob.* I can only speak about what I have done as I asked my *qhua neeb* spirits to heal him. The doctors take care of the body by checking blood and giving medicine. I heal the soul. Lost souls will continue to yearn for healing. I am ready because in healing others, I find my own life.

# 9

# Young Woman with Kidney Failure and Transplant

## A Case Story

Twenty-one-year-old Mai Neng Moua was in her junior year of college when she went to see a doctor for a physical examination in anticipation of going abroad for the summer. She had been living in the United States for thirteen years with her mother and two older brothers. Her father had died when she was three years old and her mother had never remarried. When important decisions needed to be made within the family, Mai Neng's uncle, her father's younger brother, often assumed her absent father's role. Mai Neng's immediate family converted to Christianity soon after arriving in this country, while some of the relatives, including her uncle, maintained the traditional animistic religion of ancestral reverence.

Mai Neng's mother had always taught her to be independent and strong. Although she was the only daughter in her family, Mai Neng's gender did not stop her from pursuing an education. She worked hard in school and participated in community organizations, volunteering her time to help others, working part-time, and taking part in community activities. Mai Neng dreamed of living a better life than the one her mother lived. She wanted a brighter future for herself, her family, and her community.

During the physical examination, the nurse commented to Mai Neng that she had unusually high blood pressure for someone her age. The doctor decided to do several blood tests including kidney function tests to investigate her high blood pressure. Mai Neng attributed the high blood pressure to anxiety and left the doctor's office not really worried.

Later that day, after Mai Neng returned from playing soccer, her mother told her the doctors had been calling all afternoon, demanding that she go to the hospital right away. A blood test measuring kidney function was high and the doctors were worried Mai Neng's kidneys were failing. They wanted to do further testing in the hospital.

Mai Neng and her mother were shocked by the urgency of the problem. The doctors made it sound as though Mai Neng was going to collapse and die right then. She thought, "Surely, I could not be so sick!" She had been feeling fine, just like any other twenty-one-year-old college student. Mai Neng recalled only two possible symptoms of illness. That semester she had had a decreased energy level, tiring out by midnight from a busy day, and had occasional puffiness in her face that subsided by midday. As the fatigue was more prominent during finals time she thought it was caused by her stress.

Mai Neng and her mother drove to the hospital and Mai Neng was admitted. The doctors could not explain why her kidneys were not functioning well. They needed to do more tests, including daily blood draws and a kidney biopsy. The family members agreed to the blood tests but were skeptical about the kidney biopsy. The doctor called a family conference to explain the situation to Mai Neng and her family. Because Mai Neng's command of English was very good, the hospital staff relied on her as an interpreter. She was therefore responsible for conveying the doctor's messages and her personal feelings to her family and at the same time conveying to the doctor her family's feelings.

According to the daily blood results, Mai Neng's kidneys were deteriorating fast, although she was not yet feeling physically ill. The doctors worried about Mai Neng's worsening kidney function and strongly recommended a biopsy—the sooner the better —to identify the underlying etiology and to recommend the most appropriate treatment options.

Mai Neng's family did not want her to undergo the biopsy. They believed it was too invasive, and they knew that Mai Neng was not as sick as the doctors said she was. They wanted to take her home and treat her with Hmong medicine instead.

Mai Neng decided to go ahead with the biopsy despite her family's objections because she wanted to know why her kidneys were failing. Her Hmong pastor supported her decision. The morning of her biopsy, her uncle called and told her not to go through with the procedure and to try Hmong medicine first. Mai Neng understood what her uncle and mother were saying to her, but she also understood what the doctors were saying. She wanted to live and to live meant taking what she believed was the more certain route. As Mai Neng was rolled away on a cart into the operating room, her mother sobbed on her knees, begging Mai Neng to turn back.

The biopsy results revealed that Mai Neng had IgA nephropathy, an autoimmune disease. She was told she would need to decide about dialysis soon because her kidneys would not hold out much longer, but Mai Neng could not make that decision right away. She went home and told the doctors she would let them know when she was ready for dialysis.

Over the summer Mai tried some herbal remedies. But as she became more fatigued, her doctor became concerned that the herbs might be interacting with the Western medications, and she agreed to have the herbs tested. Her mother repeatedly warned that the herbs would not work if she went on dialysis and was furious when she learned that Mai Neng had allowed her herbs to be tested. As Mai Neng's swelling increased, she decided it was time to start dialysis. Her family asked her to remain at home and not continue with school because she was sick and needed care. They worried that she would get weaker and sicker if she resumed all of her previous activities. Mai Neng did not want to let her condition alter her plans, so she went back to school and resumed her previous activities. Since there was no dialysis unit available in the college town, she performed peritoneal dialysis four times a day on herself.

Mai Neng's doctors raised the possibility of testing her brothers to determine whether either might be able to donate a kidney to her. Mai Neng's mother and uncle, however, were fearful and did not want her brothers to undergo testing; her brothers did not contest this decision. Mai Neng was placed on the kidney transplantation list and waited for a cadaver donor kidney.

Three years later, a very close European American friend, her best friend's fiancé, told Mai Neng he was willing to donate one of his healthy kidneys to her. After many lengthy discussions with each other, their parents, the pastor, and their friends, the two underwent the transplant operation. Recovery went well. While in the hospital, both were visited by their families, friends, and people they did not even know.

Since Mai Neng's kidney transplant, she has been doing well, living with her mother and brothers and working two jobs. She is under close follow-up with her doctors since rejection of the donated kidney is still possible.

## Questions for Consideration

### Questions about Culture

How do the Hmong customarily understand and treat kidney diseases?

When, according to the family, did Mai Neng become sick?

Why might Mai Neng's family have opposed a kidney biopsy? What evidence or considerations might have led them to support a kidney biopsy?

What intergenerational and gender issues are raised by this case? How do Hmong families respond to younger members who choose not to follow their families' advice?

How might the family conflict have differed if Mai Neng were married? If she had been a man? If she were a family leader? If her family had been animist rather than Christian?

What beliefs might a Hmong patient and family have to relinquish before being able to accept organ donation and transplantation? What is the significance of forgoing these beliefs?

### Questions about Cross-Cultural Health Care Ethics

What factors contributed to Mai Neng's treatment decisions and her trust in her doctors? Why did her family have less trust?

What role and obligations do families have to a sick person, according to traditional Hmong and U.S. cultures?

What risks and benefits did Mai Neng assess? How did her assessment differ from her family's?

What objections do Hmong families tend to have regarding organ removal and organ transplantation?

### Questions about Culturally Responsive Health Care

What does this case suggest about integrating traditional and Western interventions?

Why, in this case, was a trained health care interpreter never used? What assistance could an interpreter provide?

What steps might have made the family feel more respected by the physicians and health care system?

What steps might have enhanced the family's trust in the physicians and the health care system?

*Commentary*

# Endstage

*Mai Neng Moua*

It is midnight. I am driving to the hospital with my mother. I am scared and crying. I know my mother is scared too.

"Don't worry," she says. "I am still here. As long as I am alive, I won't let anything happen to you. Nothing will happen to you."

I am still scared.

My mom, my two brothers, my uncles, my cousin, who's a pharmacist, and one of my friends are all in my room now. We're waiting for the doctor to come talk to us. Everyone's worried. None of us knows people who have kidney problems. We don't even know anything about kidneys, not really.

The doctor comes in, and he tells my family he wants to do a biopsy of my kidneys. Before he can finish explaining, my uncles are already shaking their heads. The doctor looks around the room and continues anyway. He shows my family the lab results.

"Her labs are ten times the norm," he tells them but my family isn't listening. It means nothing to them. No one looks at the lab results.

"Yeah, but she was okay until now," says my youngest uncle.

The oldest uncle says, "No, we cannot have her do that."

My mother sighs. She is worried. I can see she hasn't slept much. Her eyes are puffy, and she looks like she's lost weight since that night in the emergency room. "Me, I won't let her do that," she says.

"It's a simple procedure really. She won't even have to go under," the doctor offers.

My cousin who is the pharmacist says, "It's not hard. I think it's a good idea to do it."

No one else in the room except my cousin, my friend, and I agree that the biopsy is a good idea.

"But if we don't do it, how will we know what's wrong?" I ask.

No one answers me.

"What do you want?" the doctor asks, pointing to my uncle. "What do you want?" he says, pointing to me. "Why don't we go around the room and see what everyone wants?"

We go around the room and as I had suspected, only my friend, my cousin the pharmacist, and I agree to do the biopsy.

"If you don't want to listen to us, then why are we here?" my youngest uncle says. I am thinking, "Why are you here?"

I have end-stage kidney failure. Both my kidneys work less than 10 percent. I have to do daily peritoneal dialysis (PD) in my room to maintain life. Now, on the right side of my stomach, a four-inch incision spews a six-inch catheter. Through the catheter, I drain 2.5 liters of dialysis solution into my body cavity. This fluid "dwells" in my body for several hours so that an exchange can take place between my blood and the dialysis solution, cleaning the blood of toxins that can no longer be filtered out by my kidneys. After three to eight hours, I drain out the used dialysis solution and replace it with another 2.5 liters of solution. I do this four times a day: morning, noon, evening, and before going to bed.

I am mourning the loss of my body. Shortness of breath warns of a severe asthma attack. Catch that breath. InOutInOutInOut. In the middle of the night, my calf muscles cramp suddenly like a taut rubber band. There is nothing I can do except hold my breath, grit my teeth, and wait for the moment to pass. Insomnia is boredom at three o'clock in the morning. In my head, a train goes round and round at top speed. Ideas, images, conversations, and questions flash past my eyes like fast cars on the highway. I don't know how to turn them off. My big tummy is a pregnant woman. I sleep on my side, thinking, "This is what pregnant women feel like. This is how they sleep." Weak is warm tired arms, heavy legs, and dragging steps. I see the fumes of my life force, my physical strength slip away from me like smoke from a chimney on a cold winter's day. Puffy face is the girl with slits for eyes. I can't see. I force my eyes open for minutes on end but nothing changes my narrow vision. Sometimes when I wake up in the morning, my face and eyes balloon from the undrained fluid. I want to press my cheeks in until nothing but skin remains. Fluid-filled, I no longer recognize myself. Sometimes I wonder if I am dating my current boyfriend because I need to feel I am still pretty. That someone still likes me. That someone still wants me.

The scariest thing about being on dialysis is that I feel I have no control over my body. That's hard. To feel disconnected from myself. It's strange to think my own body now is a stranger to me. I am no longer intimate with my body. I cannot get attached to it because I know I will lose more of it.

It is the first day after the peritoneal lavage tube is placed. My mom approaches me with her herbal medicines, floating in a tall glass. It did not make any difference that I was already taking Zantac, Phoslo, Procardia, Cardura, Rolcaltrol, and Neprocaps. I put down my nephrologist's book *When Your Kidneys Fail* and meet my mother in the hall, next to the bathroom.

She extends the glass to me.

"*Coj cov tshuaj no mus hauv hoob nab es muaj ib cov txhua ob ceg thiab qhov quav,*" she says and points to the bathroom.

"Mom, I'm sick on the inside, not—" How do I explain that washing myself with the herbal medicine wouldn't work for kidney failure?

"*Ab, ntxuav li ntawd thiaj zoo mas. Yog muaj no tseem yuav muab ntxuav kiag yus lub cev nas,*" she continues.

I look at her and laugh out loud. I can't help it. First it was washing my hands and feet with the herbal medicine and then scraping my toenails with a knife (to relieve the pressure inside). Now she wants me to wash between my legs with the herbal medicine. How do I tell her it doesn't matter?

"It works," she insists.

"Okay, mom," I say uncertainly, between bouts of laughter. I look at her again and laugh, but she only smiles. She is serious.

"*Kuv ntxuav los?*" she asks me.

"No, mom. I can do it myself," I say, laughing. Oh God, to be twenty-one years old and still have your mom bathe you. There is no escaping this. My mom stands there. Her outstretched hand with the herbal medicine. I take the glass and step into the bathroom. I breathe a lungful and start undressing. I sit on the cold edge of the bathtub for a long time before washing myself.

One day, my mom says, "*Wb mus xyuas* Jerusalem, *qhov chaws yug* Yesxus."

I tell her we can't go to Jerusalem, even if it is the birthplace of Jesus Christ.

"Mom, there's a war going on over there. People are bombing each other left and right," I say. She didn't know. "Besides, I can't go abroad. How am I supposed to do dialysis without my supplies?"

"*Nqa mus xwb!*" she says. "One week, no problem."

"No, mom," I say. Yeah, right! Each box of dialysis solution weighs ten pounds. Five boxes at ten pounds each. Just carry them, she tells me. I don't think so! She's never had to carry them up the stairs from the basement.

" *Ab, nram* Georgia *muaj ib lub pas dej uas cov neeg muaj mob li koj mus zoo.*"

"Mom!" It just doesn't stop. First, the birth place of Jesus Christ, now a healing pond in Georgia.

"*Es nram—*"

I am sitting on our green couch in the living room, staring at the television screen. I'd rather be by myself, but our two-bedroom apartment is so rat-hole tiny there is nowhere to go. My mother walks over and takes both of my cheeks in her hands.

"Why are you so puffy?"

I shrug. I mean, I really don't know why my face is puffy.

"And your eyes. Why are they so red? I thought I told you to put Vicks VapoRub on them. You don't want to get better, do you?"

"But mom, it's the high blood pressure. I'm already taking—"

"You never listen to me."

My whole family, nuclear and extended, is mad at me for having gone through with the biopsy and having chosen dialysis. They'd rather I try herbal medicine and if I get worse, then do dialysis.

My older brother, who is in the kitchen, overhears our conversation and comes to investigate. "You know, you are really skinny, Mai. Don't you eat?"

"Of course I eat. I've actually gained ten pounds, you know." Too bad it's only in water weight.

I want to move out and live with my college roommate. I know my mother does not want me to. She says, "*Ua cas es yuav xav mus ua tej yam qias neeg thag npauv!*"

"What 'dirty' things would I do, *niam?*" I ask her.

She thinks I'm going to invite all the men I know over and have wild parties. She's worried that other Hmong people would say bad things about me, an unmarried Hmong woman living "by herself." She's afraid that I won't have enough money to pay rent, buy food, or pay bills. She's concerned that I won't be able to take care of myself. She doesn't understand why I, a sick person, would want to move out on my own.

"Stay here. I will take care of you," she says.

I know my older brother does not want me to move out. When I ask him about it, he says, "Why do that to mom? After all she's been through, isn't it time we took care of her? Doesn't she deserve more?"

I know my uncles and relatives do not want me to move out. At a Moua family gathering, my aunt, who had heard the news from my mother, makes the announcement that I want to move out. There is an immediate rush of whispers. One of my uncles asks why I want to live by myself. I tell him the two-bedroom apartment my family lives in is too little.

"There is no room for me," I tell them. "I want to continue school, and I need a quiet place to study. I don't want to study at the kitchen table with all the dishes!"

My explanations are no good. They've already made up their minds. I am bombarded with suspicion.

"Why do you want to live by yourself?"

"Don't you love your family?"

"Don't you want to take care of them?"

"Didn't you hear about that Vang girl who was living by herself? Don't you know what people say about her?"

"You can't do that. We won't let you."

"Stay home."

It's true that the two-bedroom apartment is too little for my mom, my two grown brothers, and me. It's true that I want to go to graduate school. What I cannot tell them is that I need to move out on my own because I want to learn how to take care of myself. I want to know how to balance school, work, and dialysis. I don't want to be a burden to my family. I don't want them to worry about who's going to take care of Mai Neng, the sick one. I need to know that I pay my own bills and take care of myself. But I do not have the Hmong words for these thoughts, and so I do not say anything. Besides, they've already made up their minds. No explanation will be good enough for them anyway. I have no defenses. There is nothing I can do but cry.

I am on the waiting list for a cadaver kidney. I am told the average wait is two years but many Asians do not donate. I have to wait at least another year and a half. I may have to wait longer.

It seems kind of strange that my own family will not donate a kidney when my friends Yer, Douangta, and Eric have offered me their kidneys. I am not sure how to respond or feel about this. At first, I am skeptical. I think, "Everyone feels sorry for me. They're just trying to be nice." But when I find out that they are serious, I want to cry. I want to ask them, "How can you give me one of your kidneys? You're not my family." I want my family to give me a kidney.

Sometimes, I feel like my family is punishing me for not listening to them, for not choosing herbal medicine over dialysis, by making me wait the two years for a cadaver kidney. I don't know. I mean, I know why they don't want to. They're scared. My mom won't let my brothers even get tested because she said it was better to just have one person sick than to have two. I guess she's right. I know they're afraid, but it doesn't change the fact that I need a new kidney.

I am here again. And I am still scared. Scared of the surgery to take out the PD catheter. Will it hurt? Will it leave a scar? Scared I won't wake up after surgery. Scared of the IVs. Scared because no one is here with me. I am alone. I am sad and I don't even know why. It's too complicated. Like that passage in Richard Wright's *Black Boy,* when his mother tells him they're going to take a trip down the river. He's expecting a great boat and a great boat ride but when they finally get down to the river and the boat turns out to be an ugly old boat, he is so disappointed and angry, he starts crying. His mom asks him what's wrong and it's so complicated he can't even explain it. It goes so far back that he doesn't even know where to start. It's that kind of complicated today.

My mom is worried and angry. I am angry, too. Last night, I called her to tell her I was coming in for surgery—to take out my old PD catheter because it was probably infected and making me sick, and to put a new permanent catheter in my shoulder so I could do hemodialysis instead of peritoneal dialysis.

She said, "It's up to you. Whatever you want to do—"

What did I expect her to say? "Don't do it. I know a better way—" Shouldn't I have been glad she gave me permission to do what I wanted? All my life, it seems, I have been fighting for this exact thing. But then I think, "Please care. Tell me what to do. Don't say, 'It's up to you.'" Sometimes when she says this, I feel like she's punishing me. An angry, "Well, you chose this path, so why are you asking me what to do?" A, "Well, you didn't listen to me. See what happens?!"

My mother thinks I work too much, too hard. She's right. I do work two part-time jobs. She says, "You're working like a healthy normal person, someone who's not sick. Stop working. Go on SSI. Stay home, go to the library, read. Do a little interpreting for the doctors."

She thinks that because I have chronic renal failure, I am disabled. She sees me as a loss to her, to the family, to the Hmong community, to society in general. I mean, I can still work but I won't be able to do it as fast, as well, as hard, or as much.

She says, "A disabled person like you—who would want to marry you? A good daughter-in-law gets up early and cooks for the family. You won't be able to do that."

She's right. I wouldn't be able to do that.

And so I work two part-time jobs because working is normal. Working nine to five is normal. Normal is going to meetings with other people. Normal is teaching creative writing. Normal is going out dancing. Normal is dating. Normal is being healthy. Normal is going to school. And so in fall I went back to St. Olaf College to finish my last year, despite kidney failure and my mother's protests. I took a full load of classes; I worked ten hours a week (the maximum one could work on Work Study); I was president of the Asian Student Association; I performed with Zebra Patch, a social justice theater group; I worked with Dismantling Racism, an anti-racism group; I came home on weekends for *Paj Ntaub Voice* meetings, a literary arts magazine I started in the summer.

There were days I was so sick I just wanted to crawl into a warm corner somewhere and sleep. I didn't care who saw me, looked, or stared. Just as long as they didn't step on me. One day, I had to make it to class, but all I could think about was sleep. I managed to crawl into the Lion's Den, a room where the multicultural students had their meetings, closed the door, and lay down on the couch. I told myself it would be only ten minutes. But I could not open my eyes. There was sand in them. They were stuck together. My mind was yelling, "Get up! You must get up and go to class," but my body could not respond. I could hear my fellow students talking on their way to class, but my body felt like lead, heavy and immobile.

I am still in the waiting room at St. Joseph's Hospital. My anesthesia nurse, Jan, tells me my potassium level is too low for me to have surgery to take out the PD catheter. I will have to wait another eight hours for it to come up. I can't help but cry. There is nothing to do but cry.

"You'll feel better," Jan tells me. She is a warm woman. Her hands are warm as she hugs me and massages my back, wipes the hair away from my eyes, and holds my hands. Her eyes are gentle as she smiles. Her voice smooth as she tells me, "It's okay. You don't have to be strong." She lets me cry.

I am praying for God's guidance. "Don't leave me, Lord," I ask. "Please, I am lonely and scared. I am alone. Please, Lord, stay close to me. Don't leave me." I pray this over and over like a chant, a ritual song.

I tell Jan, "I've lost another battle. This is another loss. I have lost more of my body."

She nods, "I know. I know. It's another hurdle, huh?"

I nod through my tears and hiccups. I am crying so hard my body shakes.

"Do you want me to call someone?" she asks.

I shake my head. "Everyone is at work or busy with school," I say. I tell her my mom is at work, my older brother at school in St. Cloud, my roommate at work, my two friends at school, and my little brother? "He's sleeping. Oblivious to what's going on." We laugh.

"Yeah," she says, "I know. I have a son and a daughter, and at that age, my daughter was starting to show a kind of caretaker attitude and my son was more into himself." She continues, "He's getting better though. He's twenty-three, and he's beginning to see that things fall through when you're like that."

"Yeah. My brother is nineteen, and I keep waiting for him."

"There's hope," she says and nods.

I am still crying and she continues rubbing my back. Her one hand has not left mine. She is still at my side. She tells me, "You look like a pretty determined person."

"Yeah," I say, "a pretty tired person right now." And we laugh again. It is a good laugh. She smiles at me and squeezes my hands. "It's okay. You don't have to be strong," she tells me again.

"I'm just tired," I tell her. "I don't want to cry any more. It takes too much energy." She nods. "As much as I want my family and friends to be here—they can't really do anything for me. They don't really know what it's like, and it's hard for me to explain sometimes."

"You have a heavy burden to bear. For yourself and your family," she says. I nod.

Sometimes when I see my older relatives, they remark, "Oh, you're better!" They think I am better because I am up, walking, working, talking, and driving. I look all right. There is no open wound. Nothing is bleeding.

I want to shake them and scream, "I'm still sick!" I want to show them my catheter. I want to show them my dialysis-preoccupied mind. I want to show them my tummy of 2.5 liters of fluid, my water-filled cheeks, ankles, and legs. I want to show them my sleepless nights. I want to show them my episodes of peritonitis, when I have diarrhea and I throw up and I have chills and my tummy is so raw and sensitive it bounces back when I gently touch it. I want to show them my "I have no appetite" weeks. I want to show them all the clothes I no longer fit in. I want to show them all the medication I have to take every day. I want to show them my closet of dialysis boxes and supplies. I want to show them the bags of used plastic dialysis bags that I hide in the garbage can and pray that the garbage man never looks too closely. I want to show them my twice-a-month doctor's appointments and all the medical people I have to see. I want to show them the painful shots I have to take to stimulate my bones to make more blood. I want to show them the episodes when I don't have enough blood and I am so tired I can't get up or the periods when the dialysis machine pulled off too much water and I am so dehydrated that I can't walk down the stairs without fainting.

My friend Eric wants to give me one of his kidneys.

Is he serious? Does he understand what he's doing? What would happen if his only kidney failed? Then what would he do? Would having only one kidney affect his work as a cop? Would he be weaker and slower? What do his parents think about his decision? What does his girlfriend think? His friends? Why does he want to do this? I don't want the responsibility of all these questions.

I wave him off. How can I take him seriously when no one in my own family is willing to give me one of their kidneys? I have accepted the fact that they will not. I know how afraid they are. I don't really believe Eric is serious. How can he be? He's not my family, and he's not even Hmong! I don't trust him.

"Is it because I am white that you don't want my kidney? Is my kidney not good enough for you?" he says.

I decide to at least let him get tested.

The doctor says that Eric's kidney is not the best match but if we are still interested, we could try again in another six months. I am relieved that things did not work out. My fear about what would happen if his only kidney fails subsides. Now, maybe he would give up.

Six months later, however, he calls me.

"Eric, what happens if your one kidney fails?"

"Then my dad will give me one of his, or my two brothers, or my uncles or my cousins."

"Will it make you weaker or slower?"

"No, you only need one kidney. It can do the work of both."

"Will it affect your chances of being a cop?"

"No, I just can't be in the FBI or in the CIA."

"Well, what do your parents think about your decision?"

"It's up to me. It's my decision."

"Yeah, I know but what do they think? How do they feel about it?"

"They're happy for me. They're happy that I would want to do it."

"What does your girlfriend think?"

"She's fine with it too."

"Are you sure?"

"Yes. I want to do this. I've wanted to do this ever since I carried that box of dialysate up the stairs for you."

As I reflect back on my experiences with endstage renal failure, I feel much older than my mid-twenties. It's hard to believe that I went through all of that "stuff." Sometimes, the whole thing is surreal to me. I feel as if it's another person's story and not my own.

It has been quite a lonely journey. Many times I wanted to share my suffering (all the times I got sick from peritonitis) and my fear with my family and relatives but I did not want them to worry. I had moved out with my college roommate, and I did not want them to force me back home. It was important for me to live on my own. I needed to know that I could take care of myself. I wanted time to understand what I was going through, to try and make sense of it all. I know I have hurt and isolated many people because of my decisions, but they were the ones with which I could live.

Because Eric, my donor, is Caucasian, his decision to donate surprised and shocked the Hmong community. They did not understand why he would do it. He was not Hmong; he was not family; he was not my boyfriend or my husband. Our decision to go ahead with the transplant touched the lives of many Hmong people, especially those in my church, and has broken many stereotypes about white people.

Although I am doing very well now because of my transplant, I know many of my relatives still question my decision. Even though none of them ever talks to me about it, I know they worry about what I will do when this one fails. I worry about it too, and I wish there were a safe space for all of us to talk about these issues.

*Commentary*

# Painful Cultural Differences in a Hmong Family: The Mother's Perspective

*Phua Xiong, M.D.*

Love and trust are important issues between Mai Neng Moua and her mother, Si. This case highlights the struggles that a mother and her daughter—two very strong women—face as they seek a cure for a disease that may separate them. Independent and progressive in their actions and words, Si and Mai Neng illustrate the changing roles of women across two generations. In their journeys, both must make painful sacrifices that reveal their inner determination and strength. Both women are very much alike, yet very different. They love each other very much, yet feel tangled within the web of love, expectations, and obligations. Both desire trust, yet feel their trust betrayed. Both fight for life and seek peace.

This commentary provides cultural insight into Si's perspective on the conflicts with her daughter. In addition, it offers Hmong perceptions of kidney disorders and organ transplantation.

### Medical Diagnosis and Prognosis

Mai Neng's family and her doctors have different concepts of Mai Neng's condition and prognosis. To Si, Mai Neng did not become sick until after she took the medications the doctors prescribed. She notes that after they gave Mai Neng the kidney medicine, she swelled up badly. She thinks the medicines and the doctors made Mai Neng swell up and get sick. Like most Hmong people, Si relies on physical signs, symptoms, and energy level to assess Mai Neng's condition.

Si does not believe her daughter has a serious disease because, in her eyes, Mai Neng is well. Mai Neng has energy and is active. Only her busy schedule and intense studying make her tired. How can Mai Neng have such things wrong with her body? As a child, Mai Neng was never sick and never needed to see a doctor. Why, all of a sudden, do the doctors say Mai Neng will *die* tonight if she does not go to the hospital?

"What are the doctor's intentions when he makes such a strong statement? Does he intend to make her die? Did he do something to Mai Neng at the office so that she will die if she does not go to see him at the hospital?" Si speculates that maybe the doctor wants to kill or use her daughter to enhance his own skills. Hearing the word "die" used about her daughter is equivalent to cursing *(foom)* Mai Neng with death. Other than the doctor's causing harm, she cannot think of why Mai Neng will die so soon.

Within Hmong culture, sensitive words such as "die" have certain social, spiritual, and cultural connotations and carry a heavier and deeper meaning than physicians often intend. It behooves health care professionals to understand this cultural perspective and find ways to convey important information in culturally sensitive ways that also legally protects them. Practitioners can say that people are gravely ill, seriously ill, and need treatment quickly in order to get better, rather than sound alarmed and use the words "die," "dying," or "death." This approach strengthens the provider-patient relationship.

## Hmong Classification of Kidney Diseases

To most Hmong people, the signs and symptoms indicative of kidney disease are blood in the urine, flank pain, lower back pain, or lower abdominal pain, but not swelling in the legs, arms, or face. Without the signs and symptoms that Hmong people associate with kidney problems, it was difficult for Mai Neng's family to accept the medical diagnosis. If Mai Neng had bloody urine, however, perhaps her family would have agreed that something was wrong with her body.

Hmong people classify kidney diseases into two major categories: kidney pain *(mob raum)* and urinary pain *(mob txeeb zig)*. People whose kidneys are diseased *(mob raum)* might have blood in the urine with or without pain. They drink herbal remedies to rescue the kidney. Cure is perceived as the return of normal colored urine and the alleviation of any symptoms. *Mob txeeb zig* describes pain in the ureters, bladder, and urethra rather than in the kidneys, but it may mean different things to different people. To some, it may mean pain from a bladder infection, pain on urination, or even pain from a kidney infection. To most Hmong people, however, *mob txeeb zig* means kidney stones, which are treated with herbs to dislodge and wash them out of the body.

The Hmong do not delineate etiologies of kidney disorders in the same way that Western practitioners do. Hmong people simply see the kidneys as diseased and they focus on relieving the diseased state by employing herbs that may increase blood flow to the kidney, wash out toxins, cleanse the kidneys, or flush out stones.

## A Mother's Love

As Hmong people measure love through action, Si has shown love to Mai Neng by always taking care of her. As a single mother, Si raised Mai Neng (along with her two brothers) with her two hands, rocked her to sleep on her thighs, and cushioned her in her arms. Through the years, she has kept strong and has fought her way through many hard times. Because she loves Mai Neng, she has made sacrifices and endured suffering that other mothers might not be willing to do.

How can a mother who loves her daughter just stand there and look on as strangers—doctors who never knew Mai Neng—probe, poke, and open her body? Within a day, the results of some blood tests, and contact with one doctor, Si could lose her only daughter. Why must she feel so powerless, when she has been so powerful and strong through the years? Why can she not stand up for her daughter, as she has done for so long? It is not only that she is getting older but so many other things as well—things that come with living in a new country, among new neighbors. There are so many hurdles to overcome. This time, it may just be too hard.

Si lost her husband to the tragedies of war. Unlike many widowed Hmong women, Si chose not to remarry. Although still young, she remained single and devoted to her children. With this decision, Si defied the cultural ideal.

In Laos, when a woman's husband died, she may have been betrothed to his younger brother or cousin. This cultural practice has physical, spiritual, and social advantages for the widowed woman and her children. She and her orphaned children will have a place to stay, fields to till, a family to belong to, and a male head of household to represent them. Spiritually, the children will continue to receive ancestral protection and blessing, and sons will learn to perform religious rituals. Socially, it protects the woman from those who may attempt to take advantage of her widowed status—for example, men who may attempt to rape her, seduce her, or make up disrespectful rumors about her and her children. It also makes it possible for her to keep her children with her, for if she marries a man from a different clan, she would most likely have to leave her children with their father's family.

Despite all the advantages of this cultural practice, some widowed women and younger brothers do not want to marry each other. Perhaps they do not find each other attractive; perhaps the man already has a wife or plans to marry someone else; perhaps the woman fears her new husband will marry a second wife in the future whom he loves more. And perhaps the woman fears that her new husband will not love her children as much as his own biological children. Orphaned children have been known to suffer at the hands of their stepparents: not receive much food, work hard, receive beatings, and not get new clothes at the New Year's celebration.

Sometimes widowed women and their husbands' younger brothers want to marry and other times they do not, but feel that they must perform the duty expected of them. Some may feel it is their fate to live a life of suffering, so they accept their new roles without question. Other women marry men from another clan and leave their children. And still other women choose not to remarry at all.

Si is one of a minority of young widowed women who did not remarry. She puts all her hopes in her children and clings to them, for they are her life-sustaining lights. Since Hmong culture places great importance on having a male head-of-household, Si, as the head-of-household in her family, assumes a different social place in the community. If she carries herself well, and her behavior is deserving of respect, the community will regard her and her children with respect. If she is foolish, plays around with other men in the community, and is not able to contain her conduct and behavior within the narrow boundaries of a respectable, unmarried, widowed woman, then she may bring shame and dishonor upon herself, her children, the extended family, and clan. Throughout the past fifteen years, Si has maintained her image in the community. This image is one of honor, respect, and wisdom and is based on her love for her children.

## The Biopsy Decision

All important members of the immediate and extended family are present at the family conference to consider whether Mai Neng should have a kidney biopsy. Like most Hmong people, Mai Neng's family is fearful of the health care system in the United States. Si recalls, "a Vue family was in a car accident . . . [and] the doctors wanted to take their organs out. . . . The doctors took them away and sliced up their livers and private parts into little pieces. They hung them up like slaughtered pigs, with their heads down, hanging with their feet tied together, like animals. When did they die? Did the doctors kill the father, boy, and girl? Were they dead when the doctors sliced their livers?" Coming to the hospital with their fears, Si's family wonders what to do next. They question the doctors' motives behind the biopsy. Why the urgency? Why now and not next week? Do the doctors want to harm Mai Neng?

In the family conference, the doctors and the family look to Mai Neng as the cultural and language bridge. In a strained situation, Mai Neng has to convey her own feelings to the family, as well as to the doctors; at the same time, she has to interpret and translate the family's feelings to the doctors and the doctors' explanations to the family. Mai Neng is asked to perform a very difficult task precisely when she, herself, needs an advocate. Providing an interpreter and patient advocate for Mai Neng and her family would have eased the situation and relieved Mai Neng of a tremendous burden.

After many hours of discussion in groups, on the telephone, and in one-on-one sessions, the family decided not to consent to the biopsy. The family felt that knowing why her kidneys were failing was not as important as finding a remedy to reverse the damage, or damaging the kidney with a biopsy. They saw the best treatment option as the least invasive one, the use of herbal medicine.

Mai Neng disagreed and consented to the biopsy. But by going against her family's recommendation, she was defying cultural norms and taking a position that few Hmong women would or could. In Hmong families the sick person usually regards the family's decision as the best decision. Thus Mai Neng's action was unexpected, not well accepted, and potentially detrimental to her and her family.

Mai Neng's family felt that she did not trust them or their judgment. In their eyes, Mai Neng's counterdecision meant that she chose her own path, where the wind blows West, not East. The longer she treads this path, the farther West she will be blown. She would have further testing, more blood draws, dialysis, perhaps kidney transplantation, and other potential complications and harm.

Deviation from family recommendations may destroy or change important relationships within the family and clan. In Mai Neng's case, the older men would feel ashamed, for they would lose face in the community. If a relative asks for advice but does not follow through with the advice, the advisers are not held responsible for the consequences and may decline to respond in future situations. If Mai Neng has a bad outcome, her family might deride her for not listening to them or simply feel sad for her, wondering about what might have been had she tried the Hmong way. Some might be angry with the U.S. doctors for "using" Mai Neng. Some might be angry with Mai Neng for letting the doctors "use" her. Some might settle their feelings by reasoning that it is her fate. The relationship can be improved if the disobedient person makes a public apology and asks for the relatives' continued love, protection, and advice.

If she has a good outcome, most people will be happy. Her mother, male advisers, and other family members may acknowledge she knew more than they did. They might express happiness for her, saying it is better that she did not listen to them. Or they may never acknowledge anything.

Mai Neng might ruin her chances of finding a Hmong husband. Some families do not want a defiant, aggressive daughter-in-law; they fear their son would become the "wife" while she assumes the "husband" role. Some families do not want a daughter-in-law who cannot physically perform the duties expected of her; they fear inheriting a sick person whom they have to care for, and they fear having an infertile daughter-in-law.

## Herbal Treatments and Dialysis

Si is wise in Hmong herbal medicine, and she knows she can find herbs to cure Mai Neng. Si recounts the story of an aunt in her forties or fifties, Niam Hlob, whom the doctors said needed emergency dialysis. The family decided to try Hmong medicine first. They got some Hmong herbs from Laos and these cured her. Niam Hlob "had a lot more swelling in the face, arms, and hands than Mai Neng did. Now, she's fine. She did not need to have dialysis, like the doctor said. What if she had done what the doctor said, maybe she wouldn't be able to do what she's doing now. She might have chronic pain [*mob laug*] or might not have lived." By trusting and doing what the doctors recommended, Mai Neng's actions, to Si, are distrustful and disrespectful of her herbal treatments, profession, and tradition, as well as foolish.

At Si's urging, Mai Neng used some of the herbal remedies Si gathered for her. But when Mai Neng gave the doctors samples for analysis because they were concerned for her health and about possible interactions between Western medications, Si felt Mai Neng had betrayed her. "She does not trust my Hmong medicine," Si says. "You see, for Hmong medicine to work, you've got to believe it in your heart that it will work for you, that you will get well with herbs. If you just use it, but don't believe in it, it won't work for you." Si remains calm but sad when she says, "Mai Neng does not believe the one who gave birth to her. Who do you trust—the people who love you or the people who don't love you?"

After analyzing the herbs, the doctors decided they were harmless, and their concern over adverse interactions waned. But once Mai Neng began to receive dialysis, Si did not think the herbs would help any more. She reasoned, "We cannot do both, because if you do Hmong medicine, you cannot do dialysis. If you do dialysis, then all the Hmong medicine will come out from the blood, not stay in the body. The machine will take out the herbs. They will not stay in the blood to help her."

## Organ Donation and Transplantation

Organ donation and organ transplantation are new phenomena in the Hmong community that many people cannot comprehend physically or spiritually. Accepting someone else's organ into your body will affect you in various ways. For kidney transplants, Hmong people in the United States have the following sayings:

- If you get a white kidney, your skin will get whiter and look more beautiful.
- If you get a black kidney, your skin will become darker, like a black American.
- If you get a male kidney, you will grow a mustache and hair, your voice will deepen, and your skin will thicken.
- If you get a kidney from a good-natured person, you will have patience and a good attitude.
- If you get a kidney from a bad-natured person, you will become short-tempered and have a bad attitude.

Organ donation and transplantation have clear spiritual significance to animist Hmong. Accepting another person's organ into your body also means accepting that person's soul into your body. Doing so can cause problems with reincarnation. It may also cause problems in the land of the ancestors, for the dead person's soul may not be able to find its ancestors because it has been altered and thus is no longer recognizable. The soul will have no place to belong in the spirit world.

Even for those who have converted to Christianity, organ donation remains a difficult choice. Despite having set aside beliefs in reincarnation and spiritual existence after death in the spirit world, Christian Hmong often choose not to donate organs, perhaps because of the unknown effects on their spiritual well-being. Accepting organ transplantation, however, does not seem to be as difficult a choice for Christians in life and death situations.

## Si's Decision

Si thinks hard about the issues of kidney donation and transplantation. Although her sons are willing to be tested and willing to consider donating a kidney to their sister, she objects. "Everyone has their life to live. I cannot ask my son to give up one of his kidneys and give it to his sister. I want my family to be strong and my children to have strength to last them a lifetime. . . . I don't want two sick children. One is enough. What if something goes wrong? Will I lose two of them?"

If Mai Neng had followed Si's earlier recommendations but eventually needed a kidney transplant would Si have decided differently? She believes so. "If she had let me treat her, and she did not get well, I would have given her one of my kidneys. But, she did not want my help. Why? Mai Neng doesn't love me. My children don't love me. I tried my best to help them, but they reject me. What can I do?"

## Religious Beliefs

Si and Mai Neng are Christians but they have different concepts about how God can intervene in Mai Neng's illness. For Mai Neng, God's love for her and her faith in Him is manifested in His provision of a knowledgeable and caring health care team and the donation of a new kidney for her. "This new kidney is something God did for me because He loves me," Mai Neng says.

Si, in contrast, sees God's intervention as supernatural. God will intervene directly if it is His will that Mai Neng lives. Through human prayer and faith, God will grant Mai Neng strength and restore her kidneys to their normal function if He so chooses, without kidney transplantation. "I believe she would be okay if God lets her live. . . . Mai Neng said God and herbs couldn't help her. Only the doctors can help her. Mai Neng did not rely on God."

## The Pain of Acculturation

Mai Neng's case illustrates generational differences in the acculturation process. Young Hmong men and women strive to adapt to U.S. society, and at the same time they learn about traditional culture and change it to fit the needs of their changing identities. These processes can be emotionally draining and socially isolating, as Mai Neng's struggle illustrates.

Some Hmong parents have trouble adjusting to U.S. society. They have lost the social prestige they held in their native country, and they carry physical and psychological scars from the war. They also find themselves dependent on others, such as their children, the government, and service agencies, since they do not have basic language or job skills. Many parents feel they have become children again. They often say, "In this country, we have become children and our children have become parents" because they do not understand the United States and they cannot communicate with Americans.

Perhaps Si perceives herself in this light. First, her inability to speak, read, or write in English isolates her from non-Hmong–speaking people. Second, she lacks the skills for a well-paying job with good benefits, making her unable to provide for her children as she did in Laos and Thailand. And finally, her children reject her wisdom, knowledge, and authority.

Strong-willed women, Si and Mai Neng, continue to struggle with how to demonstrate their love for each other, challenge cultural norms, try out new ways, and pave the road for other women in their journeys.

# PART V

# Mental Illness

*Case Stories and Commentaries*

# War Veteran with Depression and Posttraumatic Stress Disorder

## *A Case Story*

Cha Va Lee, a middle-aged veteran of the war in Laos, has lived in the United States for the past twelve years. He does not speak English. His daughters have all married and left home. His thirteen-year-old son, who speaks very little Hmong, is in a gang and has been in trouble with the law. Mr. Lee worked as a janitor for five years, until he slipped and fell from a ladder two years ago. His accident left him with recurring back, leg, and arm pain. Although there is no clinical evidence for the pain, he remains disabled and walks with difficulty. He has trouble concentrating on tasks, and he sleeps only one to two hours a night. He frequently has nightmares about the war. Mr. Lee reports waking one night in sheer terror, unable to move. He felt he was being suffocated by an evil spirit. Using all his strength, he was able to throw off the evil spirit and keep it from killing him in his sleep. He remains frightened that it will return.

His medical insurer wants to find a way for him to return to work and is paying for his physical therapy sessions. Mr. Lee is not consistent about keeping appointments. Both his physical therapists, who work without an interpreter, and his primary care physician, who works with an interpreter, are frustrated and feel unsuccessful in their efforts to help Mr. Lee. His primary care physician referred him to a psychologist who specializes in posttraumatic stress disorder (PTSD) in Southeast Asian refugees.

Mr. Lee has been seeing the psychologist for four months. He told the psychologist about his many war experiences and about how angry he is at the United States. He became a soldier when he was thirteen years old and fought in the war for ten years. All the friends with whom he fought in the war are now dead. He also lost several family members during the many years they were forced to live on the run in the jungle with very little food to eat. He is deeply angry that the U.S. government does not recognize his contribution to the war effort and is not providing any veteran's benefits. He feels many promises have been broken. He attributes the problems he is having with his son to U.S. society and to his being prohibited from raising his son as he believes is best.

His anger extends to the physical therapists and others who feel he could be working. He says the physical therapists think he should be able to walk without difficulty, but they do not understand the extent of his pain and they treat him disrespectfully. He also does not know why he should continue to struggle to feel better just so that he can return to a menial job.

Mr. Lee was diagnosed with posttraumatic stress disorder and depression. He was given an antidepressant and scheduled for therapy sessions to talk about his anger, his war experience, and his future. The psychologist found a physical therapist for Mr. Lee who is knowledgeable about the Hmong and the refugee experience, and he specified that the physical therapy sessions would never again take place without an interpreter present. The psychologist attended the first appointment with Mr. Lee.

Since Mr. Lee can read and write Hmong, the psychologist encouraged him to read Hmong folktales to his grandchildren. In this way he is able to engage in satisfying activities with his grandchildren. He is beginning to sleep better and to have a more positive outlook, but he remains disabled.

## Questions for Consideration

### Questions about Culture

What are the major causes of depression and PTSD in the Hmong community?

Historically, how has depression been viewed by the Hmong? What kinds of help are Hmong patients accustomed to seeking and from whom?

How are nightmares and night terrors most commonly understood and addressed by Hmong patients? How are they most commonly understood and addressed by U.S. health care professionals?

What role might culture play in Mr. Lee's experience of pain and disability? How might Mr. Lee's being a refugee have contributed to his difficulties?

What does it mean for Mr. Lee that his only son belongs to a gang?

### Question about Cross-Cultural Health Care Ethics

What does Mr. Lee need to be able to trust in and feel respected by his caregivers?

### Questions about Culturally Responsive Health Care

How did the psychologist earn Mr. Lee's trust?

What resources and interventions might be useful for Mr. Lee given his diagnosis of PTSD?

What can health care institutions do to help patients suffering from PTSD and depression?

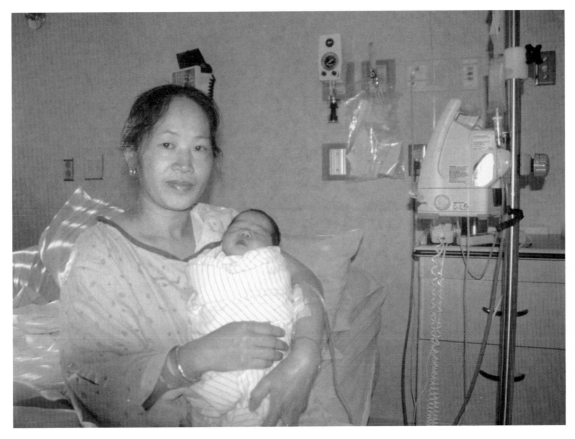

Plate 19. A woman holds her newborn infant in a hospital. She has a red cloth bracelet tied by a shaman to strengthen her soul, making her less susceptible to spiritual harm. United States 2002. (Kathleen A. Culhane-Pera [KCP])

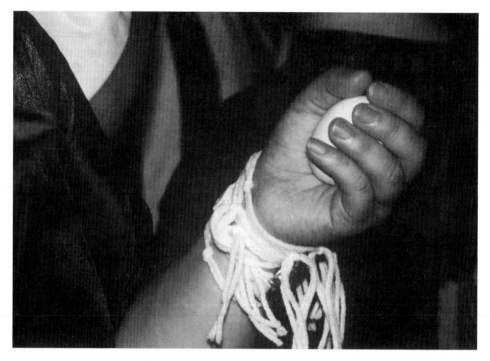

Plate 20. A man holds a boiled egg—symbolizing good wishes and love—during a wrist string-tying ceremony *(khi tes)*. United States 1996. (KCP)

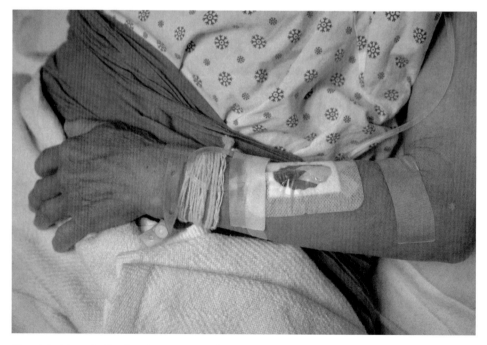

Plate 21. A hospitalized patient recovers from an operation. Note the IV in her arm and the white strings around her wrist to protect her soul during the operation. United States 2002. (KCP)

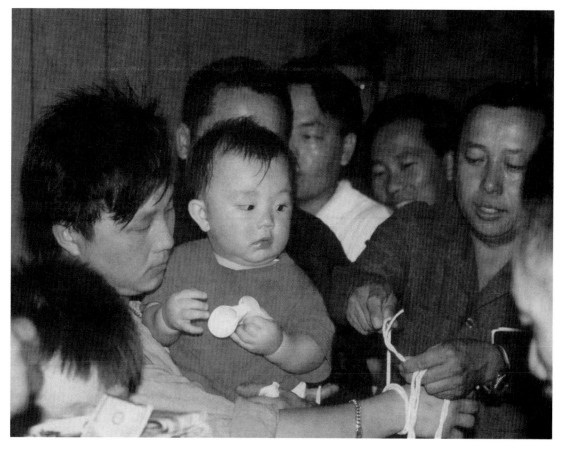

Plate 22. A father extends his hand as the soul-caller blesses him and ties strings on his wrist *(khi tes)* to strengthen his spiritual and physical health. Male family members wait their turn to offer their blessings in the string-tying ceremony. United States 1996. (KCP)

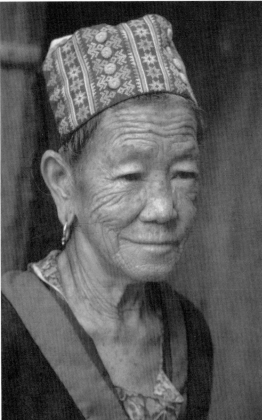

Plate 23. A medicine woman *(kws tshuaj)* wears the traditional headdress of her natal village. Thailand 2000. (KCP)

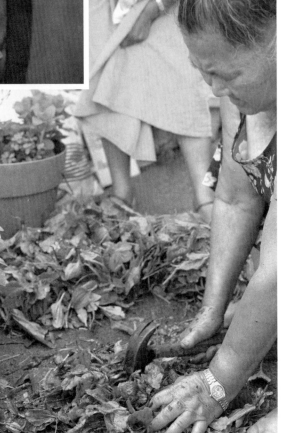

Plate 24. An herbalist *(kws tshuaj)* prepares gathered leaves by pounding them with a hammer. She will make them into a poultice. United States 1988. (Marline Spring)

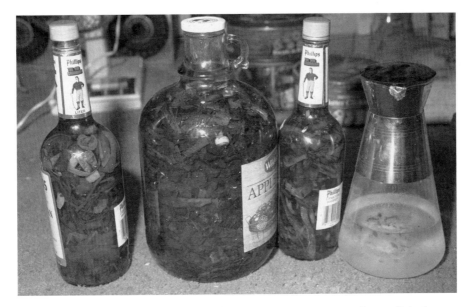

Plate 25. Herbalists cultivate or gather plants and use various parts for medicinal purposes. Plants can be pounded, steeped, or boiled. Phytochemicals may also be extracted by soaking plants in alcohol. Sick persons use botanical preparations by drinking the teas, applying the poultices, or washing their bodies with the liquid. United States 1988. (Marline Spring)

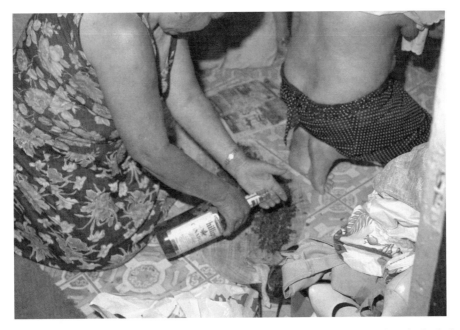

Plate 26. An herbalist *(kws tshuaj)* places crushed leaves on a cloth doused with alcohol containing extracts from other plants. When the poultice is placed on the sick woman's back, she will lie on the floor for several hours to relieve her back pain. United States 1988. (Marline Spring)

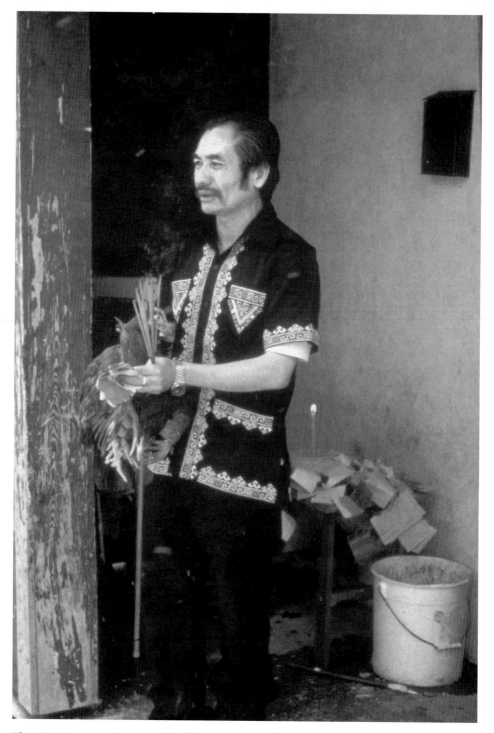

Plate 27. A man conducts a soul-calling ceremony *(hu plig)* to ensure that his family's souls are gathered together at the New Year. He stands in his doorway in front of an altar, holding a live rooster under his right arm, and incense and spirit money in his left hand. United States 1986. (KCP)

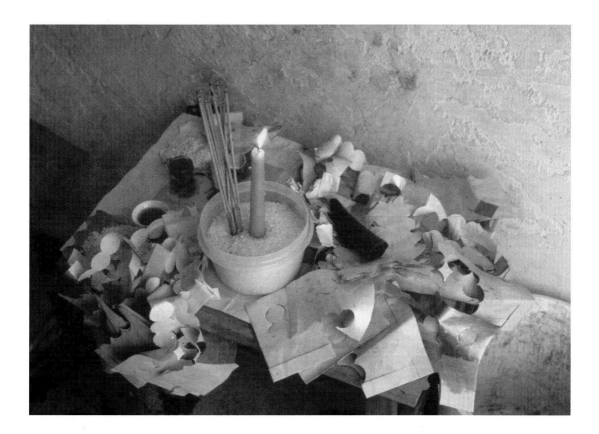

Plate 28. A spirit table is ready for a soul-calling ceremony *(hu plig)*. United States 1986. (KCP)

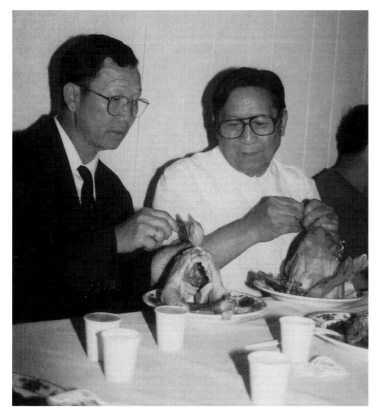

Plate 29. Men inspect the tongues and feet of two boiled chickens to divine whether the soul has returned after a soul-calling ceremony *(hu plig)*. United States 1996. (KCP)

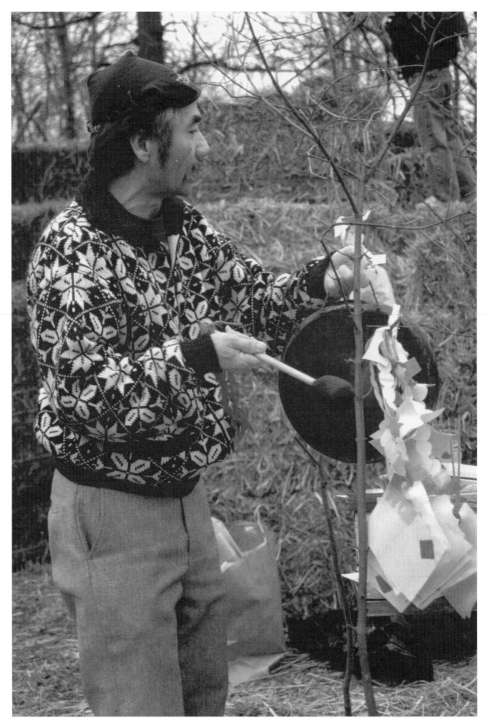

Plate 30. A shaman performs a *pauj yeem* ceremony to fulfill the promises made to spirits in a previous *fiv yeem* ceremony when someone was seriously ill. He beats a gong while chanting in front of a constructed altar including four trees at its four corners, laden with spirit money. United States 1993. (KCP)

*Commentary*

# Social and Spiritual Explanations of Depression and Nightmares

*Bruce T. Bliatout, Ph.D., M.P.H., M.S.Hyg., Dr.Ac.*

Mr. Lee, a Hmong refugee, did not recuperate from a work-related injury as well as could be expected for a man of his age and health. Explanations for his failure to recuperate include possible depression, posttraumatic stress syndrome (PTSD), and fear of nightmares or sudden unexpected nocturnal death syndrome (SUNDS). Suggestions are offered for Western practitioners on how to provide culturally appropriate mental health services to Hmong clients.

## Possible Factors Contributing to Mr. Lee's Depression

It is highly probable that depression contributes to Mr. Lee's inability to recuperate from his work-related injury. There are many factors that contribute to his depression. Being a refugee means that Mr. Lee has gone through major losses regarding family, finances, and culture. It also means that he has been relocated into a culture that is alien to him. As a refugee, he has lost his country and culture and has been resettled from a rural to an urban setting. Traditional Hmong culture is dependent on the extended family's living in close proximity to support each other economically and socially and to protect each other from outside danger. It is likely that Mr. Lee is unhappy with the loss of his culture. Without the support of the traditional extended family and village, he feels unable to raise his children in a traditional manner.

On an emotional level, his loss in economic and social status, as well as his loss of control over his family life, has likely resulted in a great loss of self-worth. While living in his homeland, Laos, and serving in the military, he commanded a good salary and a high measure of respect. Upon becoming a refugee, he found he could qualify only for menial jobs, and these jobs provide even less benefit to him and his family than does being on public assistance. He does not see any sense in struggling to better himself because he thinks it is impossible to do so in his present circumstance.

Mr. Lee probably does not have a strong educational background to help him understand or adapt to his situation. Most Hmong of his age group have limited formal education, sometimes not even as high as sixth grade, because the Hmong in Laos lived mostly in rural areas high on the mountainsides. Formal schooling was usually available only in the lowland Lao-dominated villages. So while Mr. Lee might have served in the army, and even reached prominence, the farming and military skills he developed in Laos are of little value in his new life, either to earn a reasonable living or to help him to adjust to Western culture.

Mr. Lee is most likely very unhappy with U.S. laws and customs regarding child rearing. In Laos, if a child was disobedient, the parents had the right to beat and severely punish the child until the child became compliant. Hmong children in the United States have been quick to learn that physical abuse is illegal and they threaten their parents with this fact. Many Hmong parents lack Western education and parenting skills to bring up children in this country and culture. They often do not discipline their children, allowing them to become out of control.

A major factor that may contribute to Mr. Lee's depression is his concern about his son, whom he believes to be a gang member. In traditional Hmong society, continuity of the family, clan, and Hmong tradition is ensured through having sons. In a society where there is no social security, one's sons take its place. Parents expect their sons to earn a decent living and support them fully in their old age. Hmong society is patriarchal, and only sons carry on the clan's name. Only sons (or in some cases, nephews born to one's brothers) can perform necessary religious rituals to ensure the well-being of the ancestors in the hereafter, as well as to bring about the prosperity of the current and future family and clan members. If Mr. Lee does not have a son, or has only a son who is disobedient and not willing to follow tradition, he and his wife will have no one to care for them in their old age or to bury them properly—which is the only way for them to enter the spirit world where Hmong elders hope to become ancestors and live for eternity. Nor will there be anyone to perform the appropriate ongoing rituals to have a comfortable spiritual life once they get to the spirit world.

Mr. Lee's problem is probably compounded by the lack of other close relatives such as brothers and nephews. Besides sons, the head-of-household's brothers and nephews born of true brothers can also perform appropriate burial and ancestor worship rituals. Since Mr. Lee has only a disobedient son, and no other close relatives, his concern that no one will carry on the tradition is probably a major source of his depression. He sees a bleak future in which he will have a terrible old age with no one caring for him and no one to bury him. Thus, he will be left without passage to the way to live in peace with his ancestors.

## Posttraumatic Stress Disorders, Nightmares, and Fears of Sudden Unexpected Nocturnal Death Syndrome

Mr. Lee describes nightmares of trying to fight off a spirit, presumably an ill-intentioned spirit. Nightmares are a common symptom for those suffering from PTSD, and it is possible that Mr. Lee is suffering from this syndrome. As a soldier he probably experienced a lot of combat and encountered many deaths and gruesome events. These experiences, coupled with his loss of native culture, homeland, and extended family, could contribute to PTSD.

In traditional Hmong culture, nightmares are often given more significance than in Western cultures. It is thought that there are many causes for nightmares, some of them benign and others life-threatening. Often nightmares are considered a way in which ancestors contact the living to let them know their needs and what rituals they would like to have done for them. Sometimes nightmares are interpreted as premonitions of an imminent disaster that give the family warning and time to prepare. Other times the nightmares are perceived as caused by an evil spirit trying to attack the person or family. In fact, there is a specific kind of evil spirit, known as *dab tsog,* that tries to squash the sleeping victim to death if the victim cannot fight back hard enough.

Most Hmong adults are aware that men are at risk for SUNDS, which is usually preceded by nightmares. Fear of SUNDS may contribute to Mr. Lee's terror over his nightmares, especially because his description of his nightmares matches those of other Hmong adults and elders who describe a feeling of suffocation by the *dab tsog.* In the Hmong community, in almost every large family, one or two members may have experienced this feeling, and everyone has heard of someone who has experienced it, some of whom have died from SUNDS.

In a 1982 study that included interviews with forty-five families that had experienced a member's dying of SUNDS, about 30 percent of the families felt the death had a spiritual cause (Bliatout, 1983). Only about 11 percent of the families felt they noticed behavioral changes or mental health problems immediately prior to death. This study shows that the majority of Hmong surveyed do not believe that SUNDS was associated with recent mental health problems, including depression and PTSD. It appears, however, that Mr. Lee remains concerned that his nightmares are a precursor to SUNDS.

Mr. Lee's nightmares may contribute to his depression further if he believes they are a contact from an ancestor spirit. He is probably concerned that he does not have the resources for the necessary sacrifices and rituals to appease his ancestors. If he believes an evil spirit is causing his nightmares (there are many others besides the *dab tsog*), the problem for him is even worse, since only appropriate shamanistic rituals by an experienced practitioner can be of help. Even if traditional shaman are available in the community, strict cultural protocols must be followed to obtain their services. For example, it is rarely the sick person who seeks the shaman's service. It should be a male relative who goes to the shaman's home, usually with incense and paper money, and he must kowtow to ask for help. If the shaman agrees to help, members of the sick person's family must escort the shaman to the sick person's home, helping him carry his tools. Then they must prepare a meal for the shaman before he starts his work. The shaman usually begins with a diagnostic ritual called *ua neeb saib* and then performs a second ritual, *ua neeb kho,* that is based on information obtained during the *ua neeb saib.*

This second ritual usually entails animal sacrifice, whether a pig, a cow, or some chickens. After appropriate butchering, a specific part of the animal, such as the pig's head or the cow's right front leg, must be saved as a spiritual gift for the shaman. Mr. Lee probably feels his family cannot afford a ritual of this complexity; they do not have enough appropriate people to conduct the family's parts of the ritual or enough money to buy the animal or animals, incense, paper money, and extra food. If Mr. Lee and his family converted to Christianity, he might choose to have his minister and congregation pray for him. For some Christian families, prayer seems to be an appropriate alternative to the traditional shamanistic rituals. But Mr. Lee may feel the added stress of potential isolation from his clan and community if he gives up Hmong traditional religious beliefs to convert to Christianity.

## Depression in Hmong Adults

Depression is fairly common in Hmong adults in the United States. Members of the first generation of refugees are the ones who truly make the transition from one culture to another. They must learn to walk in the middle and incorporate two vastly different cultures and belief systems while dealing with grief and struggling to survive economically. Many Hmong adults get depressed dealing with changing family roles as more wives enter the workforce and children, who are depended upon to translate English, take on more family decision-making functions.

Many adults, particularly former military personnel and their families, have the firm feeling that because of their past service and sacrifices, the U.S. government owes them some sort of assistance for many years or even for the rest of their lives. They fought what they consider to be a U.S. war. They lost family members, witnessed the destruction of their whole way of life, and, in many instances, became disabled. They helped because the U.S. government promised them that Laos would be free for them to live in, but this has turned out to be untrue. Some refugee families entered the United States on the assumption that they would indeed be on assistance for the rest of their lives. Since the standard of living provided by welfare or disability is satisfactory to some adult and elderly Hmong, they may not be motivated to adapt to Western culture or to seek education, new friendships, or gainful employment. Furthermore, some Hmong elders do not believe they have the ability to learn English, and others believe that since they are already "old," they should be supported by the U.S. government or their children and be allowed to live in retirement.

In traditional Hmong society, people usually married young, had their children young, and had grandchildren as early as in their late twenties and early thirties. Once there are grandchildren, a Hmong couple can go into semi-retirement, leaving the leadership of the family and clan to the eldest or most suited son. Thus, many Hmong who are only in their forties already consider themselves "old" and feel they should not be asked to reeducate themselves and go out to work at menial jobs. Not only do Hmong elders suffer from the trauma of the war, loss of culture and homeland, loss of status and respect, the need to adapt to a new and urban lifestyle and changing family roles, they must also adapt to a new concept of what "old age" is in their new country and put up with U.S. expectations for those who are considered only middle-aged. Should these Hmong lose their welfare or disability benefits and be forced to go to work, they are likely to become depressed. And the older the person is, the more likely there is to be a significant level of depression.

### Traditional Beliefs and Practices regarding Depression and Mental Health Problems

The Hmong are aware that at times members of their families undergo changes in behavior and that one of these changes can be depression. They believe that what causes depression is similar to what causes any other illness, including recalcitrant pain. Hmong beliefs about the cause of many illnesses is intertwined with their traditional religious beliefs. They believe, for example, that an ancestor communicating a need to the living causes benign illnesses and that nature and evil spirits co-exist in the world and if offended, or sometimes for no reason, these spirits may attack humans and cause serious and terminal illnesses. From Buddhism they have incorporated the belief that a person is reborn over and over again and what one does in past lives affects the present life. Some illnesses, including mental illness, can be due to paying a karmic debt.

Most Hmong traditionalists believe that each person has three major souls. Each soul has three more "shadow" souls. Thus, each person has twelve souls in all. All twelve souls must be intact for a person to be well both mentally and physically. The more souls that are gone and the longer the souls are gone, the sicker the person is likely to be. It is often thought that an ancestor, nature, or an evil spirit has captured one or more of a person's souls, causing illness. Sometimes trauma or extreme emotion can cause the loss of soul. When the manifestation of the loss of soul is emotional, such as depression, it is commonly and literally referred to as a "difficult" or "broken liver" problem, known as *nyuab siab* or *tu siab*. The perception among Hmong people in a situation such as this is that because the soul experienced trauma and depression for a long time, it became so unhappy that it decided to leave the body. It may or may not have been captured by a spirit. It may simply be wandering somewhere "lost."

Western practitioners should not misconstrue this "broken liver" concept to mean that the Hmong person or community believes that something is physically wrong with the liver. Rather, this is a term used to refer to a person who Western practitioners might think has mental health problems. It is not unlike the word "broken hearted" found in the English language—it describes a state of being or feeling. While English describes many feelings in terms using the word "heart," for example, light hearted, big hearted, and open hearted, the Hmong feel that the liver is the organ where emotions reside and thus use "liver" terms to describe emotional states (see Chapter 1, Tables 1.3 and 1.4.).

There are a variety of traditional Hmong healing methods for mental health problems. Usually a family will use their own resources before seeking outside help. For example, most heads-of-household or elders in a family know how to perform a simple soul-calling ceremony *(hu plig)*, which entails the sacrifice of two chickens, one hen, and one rooster. For more complicated soul calling or to communicate with ancestor, nature, or evil spirits, a Hmong shaman is required. Again, strict traditional protocol must be followed to obtain these services.

There also exists a traditional form of counseling for those with mild mental health problems. Often, family members will have elders of the family or clan talk privately with the one considered sick. Many times in conflict situations elders will mediate between family members until a compromise is reached. On rare occasions, community leaders may be sought to provide such counseling.

## Recommendations for Western Providers

Understanding that depression, nightmares, the fear of SUNDS, and the possibility of suffering from PTSD could all contribute to Mr. Lee's physical well-being, and addressing these issues in a cross-culturally appropriate way, will probably help Mr. Lee recover from his work-related injury. Understanding Mr. Lee's expectations will help the Western practitioner better map out Mr. Lee's treatment plan and be more effective. In Laos, Mr. Lee would be semi-retired, his son and daughter-in-law taking over the farm, and he would enjoy his grandchildren and help the family financially only as much as he felt willing and able to. He feels that his past service in the military gives him the right to this type of life even though he is living in a new country and culture.

Mr. Lee needs a lot of health and mental health education. Counseling and classes should be provided to help him better understand the difference in expectations between Western and Hmong culture. It should be shown in a positive way how an adult remains productive in Western culture until at least age sixty-five, and what benefits this brings to himself and his family (e.g., there is a longer life expectancy in this country, those who work usually receive better retirement packages than those on Social Security income, and many employers' medical plans are better than Medicaid).

Classes and counseling in coping with changing roles should also be provided. Many Hmong fathers have difficulty prioritizing children's needs. They often provide some things the child does not value and deny other things the child values (e.g., refusing to pay for a child to participate in extracurricular activities but purchasing a very expensive car). A comparison of what Hmong parents expect to give and receive from their children with what Western parents expect should be covered so that Mr. Lee can better evaluate his relationship with his son.

He should be reassured that a relatively low percentage of Hmong male adults actually die from SUNDS and that immediate intervention, such as getting an ambulance to the house quickly, can prevent death. Making sure he and his family are comfortable with the 911-emergency system should be part of his education.

Western practitioners working with Hmong clients should become cross-culturally sensitive and aware. If Mr. Lee knows that his caregivers understand and are at least neutral to, if not supportive of, traditional health care practices, he may feel more comfortable about seeking and complying with Western treatments. Usually the appearance of knowledge and acceptance of traditional beliefs will go a long way in earning trust among Hmong clients. Every attempt must be made to assure the client that he is being treated in the same way as any other client with the addition of cultural sensitivity. It should be clear that clients from all backgrounds have the same average waiting time before seeing the practitioner and receive the same quality of care and types of medication.

Hmong people with mental health problems usually do not go to a practitioner for counseling in the Western sense. They go to a practitioner for treatment of physical problems. If they seek counseling at all, it is from the elders in the family or community leaders. In general, if a client like Mr. Lee has access to members of his extended family or clan, he should be encouraged to strengthen those ties. If his clan has elders, he should be encouraged to seek counseling from them even if it will be primarily a support group for him. Traditional rituals and sacrifices, such as the soul-calling ceremony or the shaman's ceremonies, may be encouraged, but it behooves a Western practitioner not to unduly emphasize these practices since the family may not have the necessary resources. In general, a Western practitioner would be more tactful not to strongly urge a Hmong client to seek traditional ceremonies or counseling but gently find out whether such services are even available to the client. If the client mentions these rituals himself, however, the practitioner should be supportive.

For clients who are possible candidates for Western counseling, the psychologist or counselor should be introduced as someone who knows more about Western health problems and lifestyles and is able to help the person make a better transition. It should be carefully explained that there is a different concept of time in Western and Hmong treatment. While most traditional practitioners (e.g., shaman) give a specific time when the person will get well, in Western treatment, counseling may be ongoing as a person slowly gets more and more healthy. With education of both the client and practitioners, Western health care and mental health counseling can be made more attractive to the Hmong client, family, and community.

Clients who express an inability to access traditional healing or religion should be guided to explore other options, such as church groups, support groups, mentoring services, and other suitable agencies that can help ease the loss of support many Hmong refugees feel. The referral should not be just a name and a telephone number on a piece of paper. It is better to have the agency's contact person initiate a meeting with the client, family, and, if at all possible, the clan leader. It is important to understand that within the Hmong culture, individuals do not ask for services of this nature; the service provider should invite them in, welcome them, and offer respect.

Some Hmong persons respond better to alternative health care, such as acupuncture and herbal therapy, especially for recalcitrant pain that can aggravate mental illnesses such as depression. These kinds of services were available in Laos and of course in China where the Hmong originated. Some are familiar with and like these kinds of treatments. It may be helpful to provide the client with a list of community providers and as these treatments are rarely covered by health insurance an explanation about responsibility of payment may be necessary.

## Reference

Bliatout, B. T. (1983). *Hmong sudden unexpected nocturnal death: A cultural study*. Portland, OR: Sparkle Enterprises.

*Commentary*

# Depression and Posttraumatic Stress Disorder: Prevailing Causes and Therapeutic Strategies with Hmong Clients

*Vang Leng Mouanoutoua, Ph.D.*

Depression and posttraumatic stress disorder (PTSD) appear to be the most common psychiatric problems among Hmong refugees from Southeast Asia (Kroll, Habenicht, & Mackenzie, 1989). These emotional problems can be attributed to the fourteen years of the "secret war" in Laos, little or no prior exposure to Western culture, multiple losses of close relatives, difficulty learning survival skills in the United States, failure to have meaningful lives in their new environment, and intergenerational conflicts due to different rates of acculturation between children and parents.

This commentary explores one Hmong male veteran's perception of his depression and PTSD, the role of psychosomatic pain in his psychological problems, the influence of the Hmong belief system on his perception of his mental problems, and potential treatment. The comments reflect only this writer's experiences in dealing with the Hmong in clinical settings.

## Perception of Depression

The Hmong do not have equivalent terms for Western diagnoses of depression or PTSD. Instead they view psychological problems as evidence that a person has too many worries, too much fear, excessive distress, a troubled mind, or distraught souls or that the person is crazy *(vwm)*. Like other middle-aged Hmong refugees, Mr. Lee may perceive his depression as a form of an excessively troubled mind or disturbed souls. He may believe that his mind is so disturbed because he has had unbalanced relationships with his family, friends, environment, body, or the spiritual world. Mr. Lee has not learned English and has not attained any marketable skills. He depends on his son or daughters for translation and for making decisions about how to deal with the outside world. Also he has seen his children become Americanized and adopt many undesirable U.S. values. Mr. Lee's thirteen-year-old son has joined a gang, which may exacerbate the father's loss of hope in the future. Mr. Lee, like other Hmong fathers, may have high expectations that his son will succeed in school. He may feel very disappointed when his son does not do well at school and has trouble with the law. He likely thinks that he has failed in what he sees as his responsibility to correct his son's troubled behavior, earn a living for his family, and protect his family. His role has changed drastically, from the head of a household to a dependent member of the family. This diminishing of his familial status may intensify his feelings of helplessness and depression.

Mr. Lee's roles in the community are likely affected as well. Since he may not have skills that are transferable to his new environment or sufficient knowledge about it, he may have lost the respect of his relatives and friends and other people in the community. He may not be consulted with or visited by relatives as he and his father had been in his homeland. He may have had to relinquish his community role as an elder; community members may show more respect for young people who speak English and possess technological skills and scientific knowledge. His lack of progress in medical treatment, his feeling constrained from using physical punishment as a disciplinary tool for his out-of-control son, and his losing respect from the community may have reinforced his sense of personal deficiency and led to more social withdrawal, psychological distress, and feelings of depression.

## Psychosomatic Pain and Depression

Culturally, Hmong men are taught to tolerate life's challenges without complaining and detach themselves from their emotions, especially negative emotions such as anger, sadness, and helplessness. Psychological distress is considered very personal and private, not to be shared with people outside of the family circle. To cry, to show distress, or to lose one's temper are considered signs of weakness that humiliates not only the individual but also the family, and having a depressed or "crazy" family member can have a significant impact on the family's reputation, status, and association with the community. Hmong men rarely seek help for emotional or psychiatric problems. They do not feel it is appropriate to seek assistance from healers in the community until their emotional distress has become so severe that it affects their physical well-being.

Mr. Lee may have been depressed before he fell from the ladder. The physical pain in his back, legs, and arms may have exacerbated his depression and taxed his capacity to tolerate stress. Seeking help for pain is culturally justified. Somatizing his emotional problems therefore becomes an acceptable way of seeking help. However, presenting his emotional problems as physical ones will likely reduce his chances of being seen by appropriate mental health professionals.

## Perception of Posttraumatic Stress Disorder

PTSD has been described by the Hmong as having a "distressed and fearful mind, or frightened soul." Men who experience symptoms of PTSD usually have frequent nightmares about their past war trauma as well as a fearful and distressed mind. Many men believe that during their dreams, their souls re-visit the horrible war scenes or that decomposing bodies of deceased family members, friends, or war comrades visit them. In some dreams, malevolent spirits in deformed or decayed body forms are seen to come alive, chase after the sleeping individuals, and try to suffocate them as they sleep. Intensely fearful of dying, these men attempt to fight off the intruding spirits but are limited by their feeling of being physically paralyzed. Such a struggle usually results in total physical exhaustion, intense and lingering fear, and a sense of helplessness and hopelessness. These feelings keep the men from falling asleep, affect their interest in daily living, and take away their positive outlook in life.

In the United States, shamanic rituals are still performed to ward off malevolent spirits, create a protection zone for the client, and return the lost soul of the sick person. However, many people report that in the United States these rituals are less effective in helping them to ward off evil spirits in their nightmares than they were in Laos. The rituals seem to free them from encountering evil spirits in their dreams and to have a less distressed mind for only a few days. Others see little or no positive effect, and they come to think that the recurrent nightmares, lingering fear, episodes of fright *(poob siab)*, and agitated moods may not have a spiritual cause. As a result, they may resort to Western medicines to help them fall asleep and slow down their thought processes. In the meantime, their nightmares, intrusive memories, and other types of relived experiences continue to terrify them.

## Influence of Shamanism

The Hmong belief system deeply influences how people perceive and deal with physical and emotional problems. Hmong believe that benevolent tame spirits *(dab nyeg)* and ancestors' spirits *(dab niam txiv)* will protect the living if people treat them properly. Malevolent wild spirits *(dab qus)*, spirits of people who died a violent death and spirits of people who did not receive a proper funeral, can make people sick, capture their souls, or take their lives. Another type of spirit, the good and powerful "neng spirits" *(dab neeb)* dwell with Hmong shaman, helping them diagnose illness, negotiate with and fight off offending spirits, and heal spiritual and physical ailments.

Mr. Lee, if he has a firm belief in Hmong animism, may interpret significant changes in bodily sensations, thought processes, and emotional states as being caused by spirits. He may interpret his frequent nightmares about the war as frightening encounters of his souls with malevolent spirits. If he has already unsuccessfully tried shamanic rituals, herbal medicines, or magical rituals, he probably feels even more helpless and depressed.

## Components for Building Trust and Alliance

Service providers who wish to create and maintain trust with Mr. Lee must attend to the physical environment in which services are rendered. A proper setting is one with which Mr. Lee can identify and feel comfortable, for example, an agency or therapy room with Southeast Asian art or objects. Such a simple and often overlooked arrangement may help the client feel accepted. It may reduce any feeling of alienation, foster a less defensive stance, and create a sense of emotional connectedness with the therapeutic environment.

Another important factor is Mr. Lee's perception of the Western mental health service providers. He may see his therapists as representatives of an agency, wise men who know all about his problems, or just another set of authorities like many he has seen in the past. His expectations will guide his interaction with and reaction to providers. For example, if Mr. Lee perceives his service providers as a part of his health care and expects the providers to prescribe tangible and beneficial treatments, he may feel disappointed if the treatments do not alleviate his problems. Then he will certainly seek services elsewhere for what he believes is correct and effective treatment.

A third and closely related factor is the client's perception of his role in the treatment. Mr. Lee, for example, may expect his service providers to cure him of his physical pains, while he remains passive. Or, he may expect the providers to secure certain benefits for him, such as a disability rating or a handicapped license plate. It is crucial to work with the client early in therapy to explore his expectations of the mental health services so that he will understand his role in the treatment process and also understand what his providers can and cannot do for him.

In Mr. Lee's culture, people initiate and maintain relationships through rituals and exchanges of visits or labor. Therapists who deal with Mr. Lee might consider using a similar strategy to build a therapeutic alliance with him. For example, the therapists may make a home visit as a gesture of concern and acceptance. The therapists' participating in one or more of Mr. Lee's community or cultural events may help him see the therapists' sincerity and respect for him and his culture. However, these suggestions do not exclude the significance of empathic understanding, genuineness, and unconditional positive regard in creating a trusting alliance in the clinical setting.

In addition, non-Hmong-speaking therapists should not overlook the importance of spoken language interpretation. Incorrect and inadequate interpretation can generate a host of problems, including inaccurate description or understanding of symptoms and their severity. These in turn may lead to improper diagnoses and inappropriate treatment plans that do not engage the client in the therapeutic process. Providers should begin by ensuring a seating arrangement that best facilitates clear and comfortable communication. What is said by both client and provider must be accurately and completely interpreted. If the interpreter fails to understand what the service providers say, time must be taken to clarify the communication. It may be necessary for the interpreter to take notes to convey a lengthy message. All that is being said should be interpreted without modifying or omitting important words. Finally, debriefing time with interpreters may help providers address subtle cultural issues and concerns. Service providers' attempts to ensure the precision and quality of interpretation will enhance accurate understanding of the client's thoughts and feelings and the development of trust.

Maintaining confidentiality, as well as informing the client about confidentiality protections, may help promote trust and self-disclosure in the therapeutic relationship. My experience working with middle-aged Hmong people indicates that therapists who act with integrity, are sincere in their desire to help, and make efforts to reach out to their clients are the providers that Hmong clients come to rely on.

## Treatment Approaches

Culturally sensitive and appropriate treatment for Mr. Lee involves a comprehensive approach that helps alleviate his problems and allows him to regain his level of functioning as soon as possible. Providers should offer Mr. Lee an initial orientation that covers the possible connections between emotional problems and bodily pain, what resources are available to help him with both, the importance of his own participation in treatment, and his rights as a client. Mr. Lee's family should be helped to understand the nature and likely causes of his emotional problems and to avoid labeling him "crazy." Such education should be designed to help his family assist and support him in his treatment.

Mr. Lee needs skills and a better understanding of how to cope with his loss of status, grief over losses of relatives and colleagues, depressed feelings, agitated mood, and intense fear associated with reliving the traumatic experiences of the past. He needs to create meaningful life experiences in the United States and feel hope for the future. Some appropriate interventions that appear to achieve these goals include challenging and reframing many of his self-defeating or negative thoughts, providing support, teaching body relaxation and guided imagery, using systematic desensitization or eye movement desensitization reprocessing to help diffuse his fear responses, normalizing his memories and encouraging him to use culturally appropriate grieving processes to deal with his losses and survival guilt. Referring Mr. Lee to parenting classes may help him learn new ways both to care for and discipline his children.

Linking Mr. Lee to a support group of Hmong men who suffer similar emotional problems would help reduce his sense of isolation and sadness. Constructive projects and activities carried out by members of the support group may help him regain a sense of community and self-worth.

Participation in a job rehabilitation program is another crucial service component that will help Mr. Lee regain a sense of integrity and self-worth. Such a program would assess him in terms of his strengths, transferable skills, and preferred jobs, assist him to learn pertinent pre-employment and job skills, and encourage him to get a job as soon as possible. Research has shown that education and employment (Mouanoutoua & Brown, 1995; Westermeyer, Neider, & Vang, 1984) are significant buffers against depression and anxiety.

Case management to coordinate treatment efforts among Mr. Lee's primary doctor, physical therapist, psychotherapists, and indigenous healers, such as shaman, herbalists, and spiritual healers, would help ensure that Mr. Lee receives needed services. Providers who are new to rendering services to Hmong clients are urged to seek consultation from experienced staff or cross-cultural specialists to create a supportive and culturally appropriate environment.

Mr. Lee may perceive his suffering as encompassing the social, psychological, physical, and spiritual problems of his life. In order for him to develop a healthy sense of self, have constructive relationships with his family and community, and regain a level of physical functioning, providers must create a relationship that will engage his trust and develop a treatment plan that is culturally appropriate and has his active participation.

# References

Kroll, J., Habenicht, M., & Mackenzie, T. (1989). Depression and posttraumatic stress disorder in Southeast Asian refugees. *American Journal of Psychiatry, 146*(12), 1592–1597.

Mouanoutoua, V. L., & Brown, L. G. (1995). Hopkins symptom checklist-25, Hmong version: A screening instrument for psychological distress. *Journal of Personality Assessment, 64*(2), 376–383.

Westermeyer, J., Neider, J., & Vang, T. F. (1984). Acculturation and mental health: A study of Hmong refugees at 1.5 and 3.5 years postmigration. *Social Science and Medicine, 18*(1), 87–93.

# 11

# Domestic Violence

## *A Case Story*

Mai Pa Thao was two years old when she and her family came to the United States from a refugee camp in Thailand. She has a large, close family and is highly acculturated. She and her husband, Nhia Ger Thao, have been married for six years and have two children, aged two and five. She is now pregnant with her third child. Recently, she and her husband began having arguments, and during one especially heated episode, her husband kicked her. Fearing that he might hurt the baby, she called the police. The police referred Mrs. Thao to a local clinic, where she began working with a counselor experienced in domestic violence among Southeast Asians. She told neither her husband nor her family of her visits with the counselor.

Mrs. Thao's and her husband's families were aware the couple was having difficulty. The two families met with the couple to counsel them and asked that they be patient and try different ways to work out their problems. They disapproved of Mr. Thao's kicking his wife and of Mrs. Thao's calling the police. They suggested methods for them to talk to each other and to improve their relationship but gave no timeline for the resolution of the problems; nor did they give Mrs. Thao the option to leave.

Two weeks after the family meeting, there was another argument and Mr. Thao kicked his wife again. This time she was hospitalized. She contacted her family and told them about her work with the counselor. Her family called the counselor to find out what role she was playing and what help was being recommended to their daughter. The counselor was trying to arrange a shelter placement for Mrs. Thao. Her family was opposed to this solution and wanted her to stop meeting with the counselor. The counselor explained the importance of keeping Mrs. Thao safe and not forcing her to go back to her husband. Her family promised to intervene to help her before allowing her to return home to him.

Family leaders from both families, including uncles, brothers, fathers, and others who understood the situation, met at the home of a member of Mr. Thao's family. Mr. Thao and his family accused Mrs. Thao of having a lover and of carrying another man's child. Mr. Thao was upset and kept saying he did not trust his wife and was afraid she would leave him. He took no responsibility for their problems. His family begged her family to stop the involvement of outsiders. After a long discussion, everyone agreed that if Mr. Thao abused Mrs. Thao again, her family would "open the door" and permit her to leave the marriage. They would also support her should she wish to take additional steps, such as seek a restraining order.

# Questions for Consideration

## Questions about Culture

How is domestic violence understood and addressed in traditional Hmong families? How is it understood and addressed in mainstream U.S. families?

What are the most important stressors in the Hmong community related to domestic violence?

How has the understanding and incidence of domestic violence changed since the Hmong have immigrated to the United States?

What incentives or disincentives are there to report domestic violence to the police?

How might Mr. Thao's accusation of his wife's extramarital sexual activity influence the families' reactions to the violence? What would the families' attitudes likely be if the baby were not his?

Why might Mrs. Thao's family have been opposed to their daughter's seeking the help of a counselor? How do these reasons compare with attitudes prevalent in mainstream U.S. families?

What risks does a Hmong victim of domestic abuse take when she seeks help outside of the family?

## Questions about Cross-Cultural Health Care Ethics

What are the most important differences between the counselor's and the family's perception of best interests in this case?

What are the largest barriers to Hmong families' trust of Western-trained counselors, police, and U.S. courts?

What differences are there in family and professional roles and responsibilities in Hmong and American families struggling with domestic abuse?

## Questions about Culturally Responsive Health Care

How can health care professionals and institutions be more culturally responsive to reports of injuries due to domestic violence in Hmong families?

From whose perspective is this case successful?

What might health care professionals and institutions do to encourage Hmong families to seek assistance for problems of domestic abuse?

*Commentary*

# Traditional Hmong Concepts of Wife Beating

*Mymee Her, Ph.D., and Chue Pao Heu*

Several issues are critical to the constructive examination of this case: differences in the concept of domestic violence in mainstream American and Hmong cultures, traditional Hmong concepts of marriage, traditional social mechanisms for preventing and handling extramarital relations and wife beating, and ways in which professionals can better help Hmong families, including acculturated families, with issues of domestic violence.

## Domestic Violence

In contemporary U.S. culture, domestic violence is seen as acts of physical violence directed toward a spouse. The violent acts are seen as out-of-control behaviors that are inexcusable no matter what the reasons or the intentions may be. The aggressor is often the man, since usually he is physically stronger than the woman, and he may be held accountable for his violent behavior in a court of law.

In Hmong culture, domestic violence is understood differently. The phrase "domestic violence" is not directly translatable into Hmong. The closest translation is *ntau quas puj** (wife beating), which refers to acts of violence against a wife, but not against a husband, and includes acts of violence by a live-in boyfriend toward his girlfriend, since the Hmong consider the live-in situation a marriage. However, because a woman with a live-in boyfriend has not undergone the traditional wedding negotiation, she has little recourse in the Hmong community when she experiences violence at the hands of her boyfriend.

In "spousal abuse" (a U.S. concept) the violent behavior is seen as abusive and undesirable. "Wife beating" (a Hmong concept) does not necessarily imply abuse; it has both negative and positive connotations. According to the negative connotation, a husband's behavior may be out of control and violent, and indicative of a lack of patience, poor impulse control, and bad anger management. This type of behavior is recognized as abusive by the Hmong. According to the positive connotation, a wife

---

*Hmong terms are in the Green Hmong dialect.

may require discipline for engaging in socially undesirable behaviors, such as being lazy, being unfaithful, abusing opium, or spreading false rumors that destroy family relationships. While both forms of "wife beating" are viewed unfavorably in the Hmong community, "wife beating" as a disciplinary action is sometimes considered acceptable because it is can be seen as necessary. In this sense, "wife beating" is viewed somewhat like the Western practice of corporal punishment of children. Although not universally accepted, it is seen as sometimes justifiable by some individuals.

Wife beating is rare in traditional Hmong culture because Hmong culture has built-in social mechanisms (discussed below) that safeguard women from physical assault by their spouses. Less severe cases of wife beating can often be resolved using these social mechanisms. The cases that reach the courts and social services in the United States are usually extreme and generally do not represent the behavior of the Hmong community as a whole. Because of lack of research in this area, it is not known how often wife beating occurs among the Hmong since their arrival in United States, and it is difficult to determine the role that economic stress and acculturation have on its occurrence.

## The Traditional Hmong Marriage

The Hmong culture is patriarchal; the man is considered the head of the house. He makes sure that family members act properly and according to the expectations of the extended family and the community. This responsibility entails teaching and disciplining family members, including his wife. Mild disciplinary actions might include scolding his wife or taking her to her parents to be counseled, which is often a very embarrassing process.

When a Hmong man marries, her family collects a bridal fee. The Hmong term for marry is *yuav quas puj,* which literally translates to "buy a wife." The price is called *qe taub hau* (price of a head). When a bride is bought, she is considered "dead" of ties to her family. This means that her loyalty and duties no longer lie with her family but with her husband's family. Her family's duty is to help her realize that she no longer belongs to them, that instead she belongs to another family *(yog luas tuab neeg).* They are to teach her to adopt the ways of her husband's family and be obedient to the elders and influential members of her new family. One common phrase is, "If your family are thieves, you must become thieves like them so that you can get along with them" *(yog luas ua tub saab los yug yuav tsum tau ua tub saab es yug txhajle yuav hum luag).* This is not meant to be taken literally but is meant to illustrate to a woman the importance of complying with the ways of her husband's family.

It is costly to purchase a bride. A family may have to sell its livestock to get a wife for their son. She then becomes their most prized possession. The bridal fee cements the relationship between the two families. It stands for the commitment the husband's family makes to the wife's family to take good care of their daughter, and it may compensate the wife's family for their grief and loss.

The bridal fee also serves as collateral. If, on one hand, a wife cannot fulfill her obligations—to be dutiful, hardworking, faithful, and honorable to her husband and family—she may be sent back to her family, in return for the bridal fee her family collected. On the other hand, if the husband mistreats the bride, he is expected to send her back, without getting the money back.

The overall goal of a marriage is to remain together. It is the duty of the extended families on both sides to help the couple do so. Divorce is very rare. It is granted only if the wife's life is in danger, the wife does not fulfill her role and is formally sent back to her family (*xaa rov qaab*), or the wife has an affair and the husband no longer wants to be married to her.

## Extramarital Relationships

Although the Hmong culture is polygamous and men are permitted to have extramarital relationships, most Hmong prefer that members of their family not have them. In general, the Hmong recognize that extramarital relationships cause a great deal of distress, both emotionally and financially. Having an extramarital relationship just for pleasure is considered irresponsible and frivolous. The only time extramarital relationships are acceptable is when the man intends to marry an additional wife to better the family as a whole. He would normally do so if his first wife is unable to bear children, if extra help is needed on the farm, or if he wishes to maintain the activities of typically large families or assist his brother's widow.

Women, in contrast, are never permitted to have extramarital relationships because the woman is seen as belonging to the husband. Generally, it is the husband's duty to guard (*kaav*) her well by spending a lot of time with her and helping her. Doing this, the husband keeps himself and his wife from being unfaithful.

Infidelity is rare among traditional Hmong women, given the consequences that they must endure. If a woman has an affair and is discovered, she is met with a great deal of shame and is expected to be reprimanded. Some members of the Hmong community believe that it is appropriate or forgivable if the husband beats his wife to teach her a lesson. In some cases, a beating shows that the husband still cares for his wife and wants her back. The beating is considered a way of showing how much he cares (*mobsab*).

The wife's affair needs to be formally addressed by both her own and her husband's extended family. If the wife admits wrongdoing (*nyoo*) and asks for a pardon (*thov*), promising to be faithful from then on, the husband is expected to take her back. There are cases where husbands are so angry that they would rather get a divorce. Most of the time, however, husbands take the wives back because they have paid for their wives. If the wife decides that she would rather be with her lover, then the lover must pay the husband the bridal fee that the husband paid when they married, and divorce is granted so that the lover and the wife can be married.

If a pregnancy results from an extramarital relationship, the wife needs to decide whether she wants to remain with her husband or go to her lover. If the wife decides to remain with her husband, the lover is expected to pay a fine. A portion is meant to "fix the husband's face" (*khu tug quas yawg lub ntsej muag*), and a lesser portion is paid to the relatives involved to ensure that they will continue to assist the couple with issues related to the affair in the future, especially those that involve the child and how the child is treated by the husband.

The child is considered the husband's child, and the husband must never call the child illegitimate. Further, he must love and provide for the child as his own. This expectation is justified because the lover has given the husband money to correct the wrong to the husband. It is understandable that the husband may not feel emotionally close to this child, since it reminds him of his wife's infidelity. However, it is expected that the child's basic needs will be met.

## Social Mechanisms to Prevent Wife Beating

Traditional Hmong family and social structure has several methods for preventing the husband from abusing his authority and beating his wife. Parents and relatives commonly teach young women to "look carefully at the roots [history and background] of the young man before marrying him" *(saib luas caaj luas ceg zoo zoo tsuav maam le yuav)*. If his relatives beat their wives, it is likely that he will also beat his wife.

More formal preventative measures are implemented during the marriage proposal hearing. First, if it is known that members of the groom's family have a history of wife beating, especially of a woman from the bride's extended family, then the groom's family is reprimanded *(nplua)* and the groom and his extended family must pay a fine to the bride's family to correct the wrongdoing of his relatives. This indicates to the groom and his family that the bride's family will not tolerate wife beating, should a marriage be granted to this bride and groom.

Second, the new wife is assigned a guardian, who monitors how she is treated by the new husband's family. This person is an older man from the wife's family, an older brother or cousin. This person is usually related to the wife by blood, since it is believed that a biological relative will care more and will respond more quickly to her needs than a non-blood relative. If he sees that she is being mistreated, it is his duty to investigate. Then he must bring this problem to the attention of the wife's extended family to be formally addressed.

## Traditional Methods for Resolving Problems of Wife Beating

If wife beating occurs, the wife must issue a formal complaint. If she believes that the husband's relatives have influence over him, then the most appropriate way to deal with the situation is for her to go to her husband's relatives first, before appealing to her own relatives. This action shows that she honors her husband's relatives and increases the likelihood that they will help her in the future. It also gives the husband's family a chance to save face, by keeping the crisis in the family, and allows them a chance to intervene before the crisis goes to the wife's family, where matters would become public and cause a great deal of embarrassment.

Customarily, the wife gives her husband's family three chances to intervene. After that—if the beating continues—she appeals to her own family. Initially, she would leave her husband and go to the home of her parents or brothers, declaring that she no longer wishes to be married to her husband because he beats her. Her family, in turn, would formally request that the husband's extended family come and discuss the matter. If the husband's relatives respond, then a hearing is scheduled. If, after a certain length of time, there is no reply, it is assumed that the matter is closed. Word is sent to the husband's family indicating that, since they have not responded, her family considers the marriage dissolved.

If the husband and the relatives do respond, a hearing is held to discuss the problem. In Laos, if after three hearings the husband continues to beat his wife, the case is sent to court and no relatives from either side would remain involved. When a formal hearing occurs, the goal of the proceeding is to preserve the marriage. According to the Hmong, a marriage is like a fire. When it dims, the job of the relatives is to put more wood into it, guard it from the wind and rain that would put it out completely, and rekindle it. The hearing takes the form of mediation. One mediator from each side of the family conducts the hearing, attempting to determine what the problems are, how each person contributes to the problems, and ways each person will compromise to accommodate the needs of the other.

If the mediators determine that the wife is at fault, then she will be advised to go back to her husband and try to work things out. Typically, a wife is at fault if she is short-tempered or lazy, taunts her husband by daring him to beat her to show that he is a man, or causes family problems by her lack of involvement with her husband's family. The worst violation of the wife's role is for her to become involved in an extramarital affair. Fault against the husband includes failing to perform his role as head of the house and provider for the family. It is of utmost importance that the husband not "play around" *(ua si)*. Playing around includes frivolous affairs with no intention of marrying, neglecting responsibilities in the home, and beating his wife for no acceptable reason. If the husband is found to be at fault, then he and his relatives must formally apologize to the wife and her extended family and promise that the husband will change. The relatives are responsible for ensuring that the husband upholds his promise to change.

From a traditional Hmong perspective, three main issues must be addressed in the case of Mrs. Thao: the beatings, the alleged extramarital relationship, and the paternity of the child. Initially, Mrs. Thao's family has to insist on knowing why she is being beaten. In fact, both families have to determine whether the beating resulted from Mrs. Thao's failure to fulfill her obligations as a wife or whether Mr. Thao cannot control his temper. If the reason for the violence is simply Mrs. Thao's inability to perform her duties, Mr. Thao's beating her will be seen as drastic. He will be accused of using improper disciplinary action, since his response should fit her behavior.

In the case of Mrs. Thao, there is an allegation of infidelity. Mrs. Thao's family must determine the truth of the accusation of infidelity. Should the allegation prove to be true, Mrs. Thao would be at fault, and the beating might be considered justifiable. It is important to find out who the father is, whether he is Hmong, and whether he abides by the traditional cultural expectations. In cases where the man is not traditional Hmong, it is likely that some families will disregard the issue of paternity when paternity is uncertain, since U.S. laws do not correspond to the traditional Hmong way of handling issues of paternity. Perhaps with the advent of tests to determine paternity, some Hmong will turn to more technologically advanced means of establishing paternity and use them to resolve marital problems.

If the allegation of infidelity is proven false, then the beating is inexcusable. Mr.

Thao and his family then must formally apologize to Mrs. Thao's family for making such false accusations and Mr. Thao must promise not to beat his wife again. An older member of Mr. Thao's family, someone Mr. Thao respects and obeys, must agree to serve as a mentor to him, consulting and making sure that he does not physically harm his wife in the future. In this case, when Mrs. Thao's relatives said that they would "open the door" *(qhib hlo qhov rooj)* for her to leave the marriage, the family saw this statement as a second warning to her husband. If he beats her once more, it would be his third offense, and she would be free to do as she pleases with her family's blessing.

## Seeking Help Outside of the Hmong Community

Mrs. Thao was very young when she came to the United States. She seems quite comfortable with the U.S. culture, as evidenced by her willingness to see a U.S. counselor. However, she also appears to respect the traditional way of resolving conflicts. Thus, she struggles with whether to listen to her family or to the counselor. If she listens to her family, she may feel as though she has sacrificed her sense of individuality—a U.S. concept. If she listens to the counselor, she may lose the support of her family.

Historically, the Hmong were nomadic, moving from country to country, either because they were driven out of one country and into another by force or because they were fleeing economic difficulties. They were able to maintain some political independence in some of the countries to which they migrated. In Laos, for example, the Lao government allowed the Hmong to maintain their traditional judicial practice *(kev hais nplaub)* and take care of their own problems, unless families and village leaders asked for help. This flexibility created a separate-but-related co-existence between the Hmong and the Lao government. In the United States, most Hmong are unfamiliar with the government and its laws. They approach life in the United States the way they did in Laos, where they were allowed to handle matters within the Hmong community.

The Hmong worry that Western cultures may not understand how important the family and the extended family are to the overall functioning of the Hmong society and are afraid that Westerners will cause the family to break up. They are convinced that the U.S. system prefers to separate families rather than help them work out their problems. In the United States, the role of the service provider is to protect the weak, the ones who are physically unable to protect themselves (children and women). U.S. law assumes that it is always wrong for any man to hit his wife, whatever the reason. The law does not look at the reasons behind acts of wife beating.

A Hmong couple that seeks help from outside of the culture strays from the traditional ways of handling marital conflicts. Because a Hmong marriage is based on a whole network of verbal contracts and agreements that often involve the whole family system, going outside of the culture with marital conflicts derails the process of resolution, since the original agreements have no meaning in U.S. courts.

When a couple or one member of the couple seeks help from outside of the Hmong community, a breakdown of the family system may have already occurred, and the traditional way of resolving marital conflicts may no longer work. The couple could be too Americanized and may no longer accept the traditional process of family mediation.

## How Professionals Can Help Families Deal with Wife Beating

### Assessment

Working with families that have experienced wife beating requires a thorough, step-by-step assessment of cultural values and expectations of both the Hmong and U.S. cultures and an intervention plan that carefully integrates these values and expectations. First, the service provider should take inventory of his or her needs, attitudes, and anxieties in helping Hmong families. Not knowing what to do can make the provider feel paralyzed and inadequate. It is important, therefore, to adopt a learning attitude and allow the wife to take the role of teacher (an expert on her own culture) and ultimately, be the decision maker about her future. The Western service provider must be willing to let go of his or her need for control and allow the wife to take the lead, with the provider in the role of helper. Taking the lead empowers the wife to take responsibility for her actions and allows her to actively participate in the decision-making process with the provider serving as a guide.

Second, the provider needs to understand the woman's perception of why she was beaten. To gain this understanding, the provider may violate the customary procedures of Western intervention in domestic violence situations. Most Western domestic violence programs are based on the premise that asking why she was beaten puts the wife (labeled "the victim") at risk for self-blame and increases the likelihood that she will return to her husband ("the abuser"), where she will be subjected to abuse once again. Because people in the United States are individualistic, a U.S. woman who has been beaten may have no other social recourse. However, the Hmong social system has a built-in mechanism to deal with wife beating, so when it is appropriate, it is important to allow this system to work for the wife. Assessing the woman's perception of why she was beaten will help the service provider anticipate how the family will react to the beating and help the service provider participate in cultural proceedings and develop contingency plans, should the cultural interventions not work.

The third area of assessment is to address the woman's expectations of the service provider. How does she want the service provider to help? Is she seeking a divorce and not being supported by the culture, or is she seeking help for her family so they can stay together? Is she afraid she will lose her children by proceeding with a traditional Hmong divorce, and is she therefore turning to the "Western culture" to ensure a divorce that increases the likelihood that she will get custody of her children?

The fourth area of assessment is to conduct a thorough evaluation of the wife's support system: the availability of the immediate family for direct support and the authority of the extended family to influence change in the wife-beating problems. It is important to find out whether the family is intact or separated as a result of the war and to find out who died and who survived. If there are surviving relatives, where do the closest ones live? Do the surviving relatives have any authority to intervene? The authority to intervene in marital discord is determined by the level of respect the man holds in the community and his experience, credibility, and sense of fairness. Additionally, it is preferable that he be related by blood to the woman—typically, from the same extended family (perhaps a distant uncle or cousin)—and must be older than the husband. Members of the nuclear family (father, mother, brothers, and sisters) rarely serve as mediators because of the fear that they would be too emotionally involved and would not be objective or fair.

If there are surviving relatives, it is important to determine whether they are willing to support the woman and, should she choose to divorce her husband, to help her get started in a life independent of him. If the woman's immediate family members have died or live overseas, the service provider may be able to link her to a new set of relatives, perhaps extended relatives whom the wife did not know—for example, a distant cousin or uncle.

The fifth area of assessment is the acculturation level of the woman, her husband, and their extended families. As Hmong families become more Americanized in behavior and attitudes, they may become more individualistic in their approach to conflict resolution. They may become less group-oriented and rely less on Hmong leaders and family legal procedures for input and direction. They may be aware that the traditional problem-solving methods are not recognized by U.S. laws and therefore may be less relevant to their current situations. A useful tool is a set of questions to be answered using the Likert Scale. Ask the clients: "On a scale of zero to ten, zero meaning you are not Americanized at all, and ten meaning that you are as Americanized as your American friends, how Americanized are you?" In cases of wife beating, it may be useful to ask this question of both extended families to get an idea about how willing they are to collaborate with the U.S. system.

The sixth area of assessment focuses on the personal strengths and weaknesses of the woman who has come in for services. How well is this woman able to function independently, without the support of her family? Knowing the woman's personal strengths and weaknesses helps a service provider assist her to develop a realistic and appropriate plan of action. The needs verbalized by the woman may be different from those determined by the service provider. A Hmong woman who does not want a divorce may feel pressured to get one because Western service providers often urge women to separate. The woman will be sorry she called for help, because she believes she will have lost in the long run. When she makes decisions that do not align with the Hmong culture, will her community see her as single-minded and not respectful of her elders? If she is no longer supported by the family, will she be able to find support from outside her family? Is she willing or able to make friends outside of the Hmong community, should she be ostracized by her own community? If Western intervention fails, the woman will really have nowhere to turn. Will this be more detrimental in the long run than to have tolerated a difficult marriage?

The seventh, and probably most important area of assessment, addresses risk factors: What emotional and psychological risks will this person be taking if she forgoes the help of her family? Is she socially able to survive without her family? If she goes against her family, will her family be willing to forgive her? If they do not forgive her, can she function without them?

Providers using Western models of conflict resolution often ignore cultural implications, especially when it comes to sensitive issues surrounding women's rights. When families come for help to resolve domestic violence issues, providers may assume that the best course of action is to separate the family, so that the woman and her children will be safe. If a woman refuses to separate or divorce her abusive husband she may be labeled as "weak," "helpless," or "dependent," making her the cause of her beating. When working with a Hmong woman, it is important for service providers to respect the life from which she came. Few wish to risk losing the support of their families.

## Intervention

Initially, the response to wife beating is crisis management, and the task is to ensure the physical safety of the wife and children. At this juncture, the woman needs to decide for either traditional Hmong cultural involvement or Western involvement. If she wants to remain married and wants help from the culture, she may already have gone to the house of a relative. If she does not want culturally specific intervention, an emergency shelter (the usual U.S. approach) may be sought. Once she is safe from immediate danger, it is time to begin the long-term intervention plan, which involves responding to the needs of the family as they move beyond the initial crisis. If it is determined that the wife beating resulted from disciplinary actions, it may help to ask her whether she wishes to involve her family in a mediation process. If she wants to work things out with her husband, the service provider will need to elicit the support of the woman's extended family, who will need to take her to the home of one of her brothers to proceed with culturally appropriate mediation.

If the extended family is fragmented, the service provider may need to help the woman locate her family so she can ask for their help. This assistance is especially appropriate for a Hmong woman who may not know her culture as a result of growing up in the United States or who is not aware of her own family's whereabouts. The alliance she creates by eliciting extended family support will be helpful in the long run, after the resolution of the present situation.

If the wife beating is a result of the husband's bad temper, it is important to know how chronic and severe the problem is. It is important that the provider always help the wife decide what she truly wants, even though the service provider's values may conflict with the wife's values. Does she want a divorce or does she want to try to work out the problems if her husband gets some help? If she wants them to stay together, then the service provider must get her husband in for counseling to control his temper. He needs to be informed that wife beating (domestic violence) is a serious offense in the United States, that it is against the law, and that recent legislation has made domestic violence a deportable offense. While the husband undergoes counseling, it is important to pursue the cultural mediation process. This helps re-establish the couple's link to the extended family.

If the wife wishes to get a divorce, then the role of the service provider is to educate her about how to go about formally getting the marriage dissolved. Hmong women may not know how the U.S. system works, and the service provider may be their only link to legal services.

## Conclusion

The Hmong woman's role in her society is quite different from that of a U.S. woman. Advising her to leave her support system requires that one question how well she will adapt to an outside world. It is far more dangerous to remove a Hmong woman from her traditional support system than it appears to an outsider. Western systems often separate families and leave family members isolated and with limited long-term support. In traditional Hmong culture, couples are counseled to remain together after a wife-beating incident, and a support system is set up so that the couple would more likely be able to succeed in working out conflicts in the long run.

## Acknowledgments

Special thanks to my father, Chue Pao Heu, who has worked alongside me as a co-author of this commentary. We strove hard to be as accurate and sensitive as we could to both the Hmong and the U.S. cultures in our presentation, and my father's wisdom and knowledge is never-ending. Thank you, Father, for showing that your love and support never ends, no matter how "grown up" I become.

*Commentary*

# Changing Gender Roles and Domestic Violence in the Hmong Community: A Feminist Perspective

*Pacyinz Lyfoung, J.D.*

## Traditional Hmong Marriages

The concept of domestic violence is fairly new in the U.S. culture, but it is even more recent in the Hmong culture. Before the Hmong people came to the United States, the concept of domestic violence was unknown. Although people frowned on a husband beating his wife, families tended to fail to see the situation as a problem that required intervention or else valued women's safety less than other objectives. Perspectives on gender roles and spousal prerogatives and responsibilities are based on the traditional purposes of marriage and preserving the traditional social structure of the Hmong people.

Traditionally, the Hmong community is both patriarchal and hierarchical with a clear social order from top to bottom: clan leaders, elderly men, other men, elderly women, other women, and children. Duties to serve and obey accumulate according to one's location on that ladder; women are traditionally subservient to men. The patriarchal nature of the Hmong culture is tied to male-dominated clan structures and rituals. Men have the exclusive right to pass on the clan and family affiliations and to perform rituals marking the life cycle of the Hmong people. This social arrangement is explained by spiritual beliefs: men "lead" the ancestors' spirits, whereas women have no ties to the ancestors. It reflects the gap between men's greater and women's lesser value.

Gender disparity is reinforced by marriage customs. Because men pass on the family name and women do not, men remain with their natal homes and families, whereas women change clans upon marriage. Similarly, because men perform important rituals they must stay in their clans, whereas women can be transferred to other families. Hmong elders justify this gender division in several ways: women are too busy with their duties and men have more free time, so they can perform the rituals; men are taught the rituals, whereas women are taught only to cook and prepare the food for the rituals; and men "lead" the ancestors' spirits, so only men can perform the rituals. Because girls and women are transient members of the family, they have a secondary value, and less energy, time, money, and education are invested in them. Some consider it wasteful to nurture a daughter who will bring benefits only to her in-laws. Furthermore, because the main role for a Hmong woman is to maintain a household and raise children, women's academic education or preparation for work outside the home is less important than their training as future wives. Finally, coming from other clans, women are considered outsiders and, as a result, their husbands' clans tend to feel less attachment and loyalty to them.

After a couple settles down in the husband's village, the preservation of the clan structure continues to promote gender disparity in the marriage relationship. Along with their privileges, men have many clan and family obligations to their fathers, uncles, brothers, and cousins. Men also have obligations to their wives and families, but clan ties are stronger than marriage ties. Unless there is a shortage of men in a clan, it is considered embarrassing for a man to rely more on his in-laws than on his clan members. Since men are busy with clan and extended family duties, most of the domestic duties, such as maintaining a household and raising the children, fall to the women.

Traditional Hmong marriages do not rest on romantic love. Only recently, in the 1960s, as more Hmong people moved from the remote hills of Laos to settle in the valley of Longcheng or in the capital city of Vientiane, have they encountered Western notions of love and integrated the notion of romantic courtship and love. Before then, Hmong traditions strictly limited social contact between young men and women. The concept of eligible young men visiting young women in the safety of their homes, now an established and respectable custom, used to be unheard of. Except once a year during the New Year celebration, young people's only opportunities to catch a glimpse of each other occurred at funerals. The three-day-long marriage negotiations, which encompass all the history between the two families and clans, including settling past grievances and debts (monetary and nonmonetary) and anticipating future debts, seeks to seal the union between the families and clans. Although there is certainly a desire to form family and clan alliances and a desire to find a mate for one's child, the ultimate purpose of Hmong marriages is to continue the clan line and produce the next generation. The spouses do not need to have a romantic relationship or even a close relationship. Because spouses' lives are expected to center more on the extended family and clan than on the nuclear family, spousal relationships tend to be relatively distant. There is often both a lack of closeness and a lack of stress in the relationship.

Traditionally, there is little discussion between spouses about sexuality or reproductive options. Men do not speak about their desire but just start groping and reaching under clothes. Women do not initiate intercourse. If women do not want to participate in sex, they are not free to refuse their husbands. Nonconsensual sex and unwanted pregnancies are not considered domestic violence. They are presumed to be a wife's duties.

## Hmong Marriages in the United States

Resettlement in the United States has fostered the breakdown of extended family and clan structures, since Hmong refugees were relocated in different areas of the country and the demands of modern life conflicted with the traditional community life. As a result, individual family units have become more isolated. Individualism is emerging as the perceived need for clan and family obligation fades. Consequently, men and women are living in much more interpersonal marriages than in the past, and, with less extended family and clan to act as buffer, there is more stress between the spouses, increasing the risk of marital tension and domestic violence.

Since immigrating to the United States, many Hmong men have complained about women's rights. Now, they say, there are more family conflicts because women want their own way, want to get an education, want to work, want fewer children, do not show the proper respect for men, neglect the children, and so on. Men feel more stress and may, therefore, become more abusive, as they experience cultural and social displacement from being sole family wage-earners and sole family authorities. Other acculturation issues include the lack of familiarity with U.S. laws and lifestyles, as well as the lack of access to resources, all of which isolate and alienate Hmong refugees and new immigrants.

While communication about sex, pregnancy, and contraceptive choice has improved, tradition continues to affect the present and many people are resistant to changing the old ways. The standards and expectations set for Hmong women are so high that women cannot meet them. But many women try, and many think that it truly is their duty to meet them all. Even educated (and therefore, presumably more progressive) women strive for the traditional ideal, both to show their respect for the traditions and to compensate for having strayed from the norm when they chose to pursue an education. Their sense of duty is not limited to their husband but is extended also to their in-laws and their families. Physical and verbal abuse is often excused as a man's prerogative to discipline his wife when she fails in her duties. Hmong women have a hard time believing that they have not failed in their duties and that they do not deserve to be punished.

## Domestic Violence

In a case of serious domestic violence, the wife typically seeks help from her family and asks for an elders' council meeting to be convened to mediate or adjudicate the accusation. Since traditional Hmong perspectives on marriage have a significant impact on families' attitudes regarding domestic violence, Mr. Thao's accusation that his wife engaged in extramarital sexual activity greatly influences the families' reactions to the violence.

Accusations of infidelity are the most effective defense for a Hmong man's mistreatment of his wife. Mr. Thao needs to prove that his wife committed adultery and that the baby is not his. It must be proved that there was sexual intercourse and not merely flirting or stealing the wife's affection. The way Hmong people see it, if there was an affair, there must be witnesses, because it is impossible to meet without anyone else knowing about it. If the baby is not the husband's, then he may return his wife to her family in disgrace and ask for her bride-price to be returned. He can also force her to denounce her lover and seek reparations from him and his family.

If the husband is unable to prove infidelity, he can still seek a divorce from his wife based on his accusation, but he cannot recover the bride-price. If the wife is able to prove that there was no infidelity, she can force him to take her back and ask the families to stop the abuse, or she can ask for a divorce. If the clan system's justice is applied, the husband will be penalized for injuries, including fatal injuries, to his wife and unborn child. In Laos men have been known to give away or sell children who are the result of infidelity.

Although the Hmong people like to emphasize the clan elders' council system, which offers an opportunity for Mrs. Thao to be heard, it is more likely that with an accusation of infidelity Mrs. Thao will be perceived as having failed in her most fundamental duty: to be faithful so that the children she produces are truly her husband's and the clan's. Accused of adultery, she will be perceived as having disrespected her husband and his clan and threatened the social and spiritual order. This transgression is very serious and often has the effect of cutting off most sympathy for a wife. Although the action is not approved of, a husband thus wronged could beat his wife. Others in the family may be outraged but may choose not to intervene.

Unless the physical violence escalates to the point at which Hmong women fear for their lives, most women will not report domestic violence to their families, a counselor, or the police. There are many disincentives: the traditional lack of support from family and clan members who feel a lesser degree of loyalty to daughters and daughters-in-law, the traditional expectation that women are the ones who must sacrifice to husbands and families, the effectiveness of men's accusations that the woman must be having an affair, the large size of most Hmong families that makes it difficult for a woman to support the children on her own, lack of education and job skills sufficient for the woman to support herself and her children, and the stigma of being a divorced woman or a family with problems. As long as life is bearable, women often will sacrifice as they have been raised to do and as the community expects them to do. Other family members are very unlikely to report domestic violence. When caught in the middle of conflicting family loyalties, they are likely to shy away from getting involved in spousal disputes.

A precondition for an awareness of domestic violence is the recognition of women's rights, such as women's rights to not be beaten, to say no to sex, or to control their reproductive choices. To address domestic violence is to address issues concerning rights, roles, and responsibilities. Much of the resistance to discussions of domestic violence can be traced to the concern that redefining women's roles threatens the core traditions that hold Hmong society together.

## Turning to Counselors and the Courts

In cases of domestic abuse, there are likely to be important differences between a counselor's and a family's value commitments, approaches, goals, and definitions of a successful outcome. On the one hand, families may be deeply rooted in their cultural beliefs and traditions. Their primary concern may be to preserve the fabric of the community by avoiding the clan and family frictions that occur when spouses experience disputes, and by focusing on keeping the family together. On the other hand, the counselor is trained to focus on the client and to put the best interest and safety of the individual woman first.

Health care professionals and institutions can effectively respond to reports of injuries due to domestic violence by being sensitive to their clients' culture without compromising the fundamental mandates of their profession. In this case, the counselor should present options to Mrs. Thao only after assessing her safety and the safety of the fetus. The counselor should also make arrangements for follow-up, in case more violence occurs and the family still does not effectively intervene. Most important, Mrs. Thao should be supported and validated at all times, so that she is enabled to make her own decisions without feeling pressure or disapproval.

In terms of legal options, Mrs. Thao could seek an order of protection if she wishes legal safeguards from abuse and injuries. There is flexibility in the kind of protection that she can request from the court. She can choose to live in the same household as her husband but be safe from abuse. She can choose to exclude her husband from the premises, or keep him a safe distance from places where she works, takes the children, goes to school, and so forth.

In terms of criminal remedies, Mrs. Thao could file assault and battery charges, as well as domestic violence charges against her husband. There would be an investigation and a hearing. In both civil and criminal court, Mrs. Thao could request that the court order Mr. Thao to go through mandatory evaluation and treatment for his abusive and violent behavior. If Mr. Thao were convicted of fifth degree assault or domestic violence, he could be deported if he is still a refugee or a resident alien and has not become a citizen.

To help the extended families better understand the seriousness of domestic violence protections and penalties in the United States, the counselor can thoroughly explain those legal issues or seek the assistance of an advocate or an attorney who can explain them. These actions can help the families understand the importance of protecting Mrs. Thao from further abuse or physical injuries and help the families enforce the decrees of the elder council, such as promises to intervene or promises to free a wife from an abusive marriage.

# 12

# Woman with Psychosis

## *A Case Story*

Bao Ly, a sixty-one-year-old widow with a history of psychosis, was brought by her stepson to see her psychiatrist because she was much worse. For several weeks she had talked about demons incessantly, stating that the spirits were living in her body, eating her liver, and telling her to kill people. She had threatened her stepson and his family with a knife and then turned the knife on herself, saying that she wanted to kill the evil spirits living in her liver. Sometimes she spoke in a language the family did not understand, and sometimes she talked with people who were not there, such as her dead husband and his dead wives.

Seeking a cure, her stepson had arranged for several shaman ceremonies to protect her from the evil spirits. After each ceremony she was better, but only for several days. Her stepson was trying to arrange for a very powerful shaman to come from Laos to exorcise the evil spirits. Before he could pay for the trip, Mrs. Ly became more violent, and he sought the psychiatrist's help.

The psychiatrist knew that Mrs. Ly, a widow for two years, had been the fourth wife of a man who had had five wives. In Southeast Asia, her husband had been married to three wives concurrently. Two wives had died, and one wife had run away. By the time he married Mrs. Ly, he was a single man with six daughters. Childless herself, Mrs. Ly raised the six daughters as her own. Many years later, she and her husband decided that he would marry a fifth wife so they could have a son who would take care of them in their old age. Mrs. Ly had not known how she would react when the beautiful fifth wife gave birth to a baby boy. Enraged and jealous, she hired a sorcerer to curse the younger wife, who subsequently died in the process of giving birth to her second child, a daughter. Mrs. Ly's subsequent regret and guilt had fueled her depression for years.

As she talked with the psychiatrist at this visit, it was apparent that she was convinced that the fifth wife was taking revenge. She felt helpless and hopeless and was convinced she would be killed by the dead fifth wife or by the evil spirits or that she would kill herself. Against her wishes, the psychiatrist admitted her to the hospital, placing her on a seventy-two-hour hold to protect others and herself and to treat her psychosis.

An interpreter came to the locked in-patient psychiatric unit for thirty minutes every day, but otherwise there was no one who could speak Hmong with her. She complained to her stepson that she could not stay there and begged him to take her home. She refused to take the medications, maintaining that she was not crazy *(vwm)* but rather was possessed by spirits. The psychiatric team explained that the medicines would protect her body and mind from the evil spirits until her stepson could arrange for the definitive shaman ceremony. She reluctantly agreed, and over the next two weeks, she improved.

Before she was released, her family members expressed gratitude for the care and help she had received, but they also expressed their anger about her being called crazy and their frustration that there was no English translation for the spiritual problem causing her suffering.

## Questions for Consideration

### Questions about Culture

Typically, how are mental illnesses such as psychosis understood and treated by the Hmong? How does this approach differ from the views and practices of U.S. psychiatrists?

What is the significance in Hmong culture of placing a curse on someone?

What are the Hmong social norms and expectations regarding men married to multiple women?

What impact has Western psychiatry had on the Hmong understanding of, and openness to, the medical treatment of psychiatric disorders?

### Questions about Cross-Cultural Health Care Ethics

How (if at all) should the care of this woman differ from the usual Western approach to treating patients with her disorder?

How can Western psychiatrists explain psychosis to a family who holds different beliefs about the cause and nature of such problems?

### Questions about Culturally Responsive Health Care

What does this case reveal about disclosure and communication skills with Hmong patients?

What cultural considerations should a psychiatrist take into account before ordering a seventy-two-hour hold, over a family's objection?

How might the psychiatric team build the kind of trusting relationship that would encourage the patient and family to turn to the team, especially in times of crisis?

How might the psychiatric team and the shaman work together to relieve Mrs. Ly's distress?

From whose perspective is this a successful cross-cultural relationship?

# Commentary

# Cultural Interpretations of Psychosis

*Joseph Westermeyer, M.D., Ph.D.*

## Cultural Issues

### Hmong Understanding of Psychosis

As the anthropologist J. M. Murphy (1976) has observed, all peoples have a term for mental illness. Often these folk terms are equivalent to the English term "crazy" in that they connote a feared condition, since people do not treat or interact with a "crazy" person on equal, rational terms. The Hmong term for "crazy" is *vwm* (which sounds like "vuh" in English). Although people might use the term loosely (for example, "I was almost crazy from worry"), the application of the term to specific individuals followed certain social processes and involved the use of certain folk criteria (which bore much resemblance to psychiatric criteria). Although the prevalence of psychosis is not known among the Hmong in either Asia or the United States, the occurrence seems neither lower nor higher than that observed in other groups (Westermeyer, 1988b).

The range of concepts regarding psychosis among the Hmong in the United States today reflects the changing worldview of Hmong people, as they become acculturated to this society. However, in villages in Asia a few decades ago, the largely illiterate, animistic Hmong shared common beliefs regarding psychosis. These beliefs resembled those of adjacent ethnic groups, such as village Lao peoples (Westermeyer, 1979). Psychosis, and indeed any major illness or misfortune (such as crop failure), were likely to be caused by an angered spirit (say, the spirit of a disrespected object or place or a ghost spirit of a deceased person) and might involve the loss of one of the body's spirits or souls (say, through fright or demoralization).

Although the peoples of Laos (including the Hmong) generally viewed mental illness as having, in theory, spiritual or preternatural origins, in individual cases they looked for specific personal, interpersonal, or environmental events to "explain" the mental illness. Typical explanations included worry, stressors, loss, and insults to the brain (for example, trauma or infection). They could also include interpersonal relationships gone awry. Allegations of witchcraft growing out of interpersonal conflict could be such an explanation, since in Hmong folk theory, either spirit assault or soul loss might be induced by witchcraft.

The datum about this patient's hiring a sorcerer to harm the fifth wife warrants further attention. Although one hears allegations about sorcery often in Southeast

Asia, admitting to active sorcery efforts for homicidal purposes is extremely rare. In many settings in Asia, such efforts would be seen in the local culture as attempted murder (if unsuccessful) or murder (if death ensued). For this reason, "magic experts" *(tus ua khawv koob)* or "spirit experts" *(tus ua neeb)* would be unlikely to cooperate in such an effort since it could lead to their ruination or even death. It would be more likely that Mrs. Ly sought the services of a "magic expert" or "spirit expert" to enhance her own attractiveness, or to sway her husband toward her and away from the fifth wife. These efforts, while not especially honorable in the Hmong value system, would not constitute a major crime. Once the patient has recovered from her psychosis, this matter might be raised again; Mrs. Ly may be admitting to crimes she never committed in the midst of her psychosis. This content does suggest lingering guilt or shame with regard to the fifth wife that might be ameliorated in psychotherapy (Westermeyer, 1979).

If a person thought he or she had been cursed or if a healer made the diagnosis of a curse (as cause for an illness or misfortune), the suffering individual or family could oppose the curse through spiritual means. They would hire a "spirit expert" who would then enter the spirit world to do battle against the offended spirit who caused the problem or search after a lost spirit or soul and return it to the body.

### Polygyny and Mental Health.

Only a small minority of Hmong practiced polygyny in Laos, certainly less than 5 percent and probably less than 1 percent. Bride-price was expensive and in most cases required the combined wealth of many male relatives. Unless a man were unusually wealthy, he would ordinarily not take a second wife.

Hmong culture prescribed that, ideally, the decision to take a second wife belonged to the first or "major" wife as much as to the husband. If a decision were made to bring a second (or subsequent) wife into the marriage, the major wife often would make the choice. Often she chose a sister of her own clan, perhaps even a younger sibling or close cousin. Motivations for a second wife were often economic, since a second wife increased the potential for accumulation of wealth through poppy farming, gardening, and small animal husbandry—activities in which women participated or even took the lead. Some women wanted a younger wife to share the many chores of child-bearing, child-rearing, cooking, carrying water, carrying firewood, making clothes, and so forth. Occasionally, women recommended their spouseless friend or relative as a potential wife. Perhaps less often, women might have wanted a second wife in order to have a son. For example, the wife of a man who had eight daughters badgered him for several years beyond her own child-bearing to take a second wife. She had young, attractive relatives of hers come and stay with them for months at a time, hoping that a second marriage might develop. He resisted for several years, averring that "one wife could produce small problems, but two wives always produced big problems." As her efforts grew more frenzied (with weeping and begging), he agreed to take a second wife. Within weeks of doing so, he died in a plane crash. Several months later, the much younger second wife gave birth to a son, whom she gave to the major wife before subsequently marrying another man.

Understanding such attitudes, beliefs, and behavior is difficult for many European Americans, who are steeped in Western notions of romance, marital intimacy, and husband and wife as intimate best friends. Although passion and romance were known and idealized in Hmong society, they were often viewed as too evanescent and flimsy a basis on which to build a family. Men spent most of their time with other men, and women spent most of their time with other women. Couples might not have shared their most private thoughts with one another but would have shared them with friends and clan members. Couples might never have expressed the terms of endearment that they might fully express to their children and clan members. By the same token, many, perhaps most Hmong partners, married because of attraction to someone whom they had seen, met, or known. Even in arranged marriages, partners sometimes developed strong emotional attachments over the years with their spouse—that is, "falling in love" after marriage and even childbearing and child rearing, rather than the reverse.

Husbands did not always pursue a second or "minor" wife in this fashion but sometimes decided independently to take a minor wife and announced the decision to the first wife—rather than including her in the decision or even letting her take the lead in such a decision. Although considered legal in the Hmong context, such a move was neither sensitive nor wise and almost always led to problems. Major wives were apt to feel disrespected or to interpret this event as a message that they were no longer attractive or important to the husband. In one case, a depressed husband in a refugee camp—impotent with his wife—took a younger wife to "cure" his affliction and then discovered he was impotent with her, too. Moreover, by this course he alienated his major wife, whose love and support he wanted and needed. In this particular case, the major wife did not develop a psychiatric problem, although she clearly was angry about her husband's decision. In addition, a considerate husband would have alternated the nights he spent with each wife so as not to stimulate competition or jealousy.

Polygyny also affected women adversely. One woman who had four daughters arranged for her husband to take a minor wife so they could obtain a son. Her plan progressed as she wished: her husband did marry someone of her choosing, and the minor wife had a son. However, the minor wife did not want to surrender care of the child to the major wife. Moreover, the minor wife managed to obtain the support of the husband in this conflict (a somewhat unusual "partnership," since typically the wives would join together to sway the husband-in-common to agree with them on some intended situation or event). In this case, the major wife became progressively more withdrawn and despondent and eventually killed herself.

Since it was impossible to survive living alone in a Hmong village, polygyny was also a means for ensuring a home for all women. In a society where death in childbirth occurred with some regularity, it was also a means for ensuring continuity of child care. Furthermore, co-wives could have provided one another with much emotional and material support. As with monogamy, it was less the system that was problematic than the fashion in which partners functioned with the system.

## Cross-Cultural Health Care

### *Management*

In much clinical care, the "proof of the pudding" is in the clinical outcome, which turned out reasonably well in Mrs. Ly's case. The psychiatrist took a conservative action in hospitalizing her, since risks for suicide and possibly even homicide existed and such risks are a major indication for psychiatric hospitalization. Although the staff had limited access to a translator, they were able to educate the patient about her medications and her need for them. Their using concepts that the patient could comprehend (that the medicines "would protect her body and mind from the evil spirits") revealed their sensitivity to nuances of cross-cultural communication of complex ideas.

Taking mentally ill patients from their families can be a relief to all concerned, especially when crisis and threat exist. However, hospitalization can also constitute a crisis to family members who want to be involved in the care of their relative and to the patient who wants to be around family members during a period of great distress. For those who are unfamiliar with mainstream U.S. culture, or even with English speech and writing, hospitalization can exacerbate feelings of loneliness or abandonment, as well as the signs and symptoms of psychopathology. Consequently, at times it may be worth the risk to attempt to manage psychosis in the home or community. With patients who pose a danger to themselves or others, the following resources need to be in place if the psychosis is to be managed without hospitalization:

- A sufficient number of people to be awake and attending to the patient around the clock (twenty-four hours a day), seven days a week, until this level of close surveillance is no longer needed
- A safe place for the patient (e.g., without access to weapons or kitchen implements, not in a high building where he or she might jump)
- A sufficient number of people at all times so that the patient cannot overpower the family "watchers"
- Medication management, so that one or a few persons control the medication and keep records of times and amounts administered;
- Adequate fluids and nutrition, together with appropriate space, light, and temperature; patients receiving antipsychotic medications, lithium, or antidepressants should not be in an overly hot setting with high humidity
- Frequent, perhaps even daily, reassessment at the clinic; this may include therapeutic response (or lack of response) to medications, side effects of treatment, or complications of treatment
- A "plan B" (for example, call 911, take the patient to the emergency room) in case the situation exceeds the family's capacity to manage it

Among many, perhaps most, native-born patients in the United States, it is impossible to organize the large number of people necessary to accomplish these "hospitalization" tasks without actually hospitalizing the patients. In the United States, relatives and friends are too busy with work and other activities, expect that such care will be provided by professionals, are not accustomed to taking on such weighty responsibilities, or are concerned about the legal or financial risks of undertaking such efforts. However, organizing a large number of people is often feasible among minority, immigrant, and refugee patients, whose families are accustomed to taking on such extensive responsibilities. Although not yet within psychiatric tradition, such care can have more rapid and salutary outcomes than hospitalization. Even if intensive home care should fail, the least restrictive alternative would have been tried first.

Virtually all societies have a term like the Hmong term *vwm* or the English term "crazy." It is important that such terms not be used with patients, since they typically connote denigration, hopelessness, deviance, and chronicity. Descriptions that take into account the patient's worldview and understanding are important. Depending on the patient and the culture, patients can understand and accept being ill with other conditions, such as "illness of the heart," "illness of the spirit," or "illness of the brain." Even widely accepted terms among North Americans, such as "depression" or "anxiety," may not be understood immediately. However, clinicians can educate immigrants, even if illiterate, to appreciate better the nature of these conditions, their treatment, and the recovery process.

## Prognosis and Rehabilitation

It is not clear in this case whether a precipitating event or stressor might be present. Despite the limitations of identifying precipitants or stressful events, the effort can still be worthwhile since future recurrences are apt to occur in many (not all) patients during times of extensive life change or "stress." By avoiding excessive "life change" over brief periods of weeks or months or by helping the patient through such periods it may be feasible to reduce the frequency or the severity of recurrences.

The greater the number of the individual's "risk factors" to mood disorder the more likely that future episodes will occur. Such factors include loss of a parent during childhood, familial mood disorder or substance abuse, certain types of brain damage, as well as certain medical conditions, and a previous history of mood disorder. The absence of these factors in the presence of appreciable loss or stress suggests a better prognosis if the patient can recover from the current illness.

Improving the prognosis can be accomplished in a variety of ways. For some patients, on-going medication with lithium, the anticonvulsants tegretol or valproate, the antidepressants, and certain other adjunctive medications can be important. Certain psychotherapies have been shown to reduce the recurrence rate or at least extend the time between recurrences. Among refugees and immigrants who are failing in the tasks of acculturation, "acculturation therapy" can be important; this may consist of coaching the immigrant psychiatric patient in making a successful adjustment to the new society, providing English language instruction for those who may have learning problems, and helping the immigrant psychiatric patient in becoming employed, as well as other interventions (see more below).

## Suggestions for Improving Care

### Diagnosis

It appears that this is the patient's first episode of psychosis. Onset of psychosis late in life is unusual with the most common psychiatric disorders (such as schizophrenia, affective disorder, delusional disorder). Thus, organic causes, contributors, or precipitants for this psychosis should be vigorously investigated. A mental status exam, taking into account information that this patient could reasonably be expected to know, is an important first step (Naguib, 1991).

The co-occurrence of depressive and paranoid content is not typical. It is seen in cases of organic psychosis, long referred to as paraphrenia in the European literature. However, paranoid symptoms are commonly seen in a variety of other psychiatric conditions among patients who are migrants or minorities or otherwise in an unfamiliar setting in which distrust may exist (Kino, 1951; Prange, 1959; Westermeyer, 1989). Thus, one might discount (but not ignore altogether) the paranoid symptoms to some extent, especially given the prominence of the mood symptoms in this case.

Organic mood disorders in the elderly have been related to prefrontal stroke and other prefrontal lesions. Those on the right side seem more apt to be associated with mania, and those on the left with depression. Causes in this age group include stroke to these areas, neoplasms, collagen disease (for example, temporal arteritis or lupus erythematosis), medications (for example, steroids, certain gastrointestinal and cardiovascular drugs, certain remedies employed by Southeast Asians in the United States), trauma (for example, subdural hematoma), nutritional deficiencies (usually B vitamins), and infection (at times related to conditions common in Southeast Asia but rare in the United States, such as parasitosis, chronic tuberculosis, or leprosy).

The distinction between organic mood disorder and so-called endogenous or functional psychosis (for example, mood disorder, delusional disorder, schizophrenia, schizophreniform psychosis) is not merely an academic one. Organic mood disorder can have a good prognosis, if the organic condition is curable. If the organic condition is chronic, psychiatric treatment is complicated by factors such as the following:

- Pharmacotherapy involving medications with strong anticholinergic activity can exacerbate the condition, the so-called paradoxical psychosis with antidepressant and antipsychotic medications
- Small doses of antipsychotic medications may be effective with organic cases (whether organic mood disorder or so-called paraphrenia or organic psychosis)
- Anticonvulsants can be useful in some cases of organic mood disorder, but blood levels should be monitored and effects on blood levels of other drugs (such as antidepressants) must be followed to avoid toxicity; these drugs seem less helpful in paraphrenia cases
- Electroconvulsive therapy is sometimes necessary in such cases to reduce the severity of the psychosis and to enhance the efficacy of medications
- Even with the best of treatment, recovery may be partial or episodic

One means of narrowing down the diagnostic possibilities is to consider the patient's symptoms. Examining this woman's psychopathology, we learn she has somatic delusions (her liver is being eaten), paranoid delusions (the deceased fifth wife is trying to kill her), and auditory hallucinations (command hallucinations telling her to kill people). Her speaking "a language the family did not understand" could be any of a variety of symptoms: word salad (typical of mania), neologisms (seen with schizophrenia or paraphrenia), a mantra or magical series of sounds learned from the past, or echolalia/echopraxia (with catatonia). Speaking with the dead, especially in Asian cultures, can be a harbinger of death, whether it occurs in sleep (while dreaming) or awake (as in this case). Such experiences, usually while dreaming but occasionally in a psychotic person while awake, suggest a mood disorder. Her assaults on others can be consistent with a paranoid disorder (delusional disorder or paranoid schizophrenia), with paranoid symptoms accompanying a mood disorder (especially in immigrants and minorities), or with uncomplicated mood disorder. Women with severe depression are more apt to be self-destructive, whereas men with severe depression are more apt to harbor a homicidal intent. The suicide threat, if she failed to die at the hands of the fifth wife or the spirits, suggests a mood disorder but does not indicate whether it has an organic cause or is "endogenous."

Therapeutic trials can also aid in making a diagnosis, which can assist with setting a prognosis and deciding on subsequent care. We do know that Mrs. Ly did better on the medications, but we do not know which medications or their dosages.

### Acculturation Therapy

Some immigrants and refugees adjust poorly to the new society, although the overwhelming majority do well, including many psychiatric patients (Westermeyer, Neider, & Vang, 1984; Westermeyer, 1988a). Factors that may conduce to acculturation failure include older age, brain damage, mental retardation, and chronic or severe psychopathology of virtually any type. Failure to acculturate consists of the inability to be able to conduct age-appropriate tasks and responsibilities in the new society, to feel comfortable and competent in the society, and to achieve productivity, security, accomplishment, and health in the new society.

Helping people adjust to a new society depends on their psychosocial resources and liabilities. For many immigrants and refugees, acculturation ensues through some training in the lingua franca of the community (English in the United States), a job outside of the home, and involvement in mainstream social institutions (such as school, church, and community associations). Failure to acculturate can ensue from various psychiatric conditions, such as depression, which undermines one's energy, interest, concentration, energy, and social interaction. Likewise, failure to acculturate can precipitate or exacerbate psychiatric disorders, by isolating the patient not only from his or her ethnic peers who are acculturating but also from the society at large.

Acculturation therapy is a complex topic too large to address here. To be sure, individualization and creativity are needed to aid a variety of patients in achieving a comfortable level of acculturation. Different approaches are needed for a child and an elderly person, or for a patient with a brain lesion compared with someone without a brain lesion, or for a mentally retarded person compared with a highly intelligent person. However, regardless of the individual circumstances, patients who have failed in their acculturation tasks can be helped. This work often requires special staff and programs not available in most psychiatric settings.

A first step is to determine acculturation goals appropriate to the person. For an elderly person, learning to speak English fluently may not be a realistic acculturation goal. However, numerous other acculturation goals are feasible, among them learning the local currency, learning how to shop in a nearby store, learning how to use the telephone to contact friends, learning how to use public transportation to get around, or attaining access to clubs or associations of age-mates.

## Working with Traditional Healers

Not so many years ago, working with traditional healers was widely condemned as "consorting with quacks." Nowadays, working with traditional healers is widely praised as evidencing "cultural sensitivity" and "practicing holistic medicine." Consultation with traditional healers, or even referral to them, is practiced, or at least urged, in some quarters.

My view of traditional healers is analogous to that regarding polygyny. They are neither evil nor an unabridged asset for the patients. Perhaps a first step in working with traditional healers is to understand a people's folk healers, since they differ in certain respects from one society to the next. Hmong healers in particular resemble traditional healers in adjacent ethnic groups of Laos, but they also differ in certain respects (Westermeyer, 1988c).

Involvement of a traditional healer, whether shaman, herbal healer, spirit expert, or another type of healer, can provide great relief to a distressed patient, as did ministrations of the shaman in this case. This benefit probably accrues in a variety of ways, among them the following:

- Naming the illness and the cause of the illness in terms that are culturally and ideologically familiar to the patient and family
- Suggesting means by which a cure from the disease, or at least respite from suffering, might be achieved, thereby instilling hope (itself a great nostrum)
- Evidencing the motivation of the family to seek any help possible, especially when previous ministrations within the family have failed
- A coming-together by family members and extended kin to contract with and pay a folk healer, thereby endorsing the inherent value of the patient to the family and extended kin

By the same token, "traditional healer" care can produce certain problems (just as can the ministrations of allopathic physicians). One problem might be called "blaming the patient for lack of therapeutic benefit;" some folk healers assure patients of a cure if they believe in or carry out specific rituals exactly as described. Any subsequent failure from the treatment falls to the patient, who "did not believe" or "did not follow the prescription." Another problem may be the patient's excessive faith that the traditional therapy will alleviate the condition, so that, if the treatment fails, the patient may become demoralized and even suicidal. A third problem is the expense that folk healing often entails. This expense can exceed that of allopathic care but is usually not recompensed by third party carriers (although the Indian Health Service does recompense some folk care among the Navajo in Arizona). These considerable expenditures, borne often by the extended family, can be a major financial burden for years (Westermeyer, 1988c).

There was a time when I recommended that patients seek the help of a folk healer. On one occasion, this recommendation stimulated an unnecessary open conflict between the patient, who did not want a healer, and the family, who did want a healer. Another time, the family determined that the only known healer competent to conduct the appropriate ceremony lived in a different country, and it would require the family's entire annual income to bring him to the United States. Likewise, there have been times when one or another folk intervention was comforting to the patient and family and not too expensive. My approach in recent years has been to leave these decisions to the patient and family and to work with whatever they decide. If they are about to spend a huge sum of money that I doubt will meet with any lasting success, I might urge them to await the outcome of the treatment currently under way.

## Comment

Many immigrant groups and all refugee groups studied so far have higher rates of psychiatric disorder as compared to the general population. There is no one disorder that predominates, although major depressive disorder, posttraumatic stress disorder and various organic causes of psychiatric disorder are probably more frequent in all refugee groups and in some immigrant groups. Psychiatric disorder can account for acculturation failure, and failure to acculturate may predispose people to psychiatric disorder. Differences in family structure require that clinicians be able to set aside their own attitudes, values, and beliefs with regard to ideal family structure and relationships. Home care may be more feasible with some immigrant and refugee groups than with native-born people in the United States. However, such nonstandard and potentially risky interventions should be attempted by an individual or team that includes a psychiatrist and clinicians familiar with the particular family as well as the culture.

## References

Kino, F. F. (1951). Alien's paranoid reaction. *Journal of Mental Science, 97,* 589–594.

Murphy, J. M. (1976). Psychiatric labeling in cross-cultural perspective. *Science, 191,* 1019–1028.

Naguib, M. (1991). Paraphrenia revisited. *British Journal of Hospital Medicine, 46,* 370–375.

Prange, A. J. (1959). An interpretation of cultural isolation and alien's paranoid reaction. *International Journal of Social Psychiatry, 4,* 254–263.

Westermeyer, J. (1979). Folk concepts of mental disorder among the Lao: Continuities with similar concepts in other cultures and in psychiatry. *Culture, Medicine, and Psychiatry,* *3*(3), 301–317.

Westermeyer, J. (1988a). A matched pairs study of depression among Hmong refugees with particular reference to predisposing factors and treatment outcomes. *Social Psychiatry and Psychiatric Epidemiology, 23,* 64–71.

Westermeyer, J. (1988b). DSM-III psychiatric disorders among Hmong refugees in the United States: A point prevalence study. *American Journal of Psychiatry, 145*(2), 197–202.

Westermeyer, J. (1988c). Folk medicine in Laos: A comparison of two ethnic groups. *Social Science and Medicine, 27,* 769–778.

Westermeyer, J. (1989). Paranoid symptoms and disorders among 100 Hmong refugees: A longitudinal study. *Acta Psychiatrica Scandinavica, 80*(1), 47–59.

Westermeyer, J., Neider, J., & Vang, T. F. (1984). Acculturation and mental health: A study of Hmong refugees at 1.5 and 3.5 years postmigration. *Social Science and Medicine, 18*(1), 87–93.

*Commentary*

# Integrating Hmong and Western Approaches to Spiritual Illnesses

*Thomas Vang, M.S.*

Hmong people traditionally believe that mental illness is caused by spirits. Symptoms of mental distress may be caused by evil "wild spirits" *(dab qus)*, such as mountain, rock, and jungle spirits, or by evil "domestic spirits" *(dab nyeg)*, such as malicious ancestral spirits. It is well known in the Hmong culture that when you have intentionally killed someone, the dead person's spirit will return and cause violence or illness to you or your family members. For example, it may cause the family members to die, go crazy, or become impoverished, and it may not be satisfied until all important people in the family are dead. Only a shaman may be able to help the family by communicating with the dead person's spirit for the family. According to these beliefs, Mrs. Ly's family deals with her problems in the traditional cultural way.

Mrs. Ly started to feel guilty right after the death of her husband's fifth wife. She believed that the fifth wife had died because she had arranged the death. Her silence increased her shame, depression, and guilt and caused her to suffer from major depression and hallucinations. She probably felt that there was no one and nowhere to turn for help. Through her hallucinations, she explained to her family what she had done to the fifth wife. The family probably felt that her past actions would bring shame and harm to them and jeopardize their future. Therefore, the family decided that her illness must be treated by offering spirit money and animal souls to the offended spirit of the fifth wife.

Turning to Western health care when traditional healing fails is a common occurrence among Hmong who live in the United States. In fact, most of the first-generation Hmong refugees initially turn to traditional methods of treatment and if they are not better, then turn to Western doctors. Since Mrs. Ly did not improve with spiritual healing alone, the family realized that she must be treated with a combination of traditional and Western treatments. Western medication helped stop her violent behavior, hallucinations, and depression. A shaman helped her deal with her guilt.

Mrs. Ly, like most other Hmong people, did not seek psychiatric help or hospitalization until she and her family members had exhausted all traditional methods of treatment. Seeing a psychiatrist was their final option. It was important for the psychiatrist to respect the patient's culture and beliefs and give her time to adjust to the idea of Western medication. The hospital's staff made an excellent intervention when they suggested that medication would help her mind and body fight off the evil spirits. This also made the family members feel more comfortable and helped them trust both the doctor and the medication.

The physician's diagnosis of psychosis, often interpreted as "being crazy" *(vwm)*, caused Mrs. Ly to lose face and to be angry. The hospital needed more than an interpreter to help bridge the cultural gap. They needed a bilingual and bicultural social worker or human services counselor who could speak with Mrs. Ly and her family about the differences in the traditional and Western approaches to this kind of illness. Mrs. Ly needed frequent assurance that she was not crazy. She also needed help understanding that Western health care providers respected the traditional Hmong point of view and that some Western medicines can be very useful in dealing with angry spirits. Arranging for frequent family visits, as well as visits from a bilingual counselor, could have reduced Mrs. Ly's feelings of isolation during her hospital stay and perhaps could have aided her positive response to the medicines. The family, too, needed the assistance of the bilingual and bicultural counselor. They needed to be reminded of Western respect for their cultural beliefs and helped to add Western treatment to their belief system, rather than be pulled into what they considered an incorrect diagnosis of craziness. Encouraging Mrs. Ly to keep sacred objects, such as spirit money and incense, in the hospital might have helped her feel more secure. Since she was experiencing relief from her hallucinations and violent behavior through medication, she was almost ensured a good recovery. If this reassurance could have been provided to Mrs. Ly by a trusted person from the same cultural background, her hospital stay might have been a better experience.

Mrs. Ly also needed follow-up from a bilingual and bicultural counselor. Often Southeast Asians unfamiliar with Western medicine discontinue their medication when they start to feel better, and the symptoms can return. However, with regular follow-up from a trusted person, they can be encouraged to continue the medicine as a powerful supportive antidote to the angry spirits causing their difficulties.

# PART VI

# End-of-Life Care

*Case Stories and Commentaries*

# 13

# Hospice Patient
# with Gallbladder Cancer

## A Case Story

Cher Xiong was a fifty-four-year-old woman with ten children ranging from eight to twenty-two years of age. She and her family had been living in the United States for fifteen years. Ever since she had delivered her last child eight years ago, she had had intermittent pain in her upper right side. Her doctors diagnosed gallstones and recommended an operation to remove the gallstones (a cholecystectomy), but Mrs. Xiong was uncertain that the invasive procedure could relieve her pain. She believed the pain had been caused by nurses who, after the delivery of her last child, had vigorously massaged her uterus over her objections.

Finally, unable to tolerate the pain any longer, she agreed to the operation. Following the procedure, the family was disappointed that the physician did not show them the gallstones, as he had promised he would. The doctor informed Mrs. Xiong and her family that she had cancer of the gallbladder and recommended chemotherapy. After long discussions, Mrs. Xiong and her family decided against accepting the doctor's recommendations for chemotherapy.

A year later, the cancer obstructed Mrs. Xiong's common bile duct, her skin became yellow, and she had abdominal pain. At this point the family asked the doctors for curative therapies, including surgery, chemotherapy, and radiation. But the physicians, understanding this to be an incurable terminal illness, offered only palliative therapies. For months the doctors tried to support her with medicines for pain control, an operation to drain bile, and a feeding tube with nutritional supplements. The specialists continued to be concerned that the family was not accepting Mrs. Xiong's terminal state. When the cancer infiltrated the beginning of her small intestine obstructing her stomach outlet, the family agreed to hospice care, including DNR/DNI (do not resuscitate/do not intubate).

Mrs. Xiong was transferred to a hospice unit, where for five days she experienced good pain control and no bleeding. She was drinking small amounts. A family member brought a video camera to record her statements; she talked about how she loved her children and wanted to be their mother forever.

On the sixth day, the patient was weaker. That night, shortly after the nurse gave her an intravenous antibiotic and flushed the line with saline and then heparin, she became drowsy and barely responsive. Family members spoke with the nurse, but the communication did not go well. From the nurse's perspective, the family was upset about the patient's declining course and was not accepting her terminal state and her impending death. For their part, the family members interpreted the nurse's questions—"Why are you so upset? Don't you know she came here to die?"—and her tone of voice as meaning that the nurse wanted the patient to die. They became very upset, convinced that the nurse had harmed the patient—having poisoned or at least cursed her.

Mrs. Xiong's room filled with relatives. Her husband wanted to take her home, given that the hospice providers could not help her get better. The family wanted her to wear the ceremonial Hmong clothes she had made. They also wanted her to be with her children, to be available for family visits, to be home for Hmong New Year, to do Hmong healing practices, and to be protected from the nurses. The family took Mrs. Xiong home.

Once she was home, many people visited, including the family's Catholic priest. Family and friends kept a constant vigil around Mrs. Xiong's bed. They tried to persuade her to wake up, eat rice, and drink water, which they offered with spoons and cups. They pleaded with her not to die, saying they needed her. The Xiong house was filled with people day and night for seven days. The husband repeatedly expressed his anger that the nurse had tried to kill his wife.

A conference was held among four male family members, the family physician, and the head nurse of the hospice unit to address their concerns about the possible poisoning. After investigating, the head nurse determined that there had been a cross-cultural misunderstanding, but no evidence of poisoning.

Three shaman came to help Mrs. Xiong, performing ceremonies aimed at diagnosing and treating any lingering spiritual problems. Almost a week after coming home, she slowly woke up, to the delight of her family. Mrs. Xiong said that her dead mother had been holding her head under water; she could see and hear everyone in the room but was unable to answer them. The family rejoiced that the shaman had been successful at separating the grandmother's spirit from the ill woman.

About a week later, on the first day of the Hmong New Year, the patient experienced rectal bleeding and infection of the parotid gland. She and her husband agreed to hospitalization for blood and antibiotics as long as the nurse they distrusted was not allowed to take care of her. Two days later she again became lethargic. When her husband understood that the doctors could no longer do anything for her, he took her home. Two days later she died, surrounded by family members who wailed in grief.

At the funeral home, the family asked the undertaker to remove the staples in her abdomen from the gallbladder operation. The family dressed her in multiple layers of traditional clothes and placed her body in a wooden casket made without nails or screws, lined with a white cotton shroud, and prepared for a four-day-long ceremony.

## Questions for Consideration

### *Questions about Culture*

How did the family's and the providers' perceptions and beliefs about etiology influence ideas about appropriate treatment?

Why did the patient and her family refuse treatment for gallbladder cancer initially and then ask for treatment later?

When are pain control measures considered appropriate? Why might an ill Hmong patient refuse pain medications?

Why did the family agree to hospice care and DNR/DNI?

How are the issues of death and dying handled and discussed in traditional Hmong families? In Christian Hmong families? In Anglo-American Christian families?

In traditional Hmong culture, what counts as a "good death" and as a "bad death?" What do U.S. hospice providers consider a "good death" and a "bad death?"

What cultural values and practices may provide barriers to Hmong families accepting hospice care? Which values and practices are congruent with hospice care?

What cultural beliefs underlie the practice of dressing the dying woman in her ceremonial clothes?

Why did the family request that the staples be removed from her body after death?

### *Questions about Cross-Cultural Health Care Ethics*

Which behaviors of the U.S. providers did the most to damage the family's trust and which behaviors did the most to enhance it?

How are love, care, and concern expressed toward a dying person in traditional Hmong culture? How well does hospice's concept of "accepting" death fit Hmong beliefs about respectful treatment of the dying?

What cross-cultural differences arose regarding the disclosure and communication of health-related information?

In what way was the family's philosophy of end-of-life care in conflict with the philosophy of hospice? What accommodations is it reasonable to expect hospice to make? What accommodations is it reasonable to expect the family to make?

### *Questions about Culturally Responsive Health Care*

What aspects of this case offer examples of a good cross-cultural relationship?

How might health care professionals prevent and respond to initial refusals for early treatment of cancer?

How might traditional remedies be combined with hospice care?

How might some of the barriers to Hmong understanding and acceptance of hospice be overcome?

What factors should health care professionals take into consideration when discussing a terminally ill patient's prognosis? When pronouncing a patient dead?

What type of grief counseling might be most welcome?

What can U.S. health care professionals learn from this Hmong family that might be helpful in their relationships with other patients?

# Cultural Complications in End-of-Life Care for a Hmong Woman with Gallbladder Cancer

*Kathleen A. Culhane-Pera, M.D., M.A.*

I am privileged to have known Mrs. Xiong. She taught me a lot. First, when I was a stranger, she invited me into her home for Hmong New Year, included me in her preparations for the feast, and explained the meaning of the soul-calling ritual. Later, when I became an acquaintance, she reached out to me at Hmong gatherings to include me in the events and shared with me her family's challenges in adjusting to life in the United States. And finally, when I became her primary care physician at the end of her life, she shared with me her physical sufferings, her struggles to find meaning in her illness, and her attempts to be cured so that she could continue to be a mother to her children. I am grateful to her for opening her home and heart and for sharing her last days with me. And I am grateful to her for the lessons she taught me about the importance of culture in illness. In this commentary, I describe what I learned about her health beliefs and about culturally responsive health care.

## Abdominal Pain and Gallbladder Operation

Mrs. Xiong suffered with pain in her upper right side for years before consenting to a gallbladder operation. When I have told her story to physicians, some have asked me, "Why did she suffer rather than consent to a curative operation? Surely it would be better to have an operation than suffer from physical pain." These questions express the biomedical perspective—that pain is physically embodied and that operations can cure the pain by removing the physical source of pain. Mrs. Xiong had a different perspective.

For Mrs. Xiong, health care workers had caused the pain and she was doubtful that an invasive procedure could remove the source of pain. She recounted that after she had given birth to her last child, the nurses had forcefully massaged her uterus and had caused permanent damage to her uterus and abdomen. Proscriptive and prescriptive behaviors *(caiv)* after childbirth are important for ensuring women's short-term survival, long-term health, including fertility, and ability to produce breast milk. For example, postpartum bleeding is necessary to rid the uterus of old blood, so that the women's bodies are clean. If the old blood stays inside, women may develop infections, become infertile, and be bothered by multiple ailments for the rest of their lives. To ensure the blood flow and restoration of the uterus, women must not encounter wind, cold air, cold water, cold foods, intercourse, or rough handling of the uterus since these can cause the blood to congeal internally.

These concepts conflict with the nursing perspective that blood must stop flowing in order to prevent hemorrhage and the biomedical practice of massaging the uterus to express clots and make the uterine muscle clamp down. Hospital personnel focus on stemming the blood flow, while Hmong people focus on ensuring adequate blood flow. Nurses vigorously massage the uterus while Hmong women gently wrap the lower abdomen in a fabric binder. Compromises between these two positions can occur; for example, women can gently massage their own bodies, and nurses can accept more than the usual amount of uterine blood flow.

Mrs. Xiong tried to relieve her pain with home therapies, such as massage *(zaws hno)* and herbs *(tshuaj ntsuab)*, and sought assistance from a multitude of healers: Chinese acupuncturists and Asian grocers with their Thai and Chinese pharmaceuticals, as well as U.S. doctors and chiropractors. Finally, unable to tolerate the pain any longer, she consented to a gallbladder operation.

Still, Mrs. Xiong had fears about the operation that were similar to other Hmong people's concerns. After operations, some people have experienced long-term incisional pain and weakness that impair their abilities to return to a job, do housework, care for children, attend school, or make love for a year or more. Other people have experienced spirit loss from the fright of the operation or the "sleeping" medicine of anesthesia. Many people have been concerned that bodily mutilations can be carried into the next life. Finally, everyone has heard stories of doctors not taking good care of Hmong people and operating for their own benefit, such as learning, experimenting, or making money, or operating on Hmong people in order to harm them or kill them (Culhane-Pera, 1987; Mouacheupao, 1999). Because of these fears and concerns, Mrs. Xiong refused the operation for years, and they were still vivid in her mind when she finally agreed to have the operation.

## Gallbladder Cancer: Initial Diagnosis and Considering Chemotherapy

Mrs. Xiong and her family listened to the news about the gallbladder cancer and the doctors' recommendations for chemotherapy but never went to see the oncologist. Physicians have asked me, "Why did they not act?" "Why did they refuse chemotherapy?" In fact, the patient and her family did act, but not in a Western biomedical way. They sought Hmong healers' opinions of her health and were reassured that she was healthy. In the patient's and family's explanatory models, Mrs. Xiong was not sick; she had no signs or symptoms to indicate that anything was wrong with her. There was no pain, no weakness, no X-ray finding, and no tissue that looked abnormal. All they had was the doctor's word that she was sick. Also, they sought Hmong people's opinions of chemotherapy from their personal and familial experiences. Ultimately, the family decided they did not want her to experience hair loss, weight loss, vomiting, and profound weakness for an uncertain malady.

## Symptoms of Gallbladder Cancer

When Mrs. Xiong did become sick with jaundice and an enlarged liver, her family queried the doctors about various biomedical therapies: operations, chemotherapy, radiation, and medications. Now that she had signs and symptoms that they identified as an illness, they sought life-saving treatments. Hearing that her doctors could not help her, and thinking perhaps that her doctors did not want to help her (after all, the doctors were angry that she had refused chemotherapy initially), they pursued other options: doctors at other hospitals, Catholic priests, and traditional Hmong healers. While they agreed with the doctors' serious diagnosis and the dire prognosis, they did not accept their physicians' view that seeking a cure was futile.

Mrs. Xiong and her family wondered about the cause of her cancer. They knew that cancer was caused by the chemicals in U.S. water and food, but they routinely boiled their water and bought animals from a local Hmong farm in order to avoid these chemicals. They wondered about the staples in her abdomen from the operation; perhaps the metal had caused a serious reaction like cancer. They considered whether anyone had cursed her. They consulted their priest, went to church, and wondered whether God was punishing her for her sins. And they wondered about a spiritual cause that Christianity could not elucidate. Consulting a Hmong shaman, they learned that Mrs. Xiong's husband's father's soul was unhappy. Their father had died during the war without a funeral, without having a song to guide him to the land of the ancestors, and without a burial. Thus, his souls were in limbo, unable to fulfill their destinies of reaching the land of the ancestors, being reincarnated, and guarding over the buried body.

The family responded to Mrs. Xiong's problems, seeking to cure her as well as make her comfortable. They sought Hmong healers, gave her herbal medicines *(tshuaj ntsuab)*, massaged her swollen abdomen *(zaws)*, and tied strings on her wrist after calling her soul *(khi tes hu plig)*. They conducted a shaman ceremony *(ua neeb)* to try to rescue their father's souls. They saw doctors and gave her Western medicines for diabetes, nausea, and pain. They worked with the home nurses to create a bedroom on the first floor, complete with hospital bed, commode, and an electric nasogastric pump to administer nutritional supplements through a nasogastric tube.

In short, her family was very active in her care. Mrs. Xiong was raised in a social system that conceives of individuals as an integral part of their families, not as separate social beings. At every phase of Mrs. Xiong's illness, the men of her family—her husband, married son, husband's older brother, and husband's adult nephews—were her therapy management group. They listened to the doctors' explanations and recommendations, enlisted the assistance of Catholic priests and Hmong shaman, weighed the possible etiologies and the pros and cons of each treatment regimen, and considered whether to resuscitate her and whether to enter hospice and eventually decided to take her home from hospice. Mrs. Xiong expected and trusted her family members to make the best decisions about her care, and as far as I could tell, Mrs. Xiong agreed with her family's decisions.

## Considering Resuscitation

From her initial hospitalization for the metastases to the hospitalization for the duodenal bleeding, health care providers had recommended that Mrs. Xiong not be resuscitated or intubated, since she had a noncurable terminal illness. But the family refused these recommendations because they wanted the doctors to save her life. At one hospitalization, the doctors raised this issue again. They wanted to speak directly with Mrs. Xiong, but because she did not speak English and because a trained Hmong interpreter was not available, the doctors inquired about her desires through her married son. Her husband and son answered the question: they wanted everything done for their wife and mother. Unsatisfied, a doctor pressed them to ask Mrs. Xiong about her desire. Her son translated the doctor's question and their answer, and she replied that she agreed with her husband and her son. The doctors left the room, feeling uncertain they had heard Mrs. Xiong's true desires.

On several prior occasions, I had talked with Mrs. Xiong about her physical pain, her emotional suffering, and her desire for a cure. Mrs. Xiong had expressed ambivalence, wanting to live so her children would have a mother and wanting to die so that her pain and suffering would be over; but mostly she wanted to be cured and be a mother for her children. While she did not express any ambivalence in that hospital room, I believe that she had expressed her feelings and desires to her husband at other times.

A month later, after an episode of vomiting blood and after a CT scan indicated that a mass was invading her small intestine, the family talked about resuscitation again. Mrs. Xiong's male family members surrounded her bed, evaluated the gravity of the medical assessment, and considered their options. She turned to me, asking with begging eyes to tell her I could cure her. My heart sank. I wanted to answer her in the affirmative, as Hmong custom seemed to demand. How could I be medically accurate and not give her false information, as medical custom demanded? The family discussed the situation and ultimately decided that since neither medicines nor operation could cure her, they wanted her to receive the best supportive care that we could provide. At that bedside, the men decided to enter Mrs. Xiong in the hospice program, which included not resuscitating her. Mrs. Xiong was quiet with the solemnity of finality on her face.

## A Good Death

Through the choices they made, the actions they took, and the feelings they expressed, Mrs. Xiong and her family revealed one version of a "good death." They rejected hospital care when the hospital could no longer provide any curative assistance, and they rejected hospice care when it seemed dangerous. They decided to take care of her at home instead.

At home after she left the hospice unit comatose, Mrs. Xiong wore her traditional Hmong clothes *(khaub ncaws laus)*. When people die they travel to the land of the ancestors, live as ancestors, and relate to living people as ancestors. Wearing ancestral clothes is symbolic of this status change. At home, her family members encouraged her to eat and drink and thus expressed their love by providing for her. At home, her children cried and told her they did not want her to leave them, because she was the only mother that they had, and who would take care of them and love them if she left? At home, relatives and friends filled the house, to encourage her to get well, pay their last respects, comfort the family, and find solace for their own grief. Also, people stayed at the bedside to hear Mrs. Xiong's last words, for a dying person's last words convey wisdom and blessing on those who hear them.

The family provided her with more than just culturally appropriate supportive care, however. They also continued to seek cures from herbal therapies, from Christian prayer, and from shaman rituals. And they were rewarded in their efforts when, after many days, she woke up from her coma and lived with them for another week. When she failed again, her family and friends once again gathered around her. At the very instant that Mrs. Xiong died, the throng at her bedside began to wail *(hniaj)*, expressing their grief, all in their own words and in their own musical tune. Mingled, the voices created a powerful symphony of human emotion.

As heart wrenching as her passing was, Mrs. Xiong's death could be considered a "good death." A "bad death," in contrast, is one where a person dies alone with no one to mourn, wail, or appropriately take care of the body; where a person dies in an accident, since souls will stay at that place and take other victims in the future; where a person dies in physical agony from a violent mutilating death, which carries bad luck into the next life; or where a person commits suicide, which condemns a soul to wander in limbo for eternity.

## Hospice

The conflicts in the hospice in-patient unit were due to the nurses' and the family's different concepts of optimal care of the dying person. For the hospice nurses, optimal treatment included making Mrs. Xiong physically comfortable, telling her she was dying, verbally giving her permission to go, and not feeding her when she was comatose. These ideas conflicted with the family's cultural norms about how to care appropriately for Mrs. Xiong. To the hospice nurses, the dying patient's needs were not being met, but I suspect that Mrs. Xiong's needs were being met, since she had been socialized into her own cultural norms about appropriate behaviors toward sick and dying people. To the hospice nurses, the family was in denial; I believe that the family understood she was dying but were responding to her final days in a manner appropriate for Hmong culture. While the nurses tried to understand the Hmong concept of end-of-life care so they could adjust their care, they had difficulty embracing the Hmong approach, which, on one hand, agreed with supportive care and rejected aggressive therapies but, on the other hand, held out hope for finding a cure.

Does this mean that hospice care is inappropriate for traditional Hmong people? I do not think so. I think it means that the hospice team needs to provide support to the family and to the patient in ways that the family and the patient define as supportive, which can include taking care of a dying patient without directly communicating about dying and continuing to provide some therapies that might extend life.

## Distrust and Vulnerability

Several issues contributed to the distrust Mrs. Xiong and her family felt toward health care providers. At times their requests and desires were in direct conflict with health care providers' actions. The obstetrical nurses continued to aggressively massage her uterus after childbirth despite her protests. The surgeons did not show her the gallstones, as they had promised. The doctors refused to give her any treatment when she had symptoms from her cancer. The doctors repeatedly inquired about not resuscitating her. And the hospice nurse had wanted her to die. Distrust was fueled by communication problems. There were few trained interpreters available in the hospitals and clinics where she was seen, and when there were interpreters, providers had poor skills in working with them.

The distrust between providers and patients goes beyond the micro-level of doctor-patient communication and relationships; it extends to the macro-level of political and economic systems. As a refugee woman, Mrs. Xiong's life had been dramatically influenced by forces far beyond her control. International geopolitical and economic issues—which resulted in the Vietnam War, recruitment of Hmong soldiers, withdrawal of U.S. military forces, interim refugee camps in Thailand, and, finally, resettlement in the United States—caused feelings of vulnerability to and alienation from mainstream U.S. society.

Mrs. Xiong's own ideas about the etiologies of her cancer suggest how her suffering and her sense of vulnerability in her new country contributed to her distrust. She blamed her husband's dead father, who had not received his proper burial. The wandering soul's perpetual suffering that could not be repaired is an apt metaphor for the loss of cultural certainty that occurred when the war uprooted people from Laos and for the sense of powerlessness refugees feel. She blamed the contaminated food and water of the United States, which contrasted sharply with the untainted food the Hmong had grown and pure water they had used in Laos. She had tried to isolate herself from the contamination by boiling water or eating foods that came from Hmong farms, just as she had tried to protect herself and her family from other hazards of U.S. society; but she was unsuccessful. Perhaps sensitive to the interjection of aspects of U.S. life that are foreign, unnatural, and ultimately harmful to the Hmong people, she blamed the metal left in her body from the gallbladder operation. And by blaming the operation, which she had avoided so long, she expressed the vulnerability she felt to the potential hazards of Western health care and her fear that, after all, the surgeons may purposefully be harming Hmong people with their interventions.

Mrs. Xiong's story of suffering exemplifies the value of attending to people in the context of their lives and responding to their cultural needs as health care professionals continue the struggle to prevent and treat cancer.

## References

Culhane-Pera, K. A. (1987, April). *Hmong people's reactions to surgery.* Paper presented at the annual meeting of the North American Primary Care Research Group, Minneapolis, MN.

Mouacheupao, S. (1999, April 17). *Attitudes of Hmong patients to surgery.* Paper presented at the annual spring research forum of the Minnesota Academy of Family Physicians, Minneapolis.

# The Husband's Plea
# for Provider Honesty

*Phua Xiong, M.D.*

In 1980 when we arrived in this country, we were approached by Americans who came to our home and told us to stop having children. They said they had medicine they wanted us to take. We did not know what they were talking about or why they wanted us to stop having children. We were new. At that time we had eight children. Back in Laos, having many children was a blessing. The bigger a family, the better life was.

When we had our ninth child they came back again saying we must do something about having too many children. But we Hmong, we do not do things like Americans. We prefer natural family planning. Then we had our tenth and last child. My wife never had any problem with any of her pregnancies or deliveries. But this time, things did not go very well.

After the delivery, the nurses massaged my wife's uterus very hard, causing a lot of pain. Then she had a lot of pain with her bladder. She could not urinate, her urine path was swollen. She had so much pain in her bladder and abdomen. Her abdomen got bigger and bigger and she felt like she was going to die. Then the doctors put a plastic tube into her urine path and bladder. The urine came out and the pain went away.

Right before we left the hospital, they gave my wife a shot. They did not tell us what the shot was for or why they felt she needed it. When we got home, she started having urinary pain again. Oh, she was in pain, a lot of pain. Nothing we did would take the pain away. The pain started in her lower abdomen, then gradually radiated to her upper abdomen and continued into her chest. She was very sick, pale, and suffering much pain. We took her to the doctors and after some tests we were told it was her gallbladder that caused the pain.

We summoned several shaman, herbalists, and other Hmong healers to help my wife. They came and did their best. My wife got better, but the pain recurred. After much consideration, we decided she should have the surgery to take out her gallbladder. We agreed to the surgery on two conditions, that the doctors genuinely do

---

This commentary is based on Dr. Xiong's interview of the patient's husband.

their best to save my wife and that we get to see the "diseased" gallbladder. The doctors promised; they gave us their word. We believed they were "men of their word." We waited patiently as they rolled my wife into the operating room. Several hours passed. We were told she would be out by 1 P.M. We waited until 1 P.M. Then 2 P.M. 3 P.M. And 4 P.M. Finally, the doctors came out and said, "Everything's okay. Don't worry."

We were relieved to hear they were finally done and that she was okay. But the doctors did not let us see her right away. When she was taken upstairs we finally got to see her. She was in a lot of pain. We asked to see the gallbladder. The surgeon told us they were still examining it. "Later," he said. But later that night, we saw no gallbladder. The next morning, we asked again. We wanted to see the "thing" that caused so much pain for my wife. They told us we needed to fill out some papers before we could see it. We filled out the papers and signed our names. Still, they did not show it to us. We asked again. They replied, "Oh, we chopped it up into tiny little pieces and placed them in a glass jar. Whether you see it or not, you won't know the difference. You won't be able to tell it's a gallbladder anymore."

Whether we could tell it was a gallbladder or not, whether it was whole or chopped up into pieces, we still desired to see it. We insisted. The doctors refused. We argued with the doctors, but we were powerless. The specimen was in their hands and they kept possession of it, refusing to let us see it. We never got to see the gallbladder, the organ they claimed was the cause of my wife's pains. After much frustration and anger, we knew we had no chance. And with resignation and anger in our hearts, we gave up the fight to see the gallbladder. But, why wouldn't they let us see it? Had they done something harmful to my wife while they were in her body?

They told us they took out the gallbladder along with about three fingerbreadths of stomach. They said she had cancer. They wanted her to see the cancer doctor after she recovered from the surgery. The cancer doctor told us that with the cancer drugs, she would get weaker, her hair would fall out, and she would be sick for two months to a year. If she got better then it would mean she might be okay, but if she got worse, then it would mean, "*tag les*" (that's it!).

She had suffered so much already. We had to wait until she regained her strength so she could withstand the cancer drugs. While waiting we sought Hmong medicine to help her get better. She got better. For four months she had no pain.

Shortly after that she complained of pain in her abdomen again. We thought about possible reasons. Perhaps she lifted something heavy that caused the pain to recur at the surgical site. But she hadn't. Perhaps the pain was from the surgical scars. Or perhaps from the metal staples the doctors used.

The pain got worse and worse over the next three to four days until she could not stand it any more. We took her to a different hospital this time. We no longer trusted the doctors at the first hospital and did not want to go back to them. At this second hospital, the doctors took some X rays and told us her liver had turned into pus. "Whatever you have, wear it. Whatever you crave, eat it. Whatever you desire to do or see, do it. All that is left for you is death. You have no chance at life," they said. We all cried and begged them to help her. But they stated they had no way to make her better.

Why had the liver turned into pus? I believed it was the staples. She had twenty of them inside her. After she died, we took them out. I still have them. Twenty staples! The doctors did not use suture material. Instead, they used metal staples during her surgery. Whether the doctors had good or bad intentions, I don't know. But, I know that metal in the body can cause pain and illness. Doctors might say that staples do not cause problems, but we Hmong, we believe differently. We do not like metal in the body. We know from experience that metal can cause infection, create pus, and lead to necrosis of that part of the body. Metal in the body can cause a lot of pain, redness, and swelling and can "protrude out of the body" in your next life *(mob txhav dab)*. All metal must be removed from the body before burial to prevent this from happening.

The doctors did not tell us ahead of time they were going to use staples. They were not honest with us. They lied to us, over and over again. Frankly, I still don't really know exactly what caused my wife's abdominal pain. In my opinion, I fear that what might have happened in the operating room was this: they injured the liver while inside her body. They then turned around and told us the gallbladder and stomach had cancer, blamed the whole thing on the cancer, so that in the end, it would appear they had done nothing wrong.

Why do I say this? Because in the beginning when they took the X rays, they did not mention anything about cancer of the liver. If it truly was cancer in the gallbladder, they would have shown it to us as we requested. I am most angry with the surgeon. He did not tell us the truth and did not show us the gallbladder. If the stomach had cancer in it and they took part of it out, they should have shown it to us and let us see how it looked. Without seeing the gallbladder it is difficult to believe they actually took it out. Perhaps it was never taken out. The second set of X rays showed nothing wrong with the stomach or gallbladder; it was just the liver. It is very hard to trust the doctors. When a man gives his word, I expect him to live up to it. They made promises they did not keep. Why would they hide the truth from us? Perhaps they made false promises to placate us so we would let them use her, operate on her, study her, and make money on her.

Finally, her family doctor recommended hospice care because they could watch her closely, give intravenous fluids and medicines that would make her comfortable, and she would not suffer so much pain. Hospice was in the same hospital that she had her surgery.

She was there for three or four nights and felt okay. I went and watched her all the time, day and night. On the fourth night, when the evening nurse left, another nurse came on duty. I was tired and settled myself into the chair in the room. My wife told me she wanted to go to the bathroom. Since the nurse was in the room, I asked her to help my wife up, but the nurse said she wouldn't. "I gave her a shot of medicine already," the nurse said. I looked over to where she was and saw that the nurse had just picked up three needles to throw away. My wife told me the nurse gave her three shots of medicine into her IV. I got up from my chair and went over to my wife. Suddenly, she became nonresponsive. She did not respond to my voice or my touch. There was no answer from her.

I asked the nurse what medicines she gave my wife. She said she had not done anything wrong and rushed out the door. I believe the nurse purposely tried to kill my wife with bad medicine. The nurse thought my wife had a bad illness *(mob phem)*, and she wanted to make her die faster. I could tell by the way she treated my wife. The first nurse was kind, gentle, and friendly. This nurse was rough, hostile in her manner and her words.

Americans, they do that to us because they do not like us. We are refugees; we do not speak the language. We come here and depend on them, their money, so maybe they purposely do things like this to us. They see our people have a lot of children and do not like that, so they give us shots to stop having children without our consent. My wife never had problems with any of her children. Why did she have so many problems this last time? All the things that doctors and nurses did to my wife, I could not be sure they were done with any good intentions, without malice.

When they gave my wife the shot before we left the hospital with our tenth child, my wife never menstruated again. They never told us what the shot was for, but we figured it out. We had an aunt who was also given a shot after the birth of her twelfth child. When she got home, she started bleeding profusely and almost fainted. She went back to the hospital and they told her it was from the shot she received. They gave her another shot and that stopped the bleeding. My wife must have received the same shot except my wife never bled. The medicine interfered with her body's natural cleansing system and stopped the blood flow. After delivering babies, women need to bleed some to release all the dead blood from the uterus. If she had been able to bleed, her body might have reacted differently and she might not have had so many problems. The shot to prevent her from having anymore children harmed her. It made my wife suffer a lot, she had a lot of pain and she died.

We ask that the doctors and nurses treat us the same way they treat themselves because we all are human beings. When they help, we ask them please to help with honesty. If the situation were reversed, we would help them with all our heart. If they make a mistake we ask that they be honest with us, tell us the truth, do not keep it from us, do not make up something else to cover for their errors. When they tell us they will do something, we expect them to keep their word. Promises made from one adult to another, no matter what color you are, should be fulfilled because that is how we can trust one another. We Hmong should not have to suffer because of doctors' dishonesty, mistakes, and prejudices.

# Pregnant Woman
# with a Brain Hemorrhage

## *A Case Story*

Mao Her, a forty-year-old woman who was thirteen weeks pregnant with her eleventh child, developed a severe headache after attending a funeral. Her husband, Toua Lee Her, massaged her head and did *khawv koob*, a healing ritual, which did not relieve her headache. Recognizing the seriousness of her condition, he prepared to do *fiv yeem*, a spiritual healing ritual that promised to make an offering to the gods of the four corners of the world in return for assistance with her headache. Before he could do the ritual, Mrs. Her suddenly lost vision in one eye, and vision in her other eye began to blur. Mrs. Her's family called 911 for an ambulance to take her to the hospital.

Her husband reported that once they were in the emergency department, they waited between thirty and sixty minutes before anyone looked at his wife. Finally he prevailed on a nurse to come look at her. The nurse noticed Mrs. Her's unequal, nonreactive pupils and called a doctor. Mr. Her and his family were angry about the lack of prompt attention in the emergency department and the absence of a Hmong interpreter. They wondered whether they received poor and slow care because they were Hmong.

A CT scan of Mrs. Her's head revealed an intracerebral hemorrhage with a massive swelling that was putting pressure on the brainstem. The doctors showed the family the CT scan and recommended a cranial operation to release the pressure and remove the intracerebral blood clot. They predicted that without an operation, she would surely die, and with an operation, she would have only a 50 percent chance of living.

Her husband and her husband's male relatives (some of whom spoke English well, but none of whom had any medical training) listened to the doctors, considered their options, and decided to permit the operation, feeling that only "technology" could help her now. Once she was taken to the operating room, her husband called more of his family members and his wife's brothers to tell them about her grave condition and their decision to allow the doctors to operate. The operation proceeded without complications. The neurosurgeons found no explanation for the cause of her hemorrhage; there was no evidence of an aneurysm, a tumor, or a vascular malformation, and she had no hypertension or clotting disorder. They did send necrotic brain tissue to pathology for analysis.

In the ICU Mrs. Her did not regain consciousness and continued to need mechanical ventilation. The next day a repeat CT scan showed a stroke in the opposite hemisphere from the hemorrhage. The physicians showed these findings to the family and explained her poor prognosis during the evening hours when an interpreter was not present. That night she became hypotensive and required medication to maintain her blood pressure. Her family wanted the "technology" to save her and did not refuse or contest any of the nurses' or physicians' actions.

During her two-day hospitalization there were usually about 50 family members and friends in the visitor lounge and a steady stream of well-wishers to Mrs. Her's bedside. The nurses repeatedly described the ICU policy of no more than two visitors at the bedside at a time. The family tried to comply with the nurses' requests, but often ten or more visitors would cluster around Mrs. Her.

An obstetrician did a fetal ultrasound that showed evidence of a pregnancy but no fetus. He surmised that either she had had a miscarriage or was less than seven weeks pregnant, and he ordered blood tests twenty-four hours apart to determine the viability of the pregnancy. Mr. Her was mystified by the ultrasound picture, as his wife had definitely been pregnant for more than three months and had had no signs of miscarriage.

The family had several ideas about the possible causes of her illness. Her husband and others said she had been under a lot of stress. She had many family responsibilities in both her large nuclear and her extended family. Her teenage children were not being respectful to her; they were having trouble in school and were acting out. Also, she was pregnant again from a contraceptive failure and did not want to have another child; she already had had an abortion from a previous contraceptive failure. When she became pregnant this time, she and her husband had discussed their options, and rather than have another abortion, they decided to keep the child. From these "stresses," members of her family surmised, the blood vessel in her brain broke.

Some in the family spoke about spiritual causes. When she had considered an abortion, the soul of the fetus may have felt rejected, they speculated, and so may have taken revenge by making her sick. Perhaps this soul was the same soul that had been aborted previously and had returned to be born. Or perhaps this soul had had a conflict or complaint with Mrs. Her in a previous life and had returned to settle the conflict. Or perhaps Mrs. Her's thoughts about the abortion evoked an evil spirit who had caused her illness.

In the ICU, the family members wanted to perform several traditional treatments, including *khi hluas tes*, tying strings around her wrist to keep her soul in her body, *tshuaj noj*, an oral medicine that could dissolve the clot, and *zaws hno*, a massage followed by poking her finger with a needle to release the built-up pressure.

The family also called on a healer to perform a strong type of *khawv koob* to release the brain swelling. To burn incense as part of the ritual, they needed the doctor's permission to turn off the supplemental oxygen in her room. Knowing that he had little left to offer Mrs. Her, and conceiving of the ritual as one similar to a Catholic's last rite, the resident agreed to discontinue the oxygen during the ritual but told the family that the ritual would have to stop if she had trouble without the oxygen. The healer said he would need a day to prepare to access a powerful spirit Dab Xob, the Lightning Spirit, as he approached the very powerful evil spirit, Dab Ntuj.

Before the healer was able to perform the ceremony the next day, however, the doctors pronounced Mrs. Her brain-dead. With the assistance of a trained interpreter, the physician informed the twenty to thirty people at her bedside that she was dead. Those gathered began to wail, crying out their grief, and began to dress her in a white hemp skirt.

As required in this type of situation, the nurses asked the family about organ donation. Mr. Her's younger brothers said no and refused to ask their brother because of their cultural beliefs about the issue. A family member asked the doctors to remove the fetus so that two people would not be buried in the same grave. When shown the ultrasound picture of an empty uterus, the family members were surprised, but then interpreted the absence of the fetus as evidence of an underlying spiritual etiology: the fetus's soul had caused Mrs. Her's illness and then had left her without any vaginal bleeding.

When Mrs. Her was dressed in her Hmong skirt, the nurse extubated her, and the family removed the lines as they dressed her upper body. No one looked at the monitors. Regardless of heartbeat or blood pressure, they understood she was dead. When she was fully dressed, the family members wailed and wailed, and then one by one slowly left the room until she was alone. The husband, inconsolable in his grief, was physically supported by two men who almost carried him out of the hospital.

The pathologist reported the presence of placental tissue in Mrs. Her's brain. The physicians finally had an explanation for her hemorrhage: Mrs. Her had had a cancer of the placenta that had spread from the uterus and undeveloped fetal tissue to the brain, causing the intracerebral hemorrhage.

## Questions for Consideration

*Questions about Culture*

In what ways were the physicians' and the family's explanations for the brain hemorrhage the same; in what ways were they different?

How did perceptions and beliefs about etiology influence ideas about needed care?

How do the Hmong traditionally define or determine death? Why might the family members have believed the patient was dead while she was still breathing, her heart was beating, and she had a blood pressure?

What role did traditional healing practices play in this case?

What belief is behind the taboo about two bodies sharing one grave?

Under what circumstances might a Hmong healer agree to perform *khawv koob* in a hospital?

Within the Hmong community, what are the prevailing views of autopsy and organ donation?

*Questions about Cross-Cultural Health Care Ethics*

How well did the family and the clinicians trust and respect one another? What factors contributed to their trust and distrust?

How did the family and the clinicians differ in their evaluations of the risks and benefits to the patient?

How should the issue of organ and tissue donation be handled in the case of traditional Hmong families?

What was the resident's understanding of a good cross-cultural health care relationship?

*Questions about Culturally Responsive Health Care*

What role did negotiation play in this case?

What could the hospital have done to improve the care of Mrs. Her?

In the interest of serving culturally diverse clients, how flexible can and should hospitals be regarding such policy matters as the number of family and friends allowed in the intensive care unit, the types of traditional healing methods allowed in the hospital, definitions of death, and organ and tissue donation practices?

# Strategies for Health Care Providers and Institutions to Deliver Culturally Competent Care

*Elizabeth C. Walker Anderson, B.A.,*
*and Patricia F. Walker, M.D., D.T.M.&H.*

End-of-life care can be traumatic and difficult for patients, families, and health care providers—for different reasons. Mrs. Her's case is like a magnifying glass that concentrates the sun's energy: an acute emergency during which time is compressed and families and health care providers are brought face-to-face with dramatic contrasts of Eastern and Western health care beliefs and behaviors. In the United States (a country that is not a melting pot), illness forces ethnic and religious minorities to interact with the dominant—primarily white, male, Christian—health care delivery system. These encounters can generate alienation and mistrust across cultures; they can also inspire mutual respect and admiration among those who have been separated by language, geography, ethnicity, and religion. Health care delivery systems that respond to the acute, chronic, and emergency health needs of a diverse society in culturally competent ways can improve health outcomes.

Having tried traditional healing methods that did not work, Mrs. Her's family accessed the Western health care delivery system quickly. They did so because they recognized the gravity of her illness. But they probably came with great trepidation, fearful they would be treated poorly because they were Hmong. Despite their fear they came to the hospital because they hoped technology would save their wife, mother, sister, and cousin. They had in mind the same goal as the providers with whom they interacted: by means of the best health care, achieve the best patient outcome.

So why does the Western health care delivery system so often fail patients from diverse non-Western communities? The case story does not describe in detail the Her family's feelings when they brought Mrs. Her for care. Nonetheless, one can imagine their horror at her sudden debilitating illness, deep fear that she might die, and bewilderment over Western invasive technology, medical language, and culture. They were probably apprehensive too, that the U.S. health care providers would know little, if anything, about Hmong health beliefs and practices and that there would likely be little respect, little room for negotiation, and little hope of their influencing a good outcome for her.

The family's initial experience in the emergency department was not positive: the long wait and the lack of a Hmong interpreter must have heightened the sense of loss of control that all patients and families feel when faced with a medical emergency. Throughout Mrs. Her's brief and tragic stay in the hospital, the health care providers challenged many Hmong traditional practices: they restricted the number of visitors, they dismissed the family's explanations of the causes of her condition, they declared her dead while she was still pink "and breathing," and they invited organ donation. The inability to anticipate or prevent such cultural affronts probably heightened the family's sense of hopelessness and fear of inevitable tragedy.

Mrs. Her's case does not explore in detail the reaction of the Western health care providers to the complexities of cross-cultural health care. Her providers acted from a Western perspective, focusing on the patient's surgical emergency and health care needs. They diagnosed bleeding in the brain, performed an emergency intracranial exploration, relieved intracranial pressure, and tried to understand what happened with her pregnancy. It is significant that a resident physician also allowed a traditional healing ceremony in the patient's room.

There were many cultural misunderstandings and differences of perspective in this case. Consider, for example, the following pairs of statements, one from each cultural perspective:

Family:     Why don't the doctors help us? Can't they see my wife is sick?

Provider:     Our Emergency Department is so busy we must follow triage protocols.

Family:     Maybe the care is slow because we are Hmong.

Provider:     We treat patients based on their diseases, not on their color.

Family:     We must do our best to help her with our treatments—perform *khi hluas tes* and *zaws hno,* and give her *tshuaj*—even call on traditional healers to perform *khawv koob.*

Provider:     I can't let them burn incense in her room if oxygen is on—it's my responsibility to tell the family that I have to stop the ritual if she has trouble without the supplemental oxygen.

Family:     We must all be here as a family to show our support, to gain from her wisdom as she passes to the next life, and to help with decisions.

Provider:     Can't the family see how sick she is, and how hard it is to provide good care with so many visitors?

Family:     And then they asked us, in our inconsolable grief, to cut her body after death: what loss of souls, what horrible tragedy would befall her in her next life if we allow this?

Provider:     I've got to inform the family about the option of organ donation—it's the law.

Family:     My wife, my sister, my mother is dead. The stress broke her blood vessels. It is the new world, living with the stress of children who live with one foot in the old and one in the new world.

Provider:     The cancer in her placenta went to her brain and caused her death.

To overcome the misunderstanding and mistrust that arise for Hmong patients and others when they encounter mainstream U.S. medical culture, health care providers and institutions need to find ways to enhance cultural understanding and language and communication skills.

## Enhancing Cultural Understanding

The fundamentals of cross-cultural health care include a certain knowledge base, skills, abilities, and attitudes. Clinicians must have a basic knowledge of the patient's history and culture and geographically specific health problems. Providers need to be aware that non-Western patients often experience the Western health care system as invasive and frightening. Cultural differences may create barriers to the delivery of care and it is important that providers identify and address these barriers.

When providers learn about the history and culture of patients they serve and reflect that knowledge in simple behaviors, such as greeting people in their traditional manner, they demonstrate respect and build trust across cultures. Like all patients, Mrs. Her was unique: she carried into the hospital a history of spiritual and cultural beliefs, her own ethnic heritage, a story about her journey to the United States, and the Hmong language. To care for her well would have been to recognize, respect, and understand her needs and offer a corresponding path to assist her in regaining her health.

Among the key questions Kleinman recommends asking during a culturally competent medical history, is, "What do you think caused your illness?" (Kleinman, Eisenberg, & Good, 1978). Questions such as this may communicate respect for the patient, and the answers can help with cross-cultural understanding. If providers had learned, for example, that Mrs. Her's family believed her illness might be due to soul loss or evil spirits, they might have been more understanding of the traditional healing ceremonies the family felt were so important. Similarly, knowing that according to Hmong religious beliefs organ donation can damage patients in their next lives and can harm their families in this life, might have led health care providers to pose required questions about organ donation with greater cultural sensitivity.

Providers need to be open to combined therapeutic approaches to patient well-being. The Western view of health tends to be dualistic, offering "either/or," while the Eastern view tends to be holistic, more disposed to accept both traditional and Western healing methods, offering "and/also." Western health care delivery systems are starting to become more open to complementary health care and more "and/also" than they have been in the past.

Fundamental to good patient outcomes and satisfaction with the health care delivery system is an honest appraisal of personal health care beliefs and practices on the part of providers, patients, and families. Can providers trained in the biomedical model accept the strength and power a Hmong shaman may have in healing Mrs. Her? Can Mrs. Her's family members trust that the Western providers have her best interest in mind as they provide care? Lack of information, incomplete knowledge, or misunderstanding can contribute to lack of trust. Trust may come very slowly with new Americans who may respect Western health care providers' education but not trust their capacity or willingness to understand, empathize with, or honor patients' personal illness experiences. A quiet review of personal biases may assist both health care providers and family to accept different world views regarding health and illness and to begin to build a trusting relationship.

Insofar as hospitals aspire to serve the health care needs of particular communities, it is incumbent on them to incorporate mechanisms to hear community voices—including culturally diverse potential patients—and to plan services in partnership with them. For instance, a study of the Hmong in the Twin Cities identified cultural elements they believe are most important to retain as they adapt to U.S. society: "first, family and communal values favoring the will of the group over the individual; and second, the Hmong language" (Saint Paul Foundation, 1996).

We suggest three strategies to improve a hospital's cultural understanding. Each strategy should include a system of accountability, performance expectations and annual success measurements, and rigorous evaluation tools.

## Performance Improvement Initiatives

Hospital and health care systems continuously seek to improve care for their patients, families, and communities. Patient care, research, and program initiatives responsive to the demographics of the community can be woven into the fabric of a hospital system, internal policies, strategic plans, and procedures. Cultural responsiveness should not be presented as an add-on but instead valued as a critical component of designing and planning each new or enhanced health care service or hospital function. Hiring physician, nurse, and administrator "champions" of culturally responsive care is integral to success. For example, the dietary department would provide culturally appropriate meals to postpartum Hmong women: hot chicken soup with salt, soft steamed rice, and hot water. Information services would identify and record patients' preferred languages into relevant patient databases that would follow the patient throughout the hospital or clinic system. Pharmaceutical services would provide printed instructions in the patient's preferred language.

## Hospital Employee Education

Hospitals can develop and offer their employees a variety of educational opportunities on issues of diversity in health care and bio-medical ethics across cultures. Whenever appropriate, hospitals should link the delivery of culturally competent health care to their mission and vision statements. Hospitals can offer quarterly grand rounds, identify community educational opportunities, devote a section in the hospital library to diversity in health care, and develop on-line resources for all staff. Identifying a resource person in each department with specialized knowledge in a given cultural area is also beneficial.

*Community Partnerships and Outreach*

Partnerships between communities of diversity and health care organizations at many levels—including public health agencies, community clinics, nonprofit social services agencies, local and federal government agencies, and hospitals—produce demonstrable benefits. Partnerships offer hospitals opportunities to design programs with input from culturally diverse communities that can improve understanding by all parties. Non-Western communities in turn need accurate information about Western health care systems and practices.

Hospitals can ask communities, for example, how they can most effectively communicate the Western concepts contained in the Patients' Bill of Rights. Patients from diverse communities can and should be oriented to the Western health care system and taught how to advocate for themselves and their family members within that system. Mrs. Her's husband was upset because he waited between thirty and sixty minutes before his wife received attention in the emergency department. The hospital could have made available information on patient rights and responsibilities, along with emergency department triage policies and procedures, in the Hmong language. Educational outreach on patient rights and responsibilities in a familiar community setting would have prepared the Her family to request more prompt assistance for Mrs. Her. Proactive community collaboration also can include hiring bilingual and bicultural staff, as well as exploring whether and how policies regarding visitors, organ and tissue donation, and autopsies, for example, could be made more flexible.

Hospitals need also to ask Hmong families about their experience and level of satisfaction with the care they have received. Would Mr. Her and his extended family say that Mrs. Her received the best care possible? That their views were respected? That they felt listened to? That the nurses and doctors understood their fears? That they could ask questions? That they would recommend this hospital to their family and friends?

## Enhancing Language and Communication Skills

In Minnesota, "three-fourths (74%) of Asians over five years old speak a language other than English at home . . . [and] 46 percent of Asians. . . . rated their ability to speak English as something less than 'very well'" (Minnesota Department of Health, 1997).

The elimination or reduction of language barriers enhances mutual understanding and assists in creating respectful patient and family-centered health care environments. It also helps equalize access to health care and recognize the civil rights of all patients served by the institution. Laws that mandate such practices are ineffective, however, without appropriate standards for implementation—for example, standards for competent health care interpreters—as well as funds for implementation and monitoring.

A policy guidance issued by the U.S. Office for Civil Rights notes:

[T]he level and quality of health and social services available to persons of limited English proficiency [LEP] [may] stand in stark conflict to Title VI's promise of equal access to federally assisted programs and activities. Services denied, delayed or provided under adverse circumstances have serious and sometimes life threatening consequences for an LEP person and generally will constitute discrimination on the basis of national origin, in violation of Title VI. (U.S. Department of Health and Human Services, 2001)

All hospitals that receive federal funding (Medicare/Medicaid) must be in compliance with Title VI of the Civil Rights Act of 1964, which specifies that "[n]o person in the United States shall on ground of race, color or national origin, be excluded from participation in, be denied the benefits of, or be subjected to discrimination under any program or activity receiving federal financial assistance." Title VI carries no citizenship requirement; it applies to anyone in the United States. The policy guidance proposes specific steps organizations can take to comply with Title VI and to ensure that LEP persons have the language assistance they need to access health care services.

Currently, about 60 percent of hospitals in large urban settings contract with twenty-four-hour telephone interpretation services to facilitate communication between patients and providers. For other health care organizations, this service complements trained staff interpreters. Professionally trained staff interpreters are preferable to freelance, contract, or telephone interpreters. The hospitals that employ them must conduct rigorous assessments of their employees' knowledge and skills; in the case of interpreters, these would include independent evaluations of language proficiency, panel interviews, work history, and reference checks. The employing institution can also develop criteria-based job descriptions with outlined competencies and an ongoing evaluation cycle.

At a minimum, a competent interpreter on staff would have to be proficient in two languages, demonstrate expertise in medical terms and Western concepts of health, have knowledge of diverse health beliefs, and follow established codes of ethical and professional conduct. The interpreter must be able to listen effectively, reproduce the messages accurately, remain faithful to the spirit of the communication, and avoid personal bias. Interpreters must demonstrate consistently excellent communication and interpersonal skills with others of diverse backgrounds.

For successful interpretation to occur, clinicians must be skilled in working with the interpreters. Clinicians' respect for patients is especially crucial when there is a language gap. The presence of a professional interpreter offers cultural affinity for patients and helps reduce the apprehension often associated with asking questions of an individual in a position of power, for example, a physician.

Critical steps taken before Mrs. Her arrived at the hospital's emergency department could have improved substantially the delivery of culturally competent care for Mrs. Her and the family members who accompanied her. The ambulance service that responded, for example, could have asked, "In what language do you prefer to speak about your wife's health condition?" The response to this one question could have better prepared the emergency department staff. Throughout her experience at the hospital, Mrs. Her and her family would have benefited from the services of a professionally trained language interpreter—a Hmong staff interpreter hired by the hospital and available twenty-four hours.

Successful cross-cultural communication is often reflected in comments such as, "I felt like I was talking directly to the doctor. I forgot the interpreter was there." This relationship of respect is more difficult to establish with a freelance interpreter who is hired on an as needed basis. Using a staff interpreter provides much needed continuity between the hospital and the non-Western communities it serves.

## Conclusion

Hmong patients are often extremely grateful for positive experiences that they have with the miracles of Western medical technology, and Western health care providers have learned much from traditional, extended Hmong families with strong support systems. Providing patients and their families with dignified, respectful care across the barriers of language, culture, ethnicity, and religion is the key to success of health care delivery systems in the United States. To deliver culturally competent care, hospitals need bilingual and bicultural staff, professionally trained interpreters on staff, and providers with cultural knowledge, communication skills, and attitudes of trust and respect.

## References

Kleinman, A., Eisenberg, L., & Good, B. (1978). Culture, illness, and care: Clinical lessons from anthropologic and cross-cultural research. *Annals of Internal Medicine, 88,* 251–258.

Minnesota Department of Health, Office of Minority Health and the Urban Coalition. (1997). *Populations of color in Minnesota, health status report.* St. Paul, MN: Author.

Saint Paul Foundation. (1996). *Voices and visions: Snapshots of the Southeast Asian communities in the Twin Cities.* St. Paul, MN: Author.

U.S. Department of Health and Human Services, Office for Civil Rights. (2001). *Policy guidance: Title VI prohibition against national origin discrimination as it affects persons with limited English proficiency.* Retrieved January 27, 2003, from *www.hhs.gov/ocr/lep/guide.html*

*Commentary*

# Accommodation of Cultural Differences in End-of-Life Care

*Karen G. Gervais, Ph.D.*

In the midst of a sudden, unexplained, and tragic health care situation, Mrs. Her's family pursued both Western medicine and traditional Hmong healing practices to restore her health. Throughout, they displayed an acceptance of Western medical technology and a trusting attitude toward Western providers. While the health care professionals serving them exhibited respectful tolerance of the family's culturally based practices, itself a praiseworthy moral achievement, they missed several opportunities to accommodate the family. Accommodation, I argue, constitutes the higher moral ground for professionals and institutions in cross-cultural health care encounters. Like toleration, accommodation requires knowledge, skills, and a supportive institutional environment. But while toleration is essentially a strategy of noninterference in response to differing beliefs and values, accommodation actually promotes the expression of another's beliefs and values.

Accommodation, rooted in the ethical principle of respect for persons, requires Western caregivers and institutions to understand (though not necessarily agree with) the beliefs and values of the patient and family and to enable the patient and family to act in a manner they consider consistent with those beliefs and values. An example of accommodation is when Western health care professionals not only allow adult Jehovah's Witnesses to refuse life-saving blood transfusions but develop and offer blood-less alternatives that can save the lives of Jehovah's Witnesses who otherwise would die.

Why should health care professionals aspire to an accommodationist approach? Acts of accommodation enable families like the Hers to address tragedy in terms of their most deeply held spiritual beliefs and moral values, empowering them in the clinical situation and after to interpret and integrate this experience and loss into their lives in healing ways. The metaphysical and moral beliefs and values the Hers hold are the tools with which they make sense of life, attribute meaning to their experiences, and determine their own and others' ethical responsibilities. The healing and deathbed acts and practices that express these assumptions, beliefs, and values allow them to interpret events, to define personal and collective responsibilities, to sustain and strengthen relationships, to remain situated, and to retain a sense of control—even in the face of the dying and death of a family or clan member.

Because of her illness, Mrs. Her may have been unaware of her losses and of the losses associated with her illness that her family was suffering. Whatever her state of consciousness, however, she was a person with beliefs, values, commitments, and connections to others with definite physical and spiritual needs. Accommodating Mrs. Her and her family requires that their view of causality, which leads them to an ultimately spiritual understanding of illness, dying, and death, be facilitated in the clinical setting. To be technologically served but spiritually neglected by caregivers is a distortion of all of the sorts of healing that should occur in life-threatening situations.

The health care environment—which is unfamiliar, often frightening, and usually disempowering to patients and their families—requires health care professionals to facilitate, not simply to tolerate, the expression of cultural beliefs and values. When providers and institutions fail to empower patients and families to act in accordance with their worldviews, they risk disassociating them from their sources of meaning, belonging, and strength.

The Her family's holistic approach to healing recognized the healing power of massage, spiritual practices to address the spiritual causes of illness, and advanced medical technology to diagnose and treat the consequences of catastrophic illness. They allowed CT scans, a cranial operation, medication for hypotension, fetal ultrasound, blood tests to determine the viability of Mrs. Her's pregnancy, and the use of a ventilator and other technological supports. A family like the Hers, open to much that Western health care has to offer, presented a significant opportunity for strengthening relationships between the Hmong community and the health care system.

What evidence is there that the health care staff was less than ideally prepared for a cross-cultural encounter, that they exhibited toleration rather than accommodation? Two episodes stand out in this regard: the resident's response to the performing of *khawv koob* and the nurse's discussion of organ donation.

## Khawv Koob

When the family wanted a healer to perform the healing practice of *khawv koob,* which required turning off the supplemental oxygen, the resident allowed the practice only to the point at which Mrs. Her needed oxygen, even though Mrs. Her was known to be near death. To justify allowing this practice in the hospital, the resident resorted to the conceptual framework he already held of a terminal ritual, "conceiving of the ritual as one similar to a Catholic's last rite." The resident did not appreciate the family's expansive approach to healing and accommodate it. He tolerated their needs but did not seem to appreciate that the Hers were pursuing what was from their perspective an essential spiritual effort to heal.

The resident's decision involved disruption of the *khawv koob* and reintroduction of the oxygen in the event of respiratory distress. The implication is that his "healing" measures are privileged, even in the face of Mrs. Her's grave condition. Such an approach seems unwarranted and even potentially harmful to the family, since it disrupts their sense that they have done everything they could in order to rescue Mrs. Her.

Accommodation would have consisted of the resident's informing the family that Mrs. Her could experience respiratory crisis and that this would cause her no suffering, given her cognitive state. If respiratory distress were to ensue, would they wish the *khawv koob* to proceed or to be disrupted by the reintroduction of oxygen? The family should have been permitted to make this informed choice.

## Organ Donation

While it is required in the United States to ask families to donate the organs of their next-of-kin in the event of brain death, an ethic of accommodation requires that health care professionals refrain from making such requests of Hmong families who hold animist beliefs. In the Her case, the nurse could be said to have tolerated the younger brother's refusal to ask the older brother about organ donation in that she pressed no further to try to obtain the husband's consent for donation.

Health care institutions and professionals that regularly serve the Hmong community should have donation policies and practices in place that accommodate the distinctive beliefs of animist Hmong families concerning the spiritual significance of the integrity of the body. The Her family should not have been asked to donate, and other families should not be asked to donate in similar circumstances.

Operations have the potential to damage the soul of the deceased and thus impair its transition to the next life, render it more likely to suffer in the next life, and promote sickness in family members. The powerful assumptions about the actions of souls, their potential to harm and be harmed across generations, were an important part of the Her family's belief system as evidenced by their understanding that Mrs. Her's fatal condition was caused by the revenge of the fetus's soul from an earlier abortion.

Even if the Hers' acceptance of Western health care practices had extended to organ donation, it is disrespectful to require that all Hmong families be invited to donate the organs of a family member. The family should raise the option of donation if they are interested and choose it entirely on their own. Health care organizations and professionals should not risk engendering the Hmong community's distrust through requests for organ donation. Institutional and societal policies mandating "required request" should be revisited and adjusted for cultural differences. Such accommodation will not only promote more respectful health care encounters for families like the Hers but also will demonstrate societal respect for the deeply held beliefs of immigrant groups.

This case underscores two important points. First, illness is a personal event of both the body and the spirit, as well as a social event that disrupts and disconnects persons from their usual relationships and contexts of meaning. This disruption and disconnection happens not only for the sick person but also for those in established relationships with that person. Second, successful cross-cultural caregiving requires accommodation—that is, understanding and enabling patients and families with alternative sources of meaning to create the best possible outcome for themselves.

## Brain Death

A surprising feature of this case is the Her family's acceptance of the physicians' conclusion that Mrs. Her was dead, despite the ongoing signs of life in her ventilated body. Given the Hmong culture's customary reliance on the cessation of breathing and heartbeat to signal death, it is curious that the family seemed to acknowledge that the ventilator was now just masking death.

Even before the ventilator was removed, the family began engaging in death behaviors. The family's initiation of death practices occurred in tandem with the caregivers' removal of the technological apparati that sustained the traditional "signs of life," rather than after these signs had permanently ceased. This coincidence may have resulted more from the Hers' acceptance of Western medicine than from health care professionals' pursuit of an accommodationist approach. Perhaps though, both caregivers and family experienced a mutual sense of closure in this special moment of cross-cultural sharing.

## Conclusion

The Her family may exemplify what we may increasingly expect in health care settings in coming years: Hmong patients and families who are open to Western health care's potential benefits but who also require respect for their spiritual beliefs and moral values. This case makes clear the possibility that different belief systems can productively coexist within the same health system; the needs of patients and families are better met through creative acts of accommodation than through acts of mere tolerance. Mrs. Her's story gives us a glimpse of such a fruitful possibility.

# 15

## A Widowed Mother's Search
## for a Good Place to Die

### *A Case Story*

Mrs. Chang was a sixty-two-year-old widowed animist Hmong woman with five married daughters and one married son who, after her husband died, moved between her son's house and her daughters' houses so she could be with all of her children and grandchildren. She was in good health, never having seen a doctor or having had periodical prevention exams, when she noticed intermittent bleeding from her vagina for several months.

Finally, she talked with her daughters and agreed to see a family practice physician despite her concerns of a pelvic exam, which she had never had. During a gentle pelvic exam, the physician found a large ulcerating mass in the end of the vagina, obscuring the cervix. After the exam, the physician, with the assistance of a trained Hmong interpreter, explained to Mrs. Chang and two of her daughters that she saw a large mass that was causing the bleeding; she was not sure exactly what kind of mass it was but she knew that it could be serious and that the Pap smear she took might be helpful. She advised Mrs. Chang to see a specialist who would take a sample of the mass to look at under the microscope. The patient and her daughters listened and decided to go home to discuss the doctor's evaluation and recommendation with other family members.

When the results of the Pap smear indicated cervical cancer, the physician talked with a daughter and made an appointment for Mrs. Chang with a specialist. When Mrs. Chang missed the appointment with the specialist, her physician tried to contact her at a daughter's house. The daughter explained their mother was afraid of another pelvic exam, since she had bled a lot after the initial exam and was concerned the exams would make her bleed and be sick again. She had taken Hmong herbal medicines for vaginal bleeding and the bleeding had stopped. The daughter said she would bring her mother back to the physician and then to a specialist if her mother ever agreed to go.

Months later, the patient agreed to see a specialist, because her bleeding had returned and she was becoming weaker. At the daughters' invitation, her primary care physician agreed to escort the patient and her daughters to an appointment with a cancer doctor, a gynecology oncologist. During the appointment, Mrs. Chang told her physician she had decided to have surgery but under no conditions would she receive radiation or chemotherapy, since these therapies were poisonous and unsuccessful. The gynecology oncologist stated the mass was a cervical cancer that had spread to the middle of the vagina, so it was not amenable to surgery and responsive only to radiation therapy. Mrs. Chang begged for surgery, and the oncologist refused. The oncologist insisted on radiation therapy, and Mrs. Chang refused.

At home, Mrs. Chang, her son, daughter-in-law, five daughters, and five sons-in-law, and an elder male clan leader discussed the possible causes and possible treatments, and the pros and cons of radiation. When the clan leader said Mrs. Chang should not receive radiation therapy because all Hmong women with cervical cancer die despite receiving radiation therapy, Mrs. Chang nodded her head, and her children remained silent. The clan leader suggested traditional Hmong and Chinese medicines and shaman ceremonies. At that point, the daughters expressed their concerns that their brother was not taking proper responsibility for their sick mother: he was not taking her to live with him, was not taking her to see the doctors, and was not obtaining traditional healing methods for her. The clan leader told the son that he must be a good son and be responsible for his mother. The son quietly replied that he was a good son and would take good care of his mother.

For months Mrs. Chang continued to bleed. Three times she fainted and each time her family took her to a different emergency department where the doctors diagnosed anemia from a bleeding cervical cancer, gave her blood transfusions, and referred her to gynecology oncologists who recommended radiation therapy. Each time, she pleaded for an operation, then agreed to receive radiation but never kept her appointments. Finally, her daughters took her to a medical center in another city for another opinion, but again the doctors refused to operate, because an operation would not prolong her life.

Mrs. Chang became progressively weaker, requiring more assistance from her family. She wanted to live with her son, but he said he could not take care of her every day, so she continued to move from daughter's house to daughter's house to son's house. She wanted to stay (and ultimately die) at her son's house. She worried she would end up in a nursing home, since she was not living with her son and could not die in any of her daughters' houses. The family sought other options. They applied for public housing but the waiting list was long; they looked for apartments but they could not afford a security deposit and rent; and they continued to appeal to her son to take care of her at his house.

Her family helped her with multiple treatments, including Western medicines, Hmong medicines, and shaman ceremonies. During a shaman ceremony at her son's house, a shaman told her that her soul had been frightened away and needed to be returned; indeed, she remembered being frightened at a funeral and became optimistic that the ceremony would cure her. But she continued to become weaker and weaker.

Ultimately, she developed renal failure. The spreading cervical cancer had partially blocked both ureters and the urine could not flow to the bladder, so the kidneys could not function. The primary care physician met with the family to discuss a procedure of inserting tubes through her back into each kidney, in order to drain the urine from the kidneys. The family—her son, daughters, sons-in-law, and elder clan leaders—decided against the procedure since it would not cure the underlying cervical cancer or extend her life for long. The family wanted palliative measures. In addition, they instructed the primary care physician not to tell Mrs. Chang how severely ill she was and not to mention the procedure to her.

Discharged from the hospital, she went to her son's house. When he could not care for her any longer, she was admitted to hospice, first as a hospital patient and then as a nursing home patient. Deeply saddened by her fate of dying in a nursing home, she slowly entered a coma and died.

## Questions for Consideration

### Questions about Culture

What traditional Hmong concepts of vaginal bleeding may have influenced Mrs. Chang's response to her bleeding and the diagnosis of cervical cancer?

If Mrs. Chang wanted to get well and wanted surgery, why might she have refused radiation therapy? What type of evidence supports the claim that no Hmong woman survives cervical cancer after receiving radiation?

How do the reasons it was difficult for Mrs. Chang's son and daughters differ from the reasons it may be difficult for mainstream American sons and daughters to care for their parents in their own homes?

How are gender roles changing for sons, daughters, daughters-in-law, sons-in-law, and widows in the Hmong community?

What is objectionable for an animist Hmong or a Christian Westerner about being cared for and dying in a nursing home?

### Questions about Cross-Cultural Health Care Ethics

How did the risk-benefit assessments differ between the health care providers and Mrs. Chang and her family?

Why might a family ask a physician not to inform the patient of her end-of-life condition or of a procedure that might extend her life?

How can a physician respond to a family's request not to discuss treatment options with a patient who until now has been actively involved in treatment decisions, has requested surgical procedures, and has expressed a desire to live?

### Questions about Culturally Responsive Health Care

What might health care providers have done so that Mrs. Chang was diagnosed with cervical cancer before it had spread so far? What could health care providers have done to help Mrs. Chang obtain medical treatment for her cancer?

What can health professionals do to help relieve familial conflicts about where a patient is cared for during a terminal illness?

In what ways were the health care relationships in this case culturally responsive, in what ways were they less than optimally responsive?

# Providing a Spiritually Appropriate Place for My Mother's Care and Death

*Mrs. Chang's Daughter (Anonymous)*

My mother had five children: four daughters and one son. My mother was a single mom for a long time and she also tried to be a father figure to us. In Hmong culture, the mother should stay with one of her sons, usually the youngest son. But my mother often moved around between all of her children and helped us with cooking, baby-sitting, and even with financial problems when it became necessary. She was one of the few Hmong mothers who always knew all the current information about her children's lives. My mother cared a lot about her children and grandchildren. She put all her priority in us rather than remarry as a typical Hmong woman would. My mother loved us so much that she did not want to remarry, join a new husband's family, and leave us behind. She said she would not leave her kids just to be with a man.

In the Hmong culture, daughters are encouraged not to intervene in family problems such as finance, politics, and the well-being of the whole family since these are the responsibilities of the father and sons of a typical family. When our mother became sick with a terminal illness, my brother did not want her to stay with him. He was married and he felt that our sick mother would slow him down in life. My sisters and I did not want to place her in a nursing home because that would only make her worse. It is frightening to be cared for by others outside the family, and I know that our mother did not want to stay at any nursing home under any circumstance. My sisters and I could not do much. According to Hmong culture it was mainly our brother's responsibility to decide what to do and how to care for our mother while she was sick. However, he turned much of her care over to me and my sisters, including making arrangements for spiritual healing ceremonies *(ua neeb thiab khawv koob)* and herbal medicines *(tshuaj Hmoob)*. He claimed that since our mother moved around a lot, living with all of her children, her daughters should contribute more to help because our mother had contributed a lot of her time and money to her daughters.

My sisters and I took turns taking time off from work to take care of our mother. She was disappointed that my brother did not contribute to her care or appreciate anything we did. She stayed at my house for four weeks, but she did not get better. Many shaman told my mother and me that attempting to welcome her soul into my house for healing would not work. The household and ancestral spirits in our home come from my husband's side of the family and they would not recognize and allow my mother's soul to enter our house. My mother's soul is under the protection of ancestral spirits that are different from my husband's and mine. In order for my mother's soul to be retrieved and returned to restore her health, she had to live in a home with the proper spirits. She had two choices: live by herself in a home of her own or live in her son's home. A shaman ordered me to take her to live with my brother so they could perform a special shaman ceremony to help her. I had to explain to my brother exactly what the shaman said before he agreed to let our mother stay in his home. He insisted that one of my sisters or I had to be present at his house at all times to give her medicine, food, water, or whatever she needed.

Though my sisters and I put in as much effort as possible to help our mother, my brother and other male relatives did not fully acknowledge our help because we were daughters. It did not bother me that my husband, children, and I had to constantly watch my mother, even when she was not at our home. We were willing to do anything to make her better. What bothered me was that my brother changed his mind about our mother's staying at his house. After only two weeks, he decided to take her to a nursing home. My brother and his wife felt that having our mother stay at their house would not help her get better. They insisted that a nursing home would be better. After she was admitted to a nursing home, my family and my sisters stayed with her and took care of her twenty-four hours a day as if she was at my house or at my brother's house. Unfortunately, she passed away with a broken heart a week after she was placed in the nursing home.

I am very disappointed that I am not a son, with the authority to do whatever my mother wanted in order to make her feel better physically, emotionally, and spiritually, and to prolong her life a few more weeks. I am upset that a daughter can only do so much for her mother, no matter how much she wants to do more. Though I believe that much more could have been done, I feel I did everything I could. Several times I went against cultural rules and customs just so that I could take care of my mother. Some Hmong may judge my actions as just an optimistic plea or inappropriate conduct for a woman, but what I did for my mother was what I felt I had to do as her daughter. Many times my stomach was empty, but my mind was full.

I am not the only daughter who has faced such difficulty and sadness. I am sure that there are other Hmong daughters on the same path who are facing the same disappointments and frustrations as I. If any of you are on this path, you are not alone. Please join me and share your stories and sadness.

## Commentary

# "Please Help Me":
# A Physician Responds to a Hmong
# Woman's End-of-Life Struggles

*Kathleen A. Culhane-Pera, M.D., M.A.*

She looked up at me from her bed in her daughter's house, pleading with me to help her.* "*Thov koj pab kuv. Koj yog kuv niam. Tsis xav tuag.*" (Please help me. You are [like] my mother. I don't want to die.) Her voice was high and strained. Her eyes were full of suffering and agony. Her body leaned toward me, her hands squeezing my hands. Pleading.

"*Txhob txhawj. Kuv yuav pab koj. Peb mam pab koj. Tsis ntshais, Koj tsis tuag. Txhob hais li ntawd. Tsis ntshais li.*" (Don't worry. I will help you. We will help you. Don't be afraid. You are not dying), I replied in my Hmong way. After sixteen years of working as a physician with Hmong people, I had adopted some Hmong ways. Being present with suffering people and sharing their emotional pain. Visiting terminally ill people in their homes. Expressing my concern in culturally appropriate ways, such as saying, "You are not dying" when she and I knew that she was dying. It was not lying. It was not denying. Rather, it was expressing care in a cultural idiom of support. She and I had already talked about the terminal nature of her cancer. We had already discussed the futility of an operation, for which she had begged, and the chances of cure with radiation, which she had adamantly refused. She had already told me not to perform any procedure that would prolong her life but not cure her. When I said, "You are not dying," we understood each other; she knew I was offering her comfort for her suffering.

I understood she was pleading for help in her final days. She wanted to live at her son's house supported by her family and surrounded by her ancestral spirits. She had lived with her son and daughter-in-law after her husband died, but when they had difficulties living together in harmony, she had moved from daughter's house to daughter's house. Culturally, she should have been living with her son; both her son and her daughter-in-law should have made the necessary adjustments to accommodate her. And culturally, she should be with her ancestral spirits when she dies.

Each Hmong family's ancestral and household spirits *(dab qhuas)* accept the soul

---

*Culhane-Pera became the primary care physician when the patient was diagnosed with cervical cancer.

of a dying person only from their family; they would be angry if they had to greet the ghost of a dead person from another family in their house. If she were to die at a daughter's house, her son-in-law's ancestral and household spirits would avenge their anger by making someone in their family sick and possibly even die. Culturally, she had to die at her son's house, where her family lived, where her social identity resided, and where her ancestral spirits protected her. Traditionally, the only alternative was to be thrown away in the forest without a funeral, like a dead neonate who has not yet attained status as a full-fledged human being in the context of family. Homeless, she was afraid she would have to die in a nursing home, rejected physically, socially, and spiritually by her family. To her, the nursing home represented the worst of U.S. culture: a place where families shamelessly throw away their disgusting—but once capable and caring—parents. The nursing home represented the worst fate for a Hmong mother: cast away after caring for her children her entire life, to die in shame.

I agreed to help her. But how? I could not change her or her family's cultural beliefs. She, her daughter, and I devised a multi-option plan. I would write a letter to Section 8 public housing to appeal for an apartment for Mrs. Chang. Her daughter would investigate renting an apartment for her mother. In either of these places, with the creation of a temporary altar, her ancestral spirits could be invited to join her. And Mrs. Chang would ask her deceased husband's relatives to help her son and his wife accept their filial responsibilities *(hlub)* so she could be where she belonged during her last days.

"Grandma, the doctor is here," a girl shouted to Mrs. Chang as I knocked on the back door of her daughter's house. Inside, her daughters were cleaning up the last of the dinner plates, as other family members were gathering in the living room. By the time the male clan elder arrived, Mrs. Chang, her daughters, their husbands, and her son had arranged themselves in a circle in the living room. I thought I might have the doctor's role of explaining her cervical cancer diagnosis, the extent of the spread into the vagina, and the option of a radiation cure. But her daughter explained what the specialists had said, periodically asking for my agreement, to which I nodded. Mrs. Chang added a few specifics. Everyone sat listening quietly, except for the clan leader. He asked questions in a loud and definitive voice. Finally, when he spoke, everyone listened while barely looking at him. "The cancer is too far spread for surgery to help. Radiation will not help at all. No Hmong person has been helped by radiation. It only burns the body. It only makes the person suffer. It is not good to consider for your mother. Instead, we must look for Chinese medicines to help."

Mrs. Chang was the first one to speak, echoing his statements and assessments, and they talked for a long time about the possible Chinese medicines. He had proclaimed what she had been thinking. I wondered, if he had advised the opposite of her desires, if he had said radiation was the best way, would she have agreed? Would she have changed her mind? Would she have followed the family's decision, against her own? Or would she have spoken against his opinion and refused to follow his directive? Others spoke up, and mentioned—not argued—the possibility that radiation might help, when nothing else could cure her. But the weight of the conversation reflected the conviction of the clan leader, which agreed with Mrs. Chang's desires.

Then, finally, a daughter mentioned that her brother and his wife were not taking care of their mother the way they should. The son calmly asserted that he and his wife were not to blame. They were good children and they loved his mother. The clan elder listened attentively and slowly affirmed the cultural case. "A son and daughter-in-law must take care of his mother, the way she had taken care of him when he was young. The strength of the Hmong family stands upon familial responsibility of parents to young children and filial responsibility of sons and daughters-in-law to elderly parents. Both are necessary. To give up the cultural values now, in this country, under the difficult social and economic times is to give up completely on being human, on being Hmong. If a son does not take care of his parents, the whole Hmong society will collapse, will cave in, will perish. This is the way it must be." Again, the son quietly asserted that he was a good son, but I never heard him assert that he would take his mother home for care. Feeling uncomfortable, like an intruder, feeling as though I might increase his public shame, I politely excused myself and left out the back door.

She barely looked at me when I entered her hospital room. She had been admitted with blood clots in her urine from the tumor's invasion into the bladder. Now she was lying peacefully; we had successfully stopped the bleeding. I had just come from a family conference where her family had decided against placing tubes through her back into her kidneys to drain the urine. I thought she would agree with their decision, since it was consistent with her desires not to do things that would extend her life but not cure her disease and to have her family care for her completely. But while the family had stated they did not want to tell her about the details of the procedures, I wanted to open the door for her to consider her options. Maybe she would have changed her mind. But I did not want to go against the family's decision and betray their trust. So I said, "How are you? I just talked with your family. Do you want to hear what we said?" She spoke her refusal silently with her entire body. She closed her eyes, turned away from me, and asked for a drink of water. Her husband's male relatives entered the room behind me and told her, "Don't worry. You will be fine. The doctor has flushed your bladder, so there aren't any clots. You will be fine. You will get stronger. And you will go live with your son." At that news, she looked up at them and smiled, reassured of a peaceful death in her son's home. Her husband's male relatives—her family—had helped her son assume his filial duty. They had brought her the decision she wanted.

She grasped my hand and squeezed it hard, from her bed in her son's house. "*Kuv zoo siab koj tuaj. Zaum. Noj.*" (I am glad you came; come, sit with us, and have something to eat.) The clean, small rambler house was full of people, noise, and activity. Some of her daughters sat in the bedroom with her, talking about her health among themselves, and responding to her needs; they moved her pillows, covered her with blankets, fed her rice porridge *(kua dis)*, and walked her to the bathroom. Other daughters were in the kitchen, cooking various dishes of rice, noodles, boiled pork, and vegetables, while an aunt washed mounds of dishes. Men—her husband's relatives from California and Minnesota—sat with her son in the living room, talking about life in the United States and life as soldiers in Southeast Asia. Children sat with their parents or played with each other. Her daughter-in-law, a well-dressed young woman, was a smiling hostess to everyone, seating the men first to eat, and then the women, encouraging all the guests to eat until they were full.

The activity and interactions felt like a loving extended family. The previous conflicts of a lifetime—whatever they were—seemed nonexistent, with everyone coming together to support Mrs. Chang in the evening. At night, a teenage niece, nephew, or grandchild stayed to help her to the bathroom. During the day, her son, daughter-in-law, or a daughter stayed on a rotating schedule so they could continue their jobs and family lives, while still caring for their mother. I marveled at their dedication to Mrs. Chang and to each other. It seemed she had found the peace she desired.

The next time I did a home visit, she pleaded with me, "*Thov pab kuv. Pab kuv.*" (Please help me. Help me.) What did she want from me? What could I give her? How could I help her? She was not in physical pain; she had morphine. She was at her son's house; her family was taking care of her. But she was in emotional distress; she did not want to die. She was trying to cure her disease. She was receiving shamanic treatments and herbal treatments. Recently she had seen a Hmong healer who found her soul had been frightened at a funeral and so her family performed a soul-calling ceremony. However, she was still sick; she was afraid of dying. The agony in her voice spoke of her desire for life, for a hope of life, and hope of a cure.

How could I help someone who said she wanted to live rather than die but who had earlier refused the radiation I thought would be curative or would prolong her life significantly? In an ethical analysis, perhaps it was "easy." She was competent to make health care decisions. She and her family understood the medical ideas; there was no conflict between their decisions and her desires. They could evaluate the physical and spiritual consequences of all the options, weigh the pros and cons, and make a decision that was right for her, in her cultural context. They had the right to refuse therapy, even a life-saving therapy. I respected that. And I accepted my role as a physician: to explain the biomedical perspective, provide the care they accepted, strive to understand the parts of Hmong culture I did not understand, and be present on her journey. Still, it was difficult for me emotionally when she pleaded for help, and there was nothing more I could offer her now. I felt sad, angry, and frustrated. But eventually her suffering moved me. True, earlier she had rejected radiation, but now she wanted to live. I answered her in the only way I could. "*Tsis ntshais. Peb sawv daws mam pab koj. Kuv nrog koj nyob tau.*" (Don't be afraid. All of us will help you. I will stay with you.) Stay. Be present.

"Good morning. I am glad you have come." Her son greeted me at the door of his house. "My mother is sleeping in her room. She had a bad night and hasn't slept well." The house was quiet, in stark contrast to my first evening visit.

"Before you see my mother I want to talk with you. I cannot have my mother stay at my house any longer. My wife and I have decided she has to go to a nursing home. We have lost too much time at our jobs. We are too busy at night with everyone here. Our children are afraid to be at home for fear their grandmother *(pog)* will die. If she does die in the house, they will continue to be afraid in their own home. Also, if she does die in the house, we will not be able to sell the house. No one will want a house where someone has died; they will be afraid of the ghost. We just bought the house; we want to keep it for our family, and we want to be able to sell it later."

I felt sorry for him. The economic realities were strong, and they no longer matched the traditional social and spiritual considerations. In Laos, people had died in their homes, but because families built rather than bought their own houses, no one had to live with other families' ghosts. In Laos, children may have been present at deaths and funerals and had lived in houses where people had died, but they also stayed at other households, sheltered a bit in times of crisis.

His voice was quiet. His shoulders were sagging. Was he ashamed? Was he worried about his sisters' reactions? Did he fear his relatives' disapproval, scorn, and rejection? Or was he just tired? But he seemed determined and resolved. My heart sank at the implications for his mother.

He continued, "I know my family *(kwv tij)* will be upset with me, but I am the only son and I cannot do it all by myself. My wife, my children, our future is too important."

"Is there no other way? What about your attempts to rent an apartment?"

"Too expensive. We don't have the money for a down payment and a year's lease."

"What about the application for Section 8 public housing?

"We are still on the waiting list."

"What about other family members' homes, like your father's brothers?"

"It is only up to me because I am the son. They will not take care of her. I am the only one who can be responsible."

I considered my house, since we were moving out, but the renters would be moving in too soon.

"What about hospice respite care in a hospital?"

"OK, if we can go to a hospital or nursing home."

Disheartened, I listened to his decision and his reasons. I knew his mother would be depressed, his sisters angry, and his male relatives disappointed in his choice. But I saw that he and his wife were caught between cultures: the expectations of the old and the new. He was making an unpopular decision, against the old way and his mother and for the new way and his family. I wondered how much of his decision was a conflict between him, his mother, and his sisters, and how much was a conflict between his wife and his family. In Southeast Asia, Hmong family conflicts between mothers-in-law and daughters-in-law were legendary. Hmong family problems had been blamed on daughters-in-law *(tus nyab)* for generations. It seemed to be happening again, this time with different social and economic realities. I thought that it is so sad for women to be pitted against each other, with their son and husband caught between them. So sad that they could not figure out a way to meet everyone's needs.

Ultimately, I respected the son's fortitude and his decision. Now I had to help find a new way to take care of Mrs. Chang, of both her physical and her social needs, and let her family, her soul, or other spiritual beings address her spiritual needs.

I replied, "I will call hospice and see if we can admit her to the hospital unit for respite care." I grasped at straws as I continued, "And maybe she will die there; it is hard to know how much time she has left."

We walked back to the bedroom to tell his mother. She was thin. Her face wore lines of fatigue. Her breath smelled of renal failure. Quietly, she listened to our words. She voiced no objections; the plea was out of her voice. She seemed resigned to her sad fate *(hmoov)*.

The last time I saw her, she slept peacefully in her hospital bed, aided by narcotics to relieve her physical pain. I had come to say good-bye and to transfer her care to Dr. Phua Xiong, since I was leaving for a year in Thailand. She barely responded to me. I felt her withdrawal as anger, at her situation and at me. I felt my own disappointment, at her family for not being able to take care of her as she desired, at her culture for not being able to create new solutions to new problems that would please all family members, and at myself for "abandoning" her at the end of her life.

Because she did not die quickly, she had to leave the hospital and go to a nursing home. She audiotaped her "last words of wisdom" for her children. "Listen to each other. Help each other. If I am not alive, I will be in the clouds, watching you, protecting you like an umbrella from the rain and the sun, protecting you from the problems of life. Be good to each other. Stay together." While family members were always with her, she was ashamed that she had not raised children who appropriately cared for a dying mother. She died with her son, a daughter, and two grandchildren at her side, and with sadness in her heart.

# PART VII

# Culturally Responsive Health Care

# A Model for Culturally Responsive Health Care

*Dorothy E. Vawter, Ph.D., Kathleen A. Culhane-Pera, M.D., M.A.,*
*Barbara Babbitt, B.S.N, R.N., M.A., Phua Xiong, M.D.,*
*and Mary M. Solberg, Ph.D.*

The goal of culturally responsive health care is for patients and providers to feel respected and satisfied with both the healing methods used and the health outcomes (Jecker, Carrese, & Pearlman, 1995). This chapter presents a model of the knowledge, skills, and attitudes that support the delivery of culturally responsive health care.

The *Healing by Heart* model for culturally responsive health care, as depicted in Figure 16.1, identifies nine areas of learning and the interconnections among them. The arrows reflect the way learning in one area supports and influences learning in other areas. Table 16.1 provides a more extensive outline of the model, which is distinctive in its attention to knowledge and skills in cross-cultural health care ethics. (For examples of other models, see Betancourt, Green, & Carillo, 2002; Brach & Fraser, 2000; Campinha-Bacote, 1999, 2003; Campinha-Bacote & Munoz, 2001; Cross, Bazron, Dennis, & Isaacs, 1989; Huff & Kline, 1999a; Leininger, 1988, 1995a; Spector, 2000.)

The first section of this chapter presents practical recommendations for how health care providers can apply the *Healing by Heart* model to relationships with Hmong patients and families in the United States. Guidance is offered on cross-cultural health care ethics, communication skills, and applying such knowledge and skills to particular clinical encounters. These recommendations are consistent with the National Standards on Culturally and Linguistically Appropriate Services (CLAS) in Health Care (U.S. Department of Health and Human Services [U.S. DHHS], 2000c, 2001d).

While the model is directed primarily to practitioners in clinical settings, many of the key learning areas are also applicable to health care administrators, educators, and health policy makers working in government, insurance companies, and private organizations. The final sections of the chapter recommend ways health care administrators, educators, and policy makers can support the delivery of culturally responsive health care.

Figure 16.1. The *Healing by Heart* Model for Culturally Responsive Health Care

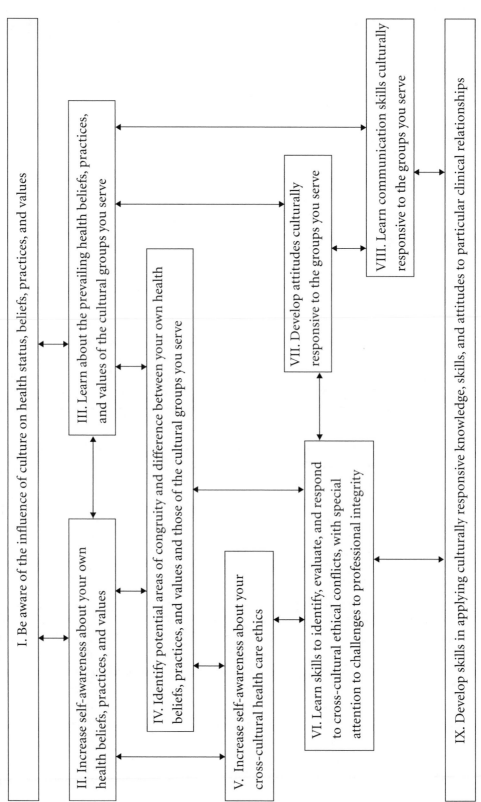

## Table 16.1. Outline of the *Healing by Heart* Model for Culturally Responsive Health Care

I. Be aware of the influence of culture on health status, beliefs, practices, and values

II. Increase self-awareness about your own health beliefs, practices, and values

    A. *Your health beliefs and practices*
   1. Your concepts of anatomy and bodily functions
   2. Your beliefs about illness causation, illness prevention, and health promotion
   3. Treatment, illness prevention, and health promotion activities you engage in

    B. *Your health care ethics*
   1. On what basis do you believe health care practitioners are to be trusted?
   2. What behaviors do you believe demonstrate respect for persons, patients, and families?
   3. What do you believe are the ideal roles, responsibilities, and prerogatives of patients, families, practitioners, institutions, and states?
   4. What types of information about a patient do you believe you should disclose, to whom, and how?
   5. What considerations do you believe are relevant when assessing a patient's best interests?
   6. What methods and criteria do you believe support good health care decision making?

III. Learn about the prevailing health beliefs, practices, and values of the cultural groups you serve

    A. *Past and present contextual influences*
   1. Politics
   2. Economics
   3. Social and family structure (gender, marriage, children, education, class)
   4. Religion
   5. Geographic location
   6. Refugee flight or immigration history
   7. Relationships with other groups (including discrimination)
   8. Culture change, acculturation, variation
   9. Access to health care systems

**Table 16.1.** *Continued*

B. *Health-related cultural beliefs and practices*
1. Traditional and changing concepts of anatomy, bodily functions, and malfunctions
2. Traditional and changing beliefs about illness causation, illness prevention, and health promotion
3. Traditional and changing practices for treatment, illness prevention, and health promotion

C. *Health-related moral practices and commitments*
1. On what basis do patients and families from this cultural group tend to trust traditional healers, health care practitioners, and institutions?
   a. What, if any, are the historical and cultural barriers to trusting practitioners?
   b. What types of trust and distrust does this group tend to have of U.S. practitioners?
2. According to this cultural group, what behaviors demonstrate respect for persons, patients, and families?
   a. What attributes are deserving of respect?
   b. How important is it to respect persons/patients/families?
   c. What behaviors demonstrate respect for persons/patients/families, and for patients of different ages and genders?
   d. What are the privacy needs and expectations of patients?
   e. What, if any, taboos are there regarding touching, disrobing, examining, or discussing parts of the body?
3. According to this cultural group, what are the ideal roles, responsibilities, and prerogatives of patients, families, traditional healers, health care practitioners, institutions, and states concerning such matters as:
   a. identifying the cause of an ailment?
   b. identifying appropriate remedies and healers?
   c. engaging in healing activities?
   d. providing and receiving information from healers and health professionals?
   e. decision making?
   f. protecting ill and vulnerable persons?
   g. conducting follow-up assessments of effectiveness and outcome?
   h. paying for services?

4. According to this cultural group, what health-related information should be disclosed, to whom, and how?
   a. What importance is ascribed to informing patients of diagnosis and prognosis?
   b. What importance is ascribed to protecting confidentiality?
   c. What, if any, topics or words are taboo?
5. According to this cultural group, what considerations are relevant to assessing a patient's best interests and the risks and benefits of treatment alternatives?
   a. What types of benefit are important?
   b. What types of risk are acceptable/unacceptable?
   c. What types of evidence are valued and relied on when assessing benefits and harms to a patient?
6. According to this cultural group, what methods and criteria support good health care decision making?
   a. Which health and non-health-related consequences are important to consider?
   b. Who needs to be involved?
   c. What is the role of the patient?
   d. What is the role of the family, friends, community members, health care practitioners, states, and proxy decision makers?
   e. What standards are proxy decision makers to use?

IV. Identify potential areas of congruity and difference between your own health beliefs, practices, and values and those of the cultural groups you serve (for example, see Table 16.2)

V. Increase self-awareness about your own cross-cultural health care ethics

   A. *What is your concept of good cross-cultural health care relationships?*
      1. Provider and patient/family have a trusting and respectful relationship?
      2. Provider and patient/family agree on interventions?
      3. The patient's best interests are secured, as the patient or family understands best interests, except when a patient/family's wish entails a significant and disproportionate ethical challenge to professional integrity? (for further examples, see Figure 16.2)

## Table 16.1. *Continued*

    B. *What are your criteria for assessing decision-making capacity in persons with diverse health beliefs?*

       1. U.S. biomedical criteria?

       2. Criteria of the patient's cultural group?

       3. Both?

VI. Learn skills to identify, evaluate, and respond to cross-cultural ethical conflicts, with special attention to challenges to professional integrity

    A. *Distinguish between types of provider objections to treatment wishes*

       1. Objections based on personal preferences

       2. Objections based on personal moral beliefs, including personal conscience

       3. Objections based on professional integrity

    B. *Learn to evaluate objections based on professional integrity*

       1. Assess the patient's or family's treatment wish

         a. Type of wish?

           • A request or a refusal?

           • A diagnostic, curative, life-sustaining, palliative, or preventative intervention?

           • A standard, prohibited, or experimental intervention?

         b. Decision-making capacity of the patient/family?

           • Child/adult with/without decision-making capacity?

           • Capacity assessment based on: biomedical criteria, criteria of patient's cultural group, or both?

         c. Source and strength of the treatment wish?

           • Deep cultural or religious beliefs or commitments?

           • Deep personal beliefs or commitments?

           • Powerful emotions?

           • Socioeconomic conditions?

           • Impaired decision-making capacity?

           • Misunderstanding or lack of knowledge?

       2. Assess the ethical challenge to professional integrity

         a. Strength of empirical support for the health claims and predictions?

         b. Type(s) of challenge to professional integrity? (see Table 16.3)

           • Violates human rights?

           • Is cruel?

- Poses significant harm to identifiable third parties?
- Poses harm that outweighs benefit?
- Poses significant risk to public health?
- Offers no health benefit?
- Offers low probability of benefit?
- Serves non-health-related objectives?

    c. Degree of professional agreement about the challenge to professional integrity?

  3. Compare the strength and source of the patient's or family's wish with the strength of the challenge to professional integrity

C. *Be aware of the range of possible responses to cross-cultural ethical conflicts*

  1. Accede

  2. Compromise

  3. Educate

  4. Build trust

  5. Persuade

  6. Transfer

  7. Refuse

  8. Override

  9. Impose

VII. Develop attitudes culturally responsive to the groups you serve

A. *Be open and nonjudgmental*

B. *Adopt cultural humility, including openness to sharing power*

C. *Demonstrate patience and empathy*

VIII. Learn communication skills culturally responsive to the groups you serve

A. *Nonverbal communication*

  1. Greetings

  2. Head movements

  3. Smiling and laughing

  4. Hand gestures

  5. Eye contact

  6. Facial expressions

  7. Tone of voice

  8. Touching

**Table 16.1.** *Continued*

---

B. *Verbal communication*

   1. Working with interpreters (see Table 16.4)

   2. Greetings

   3. Introductions

   4. Styles of address

   5. Reasons for the visit

   6. Sensitive topics

   7. Risks and benefits

   8. Bad news

   9. Compliments

IX. Develop skills in applying culturally responsive knowledge, skills, and attitudes to particular clinical relationships

   A. *Listen to the patient's or the family's responses to questions about their perspectives*

   1. "What do you [or other people] think is wrong?"

   2. "What do you [or other people] think has caused the problem?"

   3. "How has this problem affected your life?"

   4. "What are you [or other people] afraid of?"

   5. "What healing methods have you tried?"

   6. "What do you [or other people] think will help?"

   7. "Who usually makes [or, helps you make] decisions about your health care?"

   8. "What concerns do you have about seeking U.S. health care services for this problem?"

   B. *Explain the biomedical conceptualization of the problem*

   C. *Acknowledge similarities and differences between the provider's and the patient's perspective*

   D. *Recommend a course of action*

   E. *Negotiate options*

   F. *Evaluate cross-cultural ethical conflicts and appropriate responses (see Table 16.5)*

# Recommendations for Health Care Practitioners

## I.   Be aware of the influence of culture on health status, beliefs, practices, and values

The first step in delivering culturally responsive care is to appreciate that culture influences people's health status and shapes their concepts of health, illness, and healing practices. In childhood, people are molded by their families' and communities' health-related perspectives, which are influenced in turn by their history, ethnicity, religion, and socioeconomic situation. Later, formal education, geographic location, political perspectives, and interactions with the health care system influence people's beliefs, practices, and values. These cultural variables influence, but do not determine, people's understandings of normal and abnormal bodily functions, proper ways to maintain health, and appropriate responses to illness (Helman, 2000; Kleinman, 1980).

When people notice a bodily sign or symptom, they have many ideas, questions, and concerns. They wonder what caused it, how it occurred, whether it is mild or serious, and what they should do about it. They have to consider whether it is normal or abnormal; and if it is abnormal, they have to decide whether to spend time, energy, and money trying to find a remedy. In seeking assistance, they may look to their family and social group, traditional healers, or U.S. health care providers. Each of these decisions is influenced by people's cultural beliefs, values, and practices about health, illness, and healing options, as well as by social factors, such as their economic situation, social role, employment demands, and insurance availability.

Analyses of U.S. health statistics reveal that health status is not equal for all people and that many social conditions contribute to significantly worse health status for people in minority ethnic and racial groups, as well as people in low socioeconomic classes. Historical social conditions—migrant patterns and discrimination—contribute to health disparities; and current social conditions—employment status and lack of insurance—exacerbate them. Cultural and social factors not only shape patients but influence health care practitioners and institutions as well. Studies have exposed how providers' socialization and patterns of institutional care can result in discriminatory treatment (Institute of Medicine [IOM], 2001a).

## II.   Increase self-awareness about your own health beliefs, practices, and values

The recommendation that health care practitioners reflect on their own beliefs, practices, and values reinforces advice provided by many other authors (Campinha-Bacote, 1999; Campinha-Bacote & Munoz, 2001; Epstein, 1999; Gardenswartz & Rowe, 1999; Goldman, Monroe, & Dube, 1996; Jecker et al., 1995; Kune-Karrer & Taylor, 1995; Leininger, 1995a; Marshall, Koenig, Grifhorst, & Van Ewijk, 1998; Novack et al., 1997; O'Connor, 1995; Orr, Marshall, & Osborn, 1995; van Ryn & Burke, 2000).

Health beliefs developed during childhood and adulthood may change as training programs socialize practitioners into a professional subculture with its own language, norms, dress codes, and approaches to identifying and solving problems. Practitioners learn a professional language; sets of beliefs about normal and abnormal physical and mental functions, causes of illness, and determinants of health; approaches to addressing, treating, and preventing physical and mental health conditions; and a value system that guides ethical practices and influences health care decision making (Helman, 2000; Loustaunau & Sobo, 1997).

Providers committed to reflecting on and articulating their health care ethics will want to consider the six core questions presented in Table 16.1, section II.B. A host of variables influences practitioners' responses to questions of health care ethics, including their cultural background, religious orientation, personality, professional training, health care discipline, and practice venue. Practitioners also prioritize ethical commitments differently in challenging situations when not all commitments can be realized simultaneously. Their health care ethics reflect commitments based on their personal and their professional identity. Some of these moral commitments they will be open to modifying and adjusting, while others they will consider non-negotiable. In general, personal moral commitments that are non-negotiable form providers' moral conscience, and strongly held professional obligations form their professional integrity.

Reflecting on questions about their health care ethics and articulating responses may help practitioners explain their ethical perspectives to patients, families, and colleagues. Ethical self-awareness also facilitates identification of the ethical concerns of others that may be at the root of particular disagreements with patients, families, and other members of the health care team.

Providers can increase their understanding of the influence of culture on their health beliefs, practices, and values by paying attention to their reactions to cultural differences and similarities, keeping a personal journal to record their experiences and reflect on their professional group's perspectives, discussing their ideas and struggles with others, getting involved in community activities, and reading about U.S. biomedical culture and the socialization process of health care providers. They can increase their ethical self-awareness by assessing how closely they ally themselves with the health care ethics of their professional colleagues and their profession generally. What is the source of each ethical commitment? Is it a particular commitment unique to the U.S. culture and unlikely to be familiar to or shared by persons with other cultural backgrounds? Which personal or professional ethical commitments does a practitioner consider non-negotiable, and why? Which commitments are open to alternative interpretations or prioritization?

## III. Learn about the prevailing health beliefs, practices, and values of the cultural groups you serve

Practitioners who make an effort to learn about the communities they serve gain an understanding of these communities' current social, economic, and political situations, their health status, access to health care systems, and possible health disparities (see Smedley, Stith, & Nelson, 2002; Kaiser Family Foundation, 1999a, 1999b). In the process they will learn about the cultural group's history: their place of origin, their political and economic situation, their social and religious systems, how they arrived in the United States, what sort of relationships they had with other groups (particularly other Americans), and how familiar they are with various health care systems.

A cultural group's traditional and changing beliefs and practices about anatomy, bodily functions and malfunctions, disease causation, and traditional and Western approaches to treatment, prevention, and health maintenance influence people's reactions to their bodies and to U.S. health care providers' recommendations (Galanti, 1997; Helman, 2000). Chapter 1 provides much of this information about the Hmong, while Chapters 2 through 15 illustrate these health-related beliefs, practices, and values through case stories and commentaries.

Cultural groups that have no formal discipline dedicated to inquiry concerning health care ethics nevertheless have health-related moral practices and commitments. Practitioners can learn about the moral practices and commitments of the cultural groups they serve by using the core questions in Table 16.1, section III.C., as a guide.

Providers may need to tailor these core questions to their discipline and work situation. For example, providers working in end-of-life care would inquire about what behaviors convey respect for the dying person, the deceased person, and the family. What are the roles, responsibilities, and prerogatives of dying persons, their families, and practitioners? What are the best interests of dying persons and their families? These questions (coupled with inquiries into such matters as the meaning of pain, how pain is expressed, distressing symptoms, the goals of end-of-life care, criteria for determining death, and appropriate grieving) facilitate efforts to deliver culturally responsive end-of-life care. (See Crawley, Marshall, Lo, & Koenig, 2002; Kagawa-Singer & Blackhall, 2001; Vawter & Babbitt, 1997.)

Most practitioners, having crossed cultural boundaries throughout their lives, can draw on these same skills to learn about other cultures in the health care context. Cross-cultural learning about health and illness often works best when practitioners connect with people and witness and appreciate their pains and needs, their joys and desires (Kleinman, 1988; Kleinman, Das, & Lock, 1997; Leininger, 1995b). Attending community events, such as holiday rituals, and participating in family events, such as weddings and funerals, opens up opportunities for making person-to-person connections. Otherwise providers can ask interpreters, coworkers, community resource persons, and patients and their families to explain unfamiliar or confusing behaviors and choices. Books, articles, films, and videos may also deepen the practitioner's understanding.

## IV.  Identify potential areas of congruity and difference between your own health beliefs, practices, and values and those of the cultural groups you serve

Practitioners who wish to deliver culturally responsive health care should be alert to possible areas of miscommunication and misunderstanding that can arise out of differences between beliefs about what causes and cures ailments and between health-related moral practices and commitments, while being careful to avoid jumping to conclusions and stereotyping patients. There are at least six major areas of moral commitment and practice that deserve special consideration. Table 16.2 compares prevalent responses by U.S. practitioners and Hmong patients and their families to questions about trust, respect, roles, disclosure practices, best interests, and decision making.

*On what basis are health care practitioners and institutions trustworthy?*    Whereas U.S. providers generally believe their training, technical expertise, and fiduciary obligations make them trustworthy, Hmong patients and their families believe that the provider's character and expressions of genuine care and concern are more important (see Chapters 4, 7, 10, 11, and 13). The role of the United States in the Secret War in Laos and the subsequent U.S. abandonment of the Hmong set the stage for many people in the Hmong community to be deeply mistrustful and angry with Americans, especially those in positions of authority. Against the backdrop of these experiences, some in the Hmong community believe that U.S. providers intentionally sterilize, poison, hurt, and kill Hmong patients (see Kirton, 1985; Fadiman, 1997; Chapters 1, 7, and 13).

*What behaviors demonstrate respect for persons, patients, and families?*    Patients from many different cultural backgrounds say, "Just treat us with respect," but not everyone means the same thing by "respect." Not only does the importance of respectful treatment differ for U.S. providers and traditional Hmong patients but so too do the behaviors that demonstrate it and the qualities that merit it. For example, U.S. health care providers generally believe that seeking consent, honoring treatment refusals, and protecting confidentiality are among the most important ways they can show respect for patients. In contrast, Hmong patients are more likely to focus on how providers address the patient and family, their tone of voice, and their facial expressions (see Chapters 3, 4, 5, 9, and 13).

*What are the ideal roles, responsibilities, and prerogatives of patients, families, healers, health care practitioners, and institutions?*    Traditional Hmong culture defines the roles, responsibilities, and prerogatives of patients, families, and practitioners in ways that directly conflict with the value commitments of the U.S. health care community (Culhane-Pera & Vawter, 1998; Fadiman, 1997; Kirton, 1985; O'Connor, 1998; Vawter & Babbitt, 1997). In traditional Hmong culture, for example, families—not individual patients, health care providers, or the state—are responsible for making health care decisions. Patients are expected to be passive and not actively involved in healing activities and decision making. Healers participate in a patient's care only at the request of the family and are not expected to make health care decisions or to try to persuade patients and families to take a particular course of action (see Chapters 3, 5, 7, 9, 11, and 15).

*What health-related information should be disclosed, to whom, and how?*   Major cultural differences exist concerning what health-related information should be disclosed, to whom, and in what manner (see Chapters 2, 8, 12, and 15). In Hmong culture, for example, disclosing frightening diagnoses to patients is often considered harmful and disrespectful; in U.S. biomedicine, in contrast, respect for patients customarily requires that they receive this information (see Chapters 13 and 15). As Orr et al. (1995, p. 161) observe:

> When patients expect to be told the truth, withholding information may be viewed as a betrayal of trust. Conversely, if patients expect family members and physicians to be circumspect, telling the truth about an illness might be experienced as an abandonment of the healing relationship between patient and physician and the protective relationship between family members.

*What considerations are relevant to assessing a patient's best interests and the risks and benefits of treatment alternatives?*   People from diverse cultural groups may disagree sharply with the criteria U.S. providers use to assess a patient's best interests and the pros and cons of health care options. Agreeing on a therapeutic approach becomes more difficult when the patient or family and the health care professional do not have a common understanding of what has caused the condition and what risks and benefits may follow from a particular treatment.

Traditional Hmong families assess "best interest" largely in the light of what they believe has caused the health problem, its seriousness, and the most effective type of intervention (see Chapter 1). Any intervention can have effects on the person's spiritual, physical, and social well-being in this world, in death, and in future reincarnated lives, as well as on the well-being of relatives. All of this must be taken into account. A person's best interests are integrally linked with the best interests of the family and so are usually not considered independently. U.S. providers, in contrast, typically focus more narrowly on the near-term physiological effects of a proposed intervention on the individual patient (see Chapters 3, 4, 6, 7, 9, 11, and 15). Traditional Hmong families are more averse to risks associated with intervention than to risks associated with nonaction. Invasive medical procedures carry spiritual risks along with the potential risks of physical harm. Surgical interventions in particular tend to pose a larger and weightier set of risks for traditional Hmong patients than for mainstream patients in the United States (see Chapters 3, 9, and 13). The potential social risks to Hmong families can also be increased when a patient or patient's family suffers a bad outcome believed by others in the community to be the result of the family's having made a poor health care decision.

## Table 16.2. Prevalent Health-Related Moral Practices and Commitments

*On what basis are health care practitioners and institutions trustworthy?*

*U.S. Health Care Practitioners*

- Practitioners are deserving of trust as long as they exhibit expertise and act as the patient's fiduciary and advocate.
- Practitioners dedicated to serving patients who are poor, members of minority groups, women, or mentally ill give extra attention to developing trust, since historically these patients have been neglected and abused by U.S. health care institutions and providers.

*Traditional Hmong Patients*

- Practitioners earn trust primarily on the strength of their relationships with families and by providing clear evidence of being decent and compassionate persons committed to patients' and families' well-being.
- Other factors that contribute to trust of practitioners include their prior successes and good reputation in the community.
- The wisdom and experience attributed to the elderly generally warrants greater trust in older practitioners than in younger ones.
- Trust in U.S. health care institutions and practitioners has been adversely affected by experiences of prejudice and discrimination in the society at large and by the U.S. government's broken promises and neglect at the end of the Secret War in Laos.
- Distrust may be significant, ranging from expectations of second-class treatment, overtreatment due to financial incentives, and overt acts of ill-will, including poisoning and use in experimental and educational activities without their knowledge or approval.

*What behaviors demonstrate respect for persons, patients, and families?*

*U.S. Health Care Practitioners*

- Ideally all persons are respected equally, though evidence suggests that some health care institutions and providers give greater respect to persons with wealth, power, and education.
- Respect for patients refers primarily to respect for patient autonomy, i.e., respect the right of patients with decision-making capacity to consent to or refuse recommended interventions (even when the refusal seems foolish).
- Treat patients only with their consent (written, verbal, implied, or presumed consent, depending on the circumstances).
- Demonstrating respect entails listening to patients' concerns and wishes, communicating directly and honestly about their conditions and health care options, and protecting their privacy and confidentiality.
- Identify proxy decision makers to make substitute decisions or decisions in the patient's best interests for those with impaired decision-making capacity.
- Respect for families consists of turning to them as the primary source of proxy decision makers when the patient is a child or has impaired decision-making capacity.

*Traditional Hmong Patients*

- All persons are owed respect, though persons are given special respect according to their social role, age (older before younger), gender (men before women), talents, knowledge, responsibilities, and contributions to the community.
- Respect is one of the most important social values. A person who treats another with disrespect brings deep shame not only to himself or herself but also to his or her entire family.
- Respect is demonstrated through the practitioners' manner and style of relating, e.g., by being polite and formal, using good manners, speaking in a soft voice, avoiding prolonged direct eye contact, and displaying a spirit of self-sacrifice, discipline, patience, honesty, and a commitment to patients that approaches love. Other respectful behaviors include developing a personal connection with the patient before turning to health-related matters, speaking indirectly about frightening or sensitive matters, and asking patients' permission before touching them, especially their heads.
- It is disrespectful for practitioners to assert authority, imply they are more important than patients and families, threaten patients and families, shame them or cause them to lose face, and interfere with the families' responsibilities to make health care decisions on behalf of ill family members.

**Table 16.2. Continued**

*What are the ideal roles, responsibilities, and prerogatives of patients, families, healers, health care practitioners, and institutions?*

*U.S. Health Care Practitioners*

- Practitioners are expected to protect patients from harm and to pursue patients' health interests; they are expected to be active advocates for patients.
- Practitioners are expected to keep developing their expertise.
- Practitioners play many different roles, but in cases of serious illness they are expected to be directive and assertive and to take charge.
- Practitioners may be held responsible for adverse health outcomes.
- Practitioners are expected not to become too personally involved with patients or families.
- Primary relationships are between patients and the practitioners.
- Patients are expected whenever possible to take active roles in their own care and decision making.
- Families are involved in patient care and decision making only with the patient's permission or at the patient's request.
- Proxy decision makers are expected to represent the patient and not themselves.
- Proxy decision makers have limited rights to make treatment decisions; they are not to act from self-interest.
- The state has the prerogative to intercede in some health care decisions.

*Traditional Hmong Patients*

- Practitioners provide advice, service, and treatment when it is requested. It is not their role to directly persuade, override, or force people to undergo interventions they believe would be beneficial.
- Practitioners are expected to provide hope and encouragement to ill people and their families.
- U.S. health care practitioners have no expertise or power to heal problems that have spiritual causes, although their treatments may be sought to relieve related symptoms and conditions.
- Persons assume the sick role when they cannot fulfill their social roles; they are usually expected to be passive.
- Primary relationships are between families and patients. Families have responsibility for caring for the sick, consulting healers, making decisions, and paying healers.
- Families are assumed to be the decision makers and to weigh a range of factors in addition to the immediate physical health interests of their sick family members.
- Families pay Hmong healers as a sign of respect for their healing powers and helping spirits; sometimes payment occurs after desired results are achieved.
- The state has no right to interfere with the family's decision-making authority.

*What health-related information should be disclosed, to whom, and how?*

U.S. Health Care Practitioners

- Practitioners are expected to provide patients, or proxy decision makers, with the information reasonable persons would want to know about their condition and the risks and benefits of alternative treatment options.

- Practitioners are expected to disclose information about a patient to others, including family and friends, only with the patient's permission.

- Full and honest disclosures to patients are considered respectful; disclosure empowers patients to be partners in the healing process and to protect themselves from undesired intrusions and disruptions of their bodily integrity and privacy.

- Disclosures tend to emphasize the risks of interventions and non-treatment in order to underscore the seriousness of the situation, motivate patients to take action, and reduce practitioners' risk of legal liabilities.

Traditional Hmong Patients

- It is important for practitioners to share some personal or social information about themselves so that patients and families can get a feel for who practitioners are.

- Hmong healers are expected to disclose the information families need to maintain good relationships with the spirits. All practitioners are expected to offer information and recommendations necessary for families to make well-considered decisions concerning their well-being.

- When practitioners have disturbing information, they should either tell the family and leave it to them to decide whether and how the information will be disclosed to the ill family member or not disclose the information and protect the family from upset.

- Practitioners are expected to disclose information in a positive way that protects patients from frightening and sad information, that does not predict (or cause) negative events, and that provides patients and families with hope.

- Practitioners preferably disclose potentially distressing information in a soft voice, indirectly and subtly, because words have the power to break hearts, extinguish hope, cause soul loss, and become reality.

**Table 16.2. Continued**

*What considerations are relevant to assessing a patient's best interests and the risks and benefits of treatment alternatives?*

| U.S. Health Care Practitioners | Traditional Hmong Patients |
|---|---|
| • Practitioners ideally assess risks and benefits to physical health based on scientific evidence. | • Patients' best interests include spiritual, physical, and social well-being in this life, in the spirit world, and in future lives, as well as families' and clans' well-being now and in future lives. |
| • Practitioners usually assess a circumscribed set of immediate health-related risks and benefits. | • Patients' best interests are tied to families' best interests and are not considered in isolation. |
| • While the risks should not be disproportionate to the benefits, risks are acceptable. | • Families seek to secure the spiritual well-being of the family. |
| • Practitioners and patients tend to be more tolerant of risks associated with interventions than of risks associated with nontreatment and to support risk-taking in the interests of prolonged life or improved quality of life. | • Families seek to preserve the individual's ability to fulfill his or her role in and responsibility to the family and community. |
| • Proxy decision makers' decisions may be overridden by health care practitioners, or the state, if in their judgment proxy decision makers are not representing the patient's wishes or best interests. | • Determining the causes of ailments is important, since treatments fit causes, e.g., supernatural therapies are needed for spiritual problems. |
| • Practitioners are to respect patients' assessments of their own best interests unless, according to the practitioners, they entail engaging in an objectionable activity, e.g., one that is illegal, violates human rights, or violates professional integrity. | • Health care procedures offer reasonable risks and benefits when they offer benefit without risk of physical or spiritual harm. |
| | • Invasive procedures pose spiritual as well as physical risks. |
| | • Risks associated with health care interventions, especially invasive procedures, are usually assessed more negatively than risks associated with nontreatment. |
| | • It is risky for ill persons to be physically isolated from families; families protect against evil spirits and provide support and care. Personal experience, anecdotal accounts, and messages from the spirit world are consulted and relied on. |

*What methods and criteria support good health care decision making?*

U.S. Health Care Practitioners

- Patients have the authority and right to make health care decisions for themselves, though joint decision making between patients and providers is considered ideal.
- Practitioners are expected to provide information and make recommendations; in the case of acute serious illness they may actively seek to persuade the patient or proxy to follow their recommendation and may seek state involvement in the case of vulnerable patients who lack suitable proxies.
- Decisions are usually treated as discrete events and few ramifications are considered in addition to the immediate health consequences for the patient.
- Risks and adverse outcomes associated with actions are generally preferred to those associated with inaction.
- Good health care decisions are based on scientific information and reflect the authentic wishes of informed patients possessing adequate decision-making capacity.
- Family members are involved in decision making for patients with decision-making capacity only at the patient's invitation.
- Family members are involved in decision making for patients with impaired decision-making capacity, unless the patient has formally designated a non-family member to serve as his or her health care proxy or has a court-appointed guardian.
- Proxy decision makers are required to base decisions on what the patient would want, or if unknown, on the patient's medical best interests.

Traditional Hmong Patients

- Good health care decisions are well-considered decisions based on the individual's, family's, and clan's best interests. This requires careful attention to the numerous possible ramifications of a bad outcome for the patient in this life, in the spirit world, and in the next life, as well as for family members, descendants, the clan, and the community. Good decisions prevent the ancestral spirits from becoming vengeful and bringing bad luck or illness to the family and help maintain the family's reputation within the community.
- The primary responsibility for health care decision making and for caring for ill persons belongs to the family, where the family may include the nuclear family, the extended family, and the clan.
- Health care decisions are family-based decisions and the family shares responsibility for the outcomes. Patients who make decisions on their own against the counsel of their family may be blamed or left to suffer alone if there are adverse outcomes.
- Formally appointed proxy decision makers are unnecessary, because appropriate adult family or clan members make decisions.
- The decision-making process may be based on consensus or may be authoritarian.
- Risks and adverse outcomes associated with inaction are generally preferred to those associated with actions.
- Practitioners have no responsibility or authority to make health care decisions; however, their recommendations may carry significant weight.

*What methods and criteria support good health care decision making?*    People from different cultures often endorse rival methods and criteria for good health care decision making. For traditional Hmong patients, for example, good decisions are those that their extended families have carefully weighed and considered and that have gained familywide agreement. This family decision-making method considers more than the individual patient's wishes and takes more time than most U.S. providers are comfortable with. In cases of patients with impaired decision-making capacity, U.S. providers urge families to make substituted judgments based on what their sick relative would want, and when the wishes are unknown, based on the medical best interests of the patient. U.S. practices of patient consent, substituted decision making, and advance directives, however, are inconsistent with traditional Hmong decision-making practices (see Chapter 1; Berger, 1998; Fetters, 1998).

Several commentators suggest that learning about the beliefs, practices, and values of cultural groups may be of limited value—or may even be dangerous—if it leads to stereotyping (e.g., Blacksher, 1998; Koenig & Gates-Williams, 1995). They stress instead the importance of bringing a good set of questions to clinical encounters and getting to know the patient without any preconceived ideas.

While information about a group can be misused and misapplied, clinicians nonetheless can better serve if they understand the beliefs, practices, and values prevalent within the cultural groups they serve (O'Connor, 1995, 1998; Orr et al., 1995). Such knowledge can help increase insight into a particular patient's moral perspectives, help prevent misunderstandings and inadvertent expressions of disrespect, and guide providers' selection of initial questions to bring to particular cross-cultural clinical encounters. This kind of information also suggests the range of moral perspectives that patients may bring to clinical encounters.

## V.    Increase self-awareness about your own cross-cultural health care ethics

Faced with alternative cultural perspectives, practitioners vary in their willingness to learn about them, accommodate them, and adapt their own health-related moral commitments and practices (Bennett 1986, 1993; Culhane-Pera & Vawter, 1998). Some practitioners, for example, believe their health care ethics are both correct and superior to those of others. They might express their belief in statements such as, "The Hmong practice of family decision making violates my duty to respect patient autonomy." Others, after reflecting on their socialization process and becoming aware of the cultural basis of every individual's health care ethics, acknowledge that theirs is just one perspective. They might say, "While the moral practice of family decision making is not part of my own health care ethics, I support my Hmong patients' decision-making practices because they make sense within their culture."

An emerging body of literature, primarily by medical anthropologists and health care ethicists, addresses ethical issues in cross-cultural health care. Some of the literature focuses on specific issues, such as end-of-life care or international research involving human subjects, but much of it discusses the ethical issues of autonomy, consent, and truth-telling common in U.S. provider-patient relationships.*

Delivering culturally responsive health care requires attention to both the "routine" (for U.S. practitioners) ethical questions and some special ethical questions that arise in cross-cultural health care relationships. When serving patients with different cultural perspectives on illness and healing and with different moral commitments and practices, which aspects of their health care ethics are providers willing to modify or forgo? When might such modifications be inappropriate, depart too substantially from professional norms, or result in unjustifiable inequities in the delivery of health care? In some cross-cultural health care relationships, respect for persons, for example, may cause providers to modify or relinquish common U.S. moral practices concerning decision making, patient and family responsibilities, and disclosure. More specifically, providers may reconsider such common Western biomedical practices as requiring the consent of patients, securing patient signatures on consent forms, making requests for organ and tissue donation, discussing patients' prognosis for hospice admission, and conducting conversations regarding advance directives, including do not resuscitate (DNR) orders. (See Berger, 1998; Fetters, 1998; Hyun, 2002; Kagawa-Singer & Blackhall, 2001; Marshall et al., 1998; Vawter & Babbitt, 1997.)

The nature and quality of cross-cultural health care depend on how professionals understand and prioritize their obligations to respect patients and families with culturally diverse health beliefs and to protect and secure patients' best interests. Each provider must decide how he or she will determine the best interests of patients with diverse health beliefs. Does the practitioner believe that he or she is ethically required to secure a patient's best interests based on his or her own understanding, based on the patient's or the family's understanding, or based on some combination of perspectives? Despite the absence of clear consensus on these cross-cultural ethical issues, health care professionals routinely make such decisions.

*What is your concept of good cross-cultural health care relationships?*    Criteria for good health care relationships generally include that the provider and patient have a trusting and respectful relationship, are able to communicate effectively, can agree on appropriate therapeutic measures, and are satisfied with the outcome. Additional criteria are necessary, however, to guide the resolution of cross-cultural ethical differences or conflicts. For example, different acute care providers might adopt one or another of the examples of criteria for good cross-cultural health care relationships

---

*See Berger, 1998; Blackhall, Frank, Murphy, & Michel, 200l; Blackhall et al., 1999; Blackhall, Murphy, Frank, Michel, & Azen, 1995; Blacksher, 1998; Caralis, 1993; Carrese & Rhodes, 1995; Clouser, Hufford, & O'Connor, 1996; Crawley, Marshall, & Koenig, 200l; Crawley et al., 2002; Culhane-Pera & Vawter, 1998; Dula & Goering, 1994; Fetters, 1998; Flack & Pellegrino, 1992; Gervais, 1998; Gostin, 1995; Hern, Koenig, Moore, & Marshall, 1998; Jecker et al., 1995; Kagawa-Singer & Blackhall, 2001; Kaufert & O'Neil, 1990; Kleinman, 1995; Klessig, 1992; Kunstadter, 1980; Lane & Rubinstein, 1996; Lieban, 1990; Lock, 2002; Macklin, 1999; Marshall, 1992; Marshall & Koenig, 1996; Marshall, et al., 1998; Meleis & Jonsen, 1983; Muller & Desmond, 1992; Nie, 2000; O'Connor, 1995; Orona, Koenig, & Davis, 1994; Orr et al., 1995; Pellegrino, 1992; Perkins, Supik, & Hazuda, 1993, 1998; Vawter & Babbitt, 1997; Veatch, 1989, 2000; Yeo, 1995.

in Figure 16.2. These examples reflect a range of possible criteria, starting with the most ethnocentric at the top to the most ethnorelative at the bottom.

We recommend that practitioners make a commitment to respect patients' and families' wishes—except when a treatment decision poses a significant and disproportionate ethical challenge to professional integrity. This intermediate criterion commits neither the error of radical cultural relativism nor the error of radical ethnocentrism. It acknowledges that neither all challenges to professional integrity nor all patient or family treatment wishes have equal moral strength (see pp. 323–27 below). Being aware that there are different understandings of what constitutes good cross-cultural health care relationships can also offer insight into possible sources of conflicts with other team members.

*What are your criteria for assessing decision-making capacity in persons with diverse health beliefs?*     Patients from some cultural groups think about health and illness in ways so unfamiliar to and different from those of their U.S. providers that providers may doubt that their patients possess decisional capacity. For example, the explanations of health problems and possible interventions by traditional animist Hmong patients frequently are not germane to the beliefs of U.S. providers (Culhane-Pera & Vawter, 1998; see Chapters 4, 5, 6, 7, 8, 9, 10, and 15). In this situation, is it

## Figure 16.2. Criteria for Good Cross-Cultural Health Care Relationships

Ethnocentric
Ethnorelative

- The practitioner treats the patient with the same interventions as any other patient with the same problem, without regard for the patient's culture.
- The practitioner does not permit the patient's or family's cultural beliefs to interfere with providing life-saving or palliative interventions to any patient (adult or child).
- The practitioner does not permit the family's cultural beliefs to interfere with providing life-saving or palliative interventions to any child.
- The patient's best interests are secured, as the patient or family understands best interests, except when a patient or family wish entails a significant and disproportionate ethical challenge to professional integrity.
- The patient's best interests are secured, as the patient or family understands best interests, except when the course of action is prohibited by law or violates the patient's human rights.
- The patient's best interests are secured, as the patient or family understands best interests for any adult patient.
- The patient's best interests are secured, as the patient or family understands best interests for any patient (child or adult).

appropriate to assess the patient's decision-making capacity based on his or her appreciation of the Western biomedical explanations? Or should the criteria for assessing decision-making capacity accommodate persons with health beliefs unfamiliar to U.S. providers? And if the customary criteria should be modified, how can providers ensure that they can identify and adequately protect those people with impaired decision-making capacity?

Assessments of decision-making capacity can play a key role in whether practitioners honor or override patient wishes. When providers believe a patient's or family's wishes may reflect impaired decision making, it is their responsibility to assess decision-making capacity. If the providers judge that the patient's or the family's capacity is impaired, they have the prerogative—and in some circumstances may even have the obligation—to override such treatment wishes.

Mistaken judgments regarding patients' decision-making capacity can be dangerous, disrespectful, and unfair to patients. Two mistakes can occur: overriding patient or family refusals based on a mistaken judgment of impaired decision-making capacity, or honoring inauthentic and uninformed risky treatment decisions based on a mistaken assumption of intact decision-making capacity.

Although decisions about which criteria to use to assess decision-making capacity can be crucial, the current criteria are variable and commonly noted to be less than optimal. One approach considers patients' abilities to understand information relevant to the decision about treatment, to appreciate the significance for their own situation of the information disclosed about the illness and possible treatments, and to manipulate the information rationally (or reason about it) in a manner that allows them to make comparisons and weigh options (Grisso & Appelbaum, 1995, p. 1033). A similar set of criteria considers the patients' ability to understand a therapy, to deliberate about major risks and benefits, and to make a decision in the light of this deliberation (Beauchamp & Childress, 1994, p. 136).

Many patients and families in the case stories in Chapters 2 through 15 might fail to meet these customary criteria of decision-making capacity. They do not understand or agree with the biomedical explanation of the problem, the proposed treatment, or the predicted consequences of forgoing the recommended intervention.

Such serious differences in understanding are sometimes due to Hmong patients and families' believing in causes that are alien to U.S. health care professionals. When a spiritual cause is identified, for example, families tend to believe the problem requires a spiritual rather than a biomedical intervention. For example, Culhane-Pera and Vawter (1998) describe a case in which an older Hmong woman and her family requested that an endotracheal tube placed to help her overcome an acute breathing problem be removed. Their request came after her family had addressed the spiritual causes of her ailment, resolved their familial conflict, ascertained that her physical condition had improved, and understood that the endotracheal tube could harm her trachea. Her physicians refused to comply with the request because they believed neither she nor her family understood their warnings that she would die if they withdrew the tube.

Approaches to assessing decision-making capacity that presuppose particular cultural perspectives on health and turn on whether the patient understands and embraces the provider's perspective on the illness and treatments reveal inadvertent and perhaps unavoidable cultural biases. They can also unfairly disadvantage persons with unfamiliar health beliefs and cultural values.

> In attempting to gauge understanding, the values of the tester play an insidious and probably unavoidable role. Not only does the tester's view of what constitutes understanding affect the determination, but the initial selection of the information the patient is to be tested on reflects the importance the tester attaches to that information. (Appelbaum, Lidz, & Meisel, 1987, p. 85)

Providers may be unable or unwilling to eliminate all cultural bias in their assessment criteria. They can decide, however, whether to (1) assess decision-making capacity by applying criteria developed by and for members of the mainstream culture to all patients uniformly or (2) amend these criteria so that persons who are unfamiliar with or unwilling to accept biomedical perspectives on illness and healing are less likely to be judged to be impaired. We recommend the latter option and suggest including criteria such as these:

- Whether the patient's or family's health beliefs, reasoning, and treatment decision are consistent with those of others from the patient's cultural group
- Whether the patient's decision "is stable over time, . . . consistent with the patient's values and goals, . . . [and does] not result from delusions or hallucinations" (Lo, 1995, p. 85) as evaluated by others in his or her community
- Whether the patient "has previously behaved in ways consistent with these beliefs" (Lo, 1995, p. 85)
- Whether members of the patient's cultural group believe the patient or family possess decision-making capacity
- Whether the decision is idiosyncratic
- Whether the patient's "choices are based on distorted or irrational beliefs that are part of a mental disorder or psychological dysfunction . . . [and] presumably do not reflect the judgments that [he or she] would otherwise have made" (Grisso & Appelbaum, 1998, p. 48)

These criteria can help providers to determine that patients and families with divergent cultural perspectives possess decision-making capacity and identify persons whose reasoning is impaired because of a mental disorder or psychological dysfunction.

Deciding that a patient lacks decision-making capacity, however, is only one rationale for providers to override treatment wishes that they judge to be unreasonable. The treatment wishes of patients or families are sometimes objectionable to providers for other reasons. Deciding that a patient or family possesses decision-making capacity does not require that providers accede in every case to the patient's treatment wish (Brock & Wartman, 1990).

## VI.  Learn skills to identify, evaluate, and respond to cross-cultural ethical conflicts, with special attention to challenges to professional integrity

Providers in cross-cultural health care experience many conflicts as simply unusual, interesting, annoying, or inconvenient. More serious conflicts arise, however, when negotiations fail to find options that adequately respect both the core values of patients and families and the professional integrity of the practitioners. These conflicts cannot be resolved easily through further discussion and education, because they arise from different health-related moral practices and commitments. Conflicts may involve procedural matters, such as honoring patient or family requests to not tell the patient "the truth" about a terminal diagnosis, or they may involve the substance of treatment decisions, such as respecting a patient's or a family's decision to forgo interventions that the provider believes are life-saving or will ease the dying process (see Chapters 3, 5, 7, 13, and 15). When these cross-cultural challenges arise, appropriate responses require skills to distinguish among different types of provider objections to patient or family treatment wishes as well as an effective method to assess the degree of challenge to professional integrity.

### Distinguish between types of provider objections to treatment wishes

Providers who participate in cross-cultural health care relationships experience an array of personal responses. Some may be positive, such as excitement, intellectual interest, and pleasure. Others may be more equivocal or negative, such as confusion, frustration, or anger. These emotions can be triggered by challenges to health care providers' personal concerns or preferences, cultural or spiritual beliefs, moral beliefs, or their professional integrity.

Not all challenges are ethical challenges. And not all ethical challenges are equally serious. Indeed most cross-cultural differences are minor and cause little emotional discomfort or ethical conflict for those involved. U.S. providers are unlikely to experience emotional or personal moral concern, for example, when Hmong families and friends ceremonially tie strings around the wrists of ill persons or when families replace the hospital gowns of dying family members with traditional Hmong clothes.

In some situations, providers are justified in refusing to accede to or in overriding the treatment decisions and wishes of persons with culturally diverse health beliefs, but these situations need to be carefully circumscribed. The most serious cross-cultural ethical conflicts challenge a provider's moral conscience or his or her professional integrity. When a provider experiences negative reactions to treatment wishes, it is important to clarify which types of objection he or she has.

*Objections based on personal preferences*   Cross-cultural health care relationships frequently challenge providers' personal preferences. Some clinicians may become frustrated with parents who are loathe to displease their children by requiring them to take unpleasant medications; some may discourage women in labor from leaving the hospital to go home briefly to conduct a traditional ceremony to ensure a safe birth; and some may refuse to allow or accommodate traditional healing practices in a hospital.

In general, providers should be prepared to accommodate patient or family wishes that challenge their personal, spiritual, and cultural preferences. Those who find themselves overwhelmed by strong personal concerns or prejudices or by other strong negative reactions to patients with culturally diverse health beliefs and practices may want to discuss their feelings with other health care professionals, seek personal advice and counseling, or transfer care to other providers.

*Objections based on personal moral beliefs, including personal conscience*    Challenges to a health care professional's personal moral beliefs may elicit feelings ranging from slight moral concern or disquietude, to moderate discomfort, to serious threats to personal conscience.

For example, a hospice nurse may disagree with the patient's and family's preferences not to plan for death and personally believe it is morally important to speak directly about a young mother's impending death so that she can decide who will care for her children after she dies. A physician may have personal moral objections to a family's plans to conduct a spiritual healing ceremony that involves animal sacrifice. Neither of these cases requires a provider's direct participation in procedures or interventions so objectionable that the providers "could no longer live with themselves" if they participate in the care of the patient.

Stronger challenges to providers' moral beliefs can threaten personal conscience. Objections based on personal conscience arise from a person's deepest identity-conferring ethical convictions about what it means to be a good person (Benjamin, 1995). Providers who experience such objections are so deeply disturbed by the patient's or family's wishes that they "would be unable to live with themselves" if they were to directly participate in the objectionable intervention. Some providers may object, for example, to legally available interventions, such as pregnancy terminations, operating on patients with do not resuscitate (DNR) orders, withdrawing life-support from conscious non-terminally ill patients, and participating in physician-assisted suicide. When the only objection a practitioner raises is that the patient's treatment wish challenges his or her personal conscience, the practitioner should seek to transfer care or request to be excused from participating in the specific intervention or procedure. A decision to override a patient's treatment wish solely because the provider has an objection based on personal conscience is not justified.

*Objections based on professional integrity*    The most ethically compelling objections that health care professionals may have to patients' and families' treatment wishes involve threats to professional integrity, that is, challenges to the core professional roles, responsibilities, and obligations by which health care providers define themselves. When clinicians talk with adult patients about patients' preferences regarding such moral practices as who is to receive health-related disclosures and who is responsible for health care decision making, clinicians usually find that the cross-cultural challenge to their professional integrity is manageable and not excessive. More difficult challenges to professional integrity concern the substance of treatment decisions. The sources of such conflicts usually include some combination of health-related beliefs and practices involving the type, cause, and severity of the ailment, appropriate interventions, and valued outcomes, as well as moral commitments concerning what is in the best interests of a patient with this condition and what constitutes a relevant and appropriate risk/benefit assessment. Conflicts of this kind may occur, for example, when a patient or family decides to forgo interventions that the provider believes are necessary to protect the patient from serious, avoidable, and irreversible harm (see Chapters 3, 5, 6, 7, 11, and 13; see also Orr et al., 1995; Culhane-Pera & Vawter, 1998). Other examples involve treatment requests that challenge the practitioner's professional obligation to provide only interventions that offer a chance of benefit (see Chapters 13–15).

Objections based on professional integrity in some cases may justify overriding the treatment wishes of a patient or family. Whenever a treatment wish challenges a provider's professional integrity, however, further analysis is required before selecting a response.

### Learn to evaluate objections based on professional integrity

There are three general strategies for evaluating cross-cultural ethical challenges to professional integrity: the provider's perspective always prevails, the patient's or family's perspective always prevails, or assess each conflict case by case (Jecker et al., 1995).

The strategy a provider chooses tends to correspond with the provider's choice of criteria for good cross-cultural health care relationships (see pp. 317–18 above). Those who choose, as recommended, to secure the patient's best interests as the patient or family understands best interests (except when a patient or family wish entails a significant and disproportionate ethical challenge to professional integrity) are likely to adopt a case-by-case approach to discern whether the moral strength of the patient's or family's wish outweighs the ethical challenge it poses to professional integrity and how best to respond.

The case-by-case approach we recommend for evaluating cross-cultural ethical challenges to professional integrity rests on our observation that both the moral strength of patient wishes and the strength of ethical challenges to professional integrity vary from case to case. A default position regarding whether the patient's or the provider's perspective should trump in every case is unlikely to be either effective or appropriate.

Table 16.1, section VI.B., offers points to consider when evaluating whether the patient's or family's wish should be respected and honored in a particular case or whether the wish poses a significant and disproportionate ethical challenge to the practitioner's professional integrity.

*Assess the patient's or family's treatment wish*     Assessing the patient's or family's treatment wish calls for three sets of considerations. The first set concerns the type of wish involved. Is it a refusal of an intervention? In general, providers are less obligated to provide requested interventions and they are more obligated to honor treatment refusals. For example, providers refused to provide requested operations, chemo-therapy, and radiation to patients in the case stories in Chapters 13 and 15, though they acceded to the patients' treatment refusals. Much also depends on the status of the interventions that are requested. Are the requested interventions standard treatment? Are they diagnostic, curative, life-saving, palliative, or preventive? Are they prohibited procedures (e.g., participating in physician-assisted suicide, prescribing steroids for athletes, or performing female genital mutilation) or are they experimental?

The second set of considerations concerns the decision-making capacity of the patient or family and the criteria used to assess capacity. Is the patient an adult with intact or impaired decision-making capacity? Is the patient a child? In general, the wishes of adults with decision-making capacity have greater weight than treatment wishes by family or surrogates on behalf of persons without such capacity, especially young children. The criteria practitioners use to assess the patient's or family's decision-making capacity—U.S. biomedical criteria, the criteria of the patient's cultural group, or both—can be crucial, since some criteria are more culturally biased than others, and hence more likely to result in providers' judging patients and families with diverse health beliefs as lacking decision-making capacity and then overriding their treatment wishes (see pp. 318–20).

The third set of considerations is the source and strength of the treatment wish. From an ethical perspective, the strongest sources are deep cultural or religious beliefs and values. And when such deep beliefs and values are identity-defining for the patient and family, they are morally the weightiest. Other less morally weighty sources of treatment wishes include personal values, emotions, socioeconomic realities, impaired decision-making capacity, and lack of knowledge.

Since not all treatment wishes have equal moral weight, it is important to learn about the source of the patient's or family's particular wish and how strongly it is held. Simply knowing that a treatment wish stems from a deep cultural or religious belief is not enough information, since the particular patient or family may or may not be strongly committed to this belief. Practitioners can try to determine how strongly the belief is held and how likely the patient or family is to be amenable to compromise or to reinterpreting the belief (O'Connor, 1995; see also Chapters 3, 4, 6, 8, 11, 12, and 15; Hyun, 2002).

*Assess the ethical challenge to professional integrity*    After assessing the source and strength of the patient's or family's wishes, it is important to engage in a similar assessment of the provider's perspective and assess the strength of the ethical challenge the treatment wish poses to the provider's professional integrity.

This assessment involves inquiry into three matters. First, how strong is the empirical support for the provider's health claims and predictions about what benefits and harms may befall the patient were the provider to abide by the patient's or the family's wishes? Clearly, predictions based on evidence-based medicine tend to be stronger than predictions based on professional judgment or best guesses.

Second, what type of challenge does the treatment wish pose to the provider's professional integrity? While it is often assumed that any challenge to professional integrity has equal moral importance and deserves to be rebuffed, some challenges to professional integrity are graver than others (Vawter, 1996). The most significant challenges to professional integrity are treatment requests that violate a patient's fundamental human rights (Kleinman, 1995). Other serious challenges to professional integrity come from treatment wishes that the provider believes are cruel, that is, interventions that provide no health benefit and are so harmful as to be inhumane and abhorrent. Such patient and family treatment wishes violate the provider's strongest professional obligations: respect for persons and nonmaleficence. These wishes pose morally weightier challenges to professional integrity than do those that, while not harmful, offer only a low probability of benefit or no benefit. The major types of challenge to professional integrity in Table 16.1, section VI.B.2.b., are listed in roughly descending order of moral importance, beginning with the most important, "Violates human rights." Table 16.3 presents a more detailed list of types of challenge to professional integrity.

The final point to consider is the agreement among U.S. health care professionals that the particular case presents a strong challenge to professional integrity. The goal of this hypothetical exercise is to assess whether the degree of professional agreement is strong, moderate, or weak.

*Compare the strength and source of the patient's or family's treatment wish with the strength of the challenges to professional integrity*     Once the provider has assessed the source and strength of the treatment wish and the strength of the challenge it poses to professional integrity, the two can be compared. According to our recommended criteria for good cross-cultural health care relationships, if the provider finds the strength of the challenge to professional integrity to be significant, the next question is whether the strength of the challenge is disproportionate to and outweighs the moral weightiness of the patient's or family's wishes. When the challenge to professional integrity is either insignificant or does not outweigh the patient's or family's treatment wish, then the patient's perspective should prevail. When the challenge to professional integrity is significant and it outweighs the source and strength of the patient's or family's treatment wish, then the provider's perspective should prevail. When the patient's wishes and the challenges to professional integrity are both strong and neither outweighs the other, then the general presumption should be that the patient's perspective prevails, though admittedly there is as yet no firm consensus on these ethical matters.

Increased experience with providing culturally responsive health care may result in expanded understandings of professional integrity and what it requires of and allows health care providers. With increased appreciation for the health beliefs, practices, and values of patients from different cultural backgrounds, providers may discover ways to reinterpret "professional integrity" and increasingly conclude that challenges to professional integrity are not always the most important ethical issue— other ethical considerations should sometimes take precedence.

Martin Benjamin (1990; see especially pp. 36–38, 130) offers several reasons why health care professionals may conclude that compromising or acceding to a patient's

## Table 16.3. Practitioner Objections to Patients' or Families' Treatment Wishes Based on Professional Integrity

Treatment disrespects patient
- Violates patient's human rights
- Violates competent patient's treatment wishes
- Undermines patient's ability to make autonomous decisions
- Violates patient dignity

Treatment is cruel
- Is inhumane, abhorrent
- Mutilates, destroys body image without benefit
- Provides no benefit and imposes significant and preventable pain or suffering

Treatment poses significant harm to identifiable third parties

Potential harm of treatment outweighs potential benefit
- Risks of physical harm are predicted to be significant and to far exceed benefits
- Prolongs the dying process
- Entails pain, mutilation, or loss of function disproportionate to benefit
- Safer and more effective alternative exists

Treatment poses significant risk to public health

Treatment offers no health benefit
- Death is imminent and unavoidable
- Well-designed studies prove it does not work
- Will not achieve physiologic objective; no physiologic or pharmacologic rationale
- Will not heal, promote health, preserve or restore functioning, or alleviate suffering

Treatment offers low probability of benefit
- Unlikely to restore quality of life satisfactory to patient
- Conflicts with well-established practice guidelines
- Unlikely to heal or promote health
- Unlikely to achieve patient's objective
- Health professional does not possess requisite expertise

Treatment serves non-health-related objectives
- Serves state's investigatory, disciplinary, or punitive objectives
- Directly conflicts with preserving life, health, function, and bodily integrity
- Violates professional taboos
- Supports the patient's or family's hope for a miracle
- Responds to the patient's or family's fear of abandonment and distrust
- Serves the patient's or family's cultural or religious beliefs, practices, or values regarding health, illness, well-being, life, death, or respectful behavior toward ill family member, clan, and tribe
- Would not be wanted by reasonable persons in mainstream culture

or family's treatment wish may be more integrity preserving than any available alternative. Providers may relax their understanding of what professional integrity requires and allows of them because they

- appreciate the full complexity of the nature and circumstances of the disagreement and see matters from the other's point of view,
- recognize that the matter does permit a plausible difference of opinion,
- value relationships, preservation of trust, and continuing communication,
- have compassion for psychological and spiritual suffering, as well as physical suffering,
- prefer not to settle disputes by force or by unilaterally asserting authority, or
- distinguish between what they believe should be done and what they judge ought to be done, all things considered.

### Be aware of the range of possible responses to cross-cultural ethical conflicts

The responses that providers focus on are influenced by such factors as the culture and politics of the organization where care is being provided, as well as the providers' training, creativity, experiences, attitudes, and cross-cultural health care ethics (U.S. DHHS, 2000c). Are the practitioners' criteria for good cross-cultural health care relationships (Figure 16.2) and criteria for assessing decision-making capacity in patients with unfamiliar health beliefs strongly ethnocentric, strongly ethnorelative, or in between, representing a balancing of patients' and providers' health-related moral commitments and practices? Each of these cross-cultural ethical decisions reflects providers' prioritization of their moral commitments to protect and serve patients' physical health interests, preserve trusting and respectful relationships with patients and families, and preserve professional integrity.

The scant literature on responding to ethical conflicts in cross-cultural health care advises providers to do more than simply assert "moral superiority on the basis of membership in the dominant white culture of the United States" (Orr et al., 1995, p. 163). It suggests that providers engage in "reciprocal participatory engagement" (Kleinman, 1995, p. 1672) and respectful negotiation and compromise (Crawley et al., 2002; Kagawa-Singer & Blackhall, 2001; Kleinman, 1995; Marshall et al., 1998; O'Connor, 1995; Orr et al., 1995). A few authors suggest that there are limits to professional obligations to compromise and that not all conflicts can be resolved through negotiation and compromise (Jecker et al., 1995; Kleinman, 1995; Koenig & Gates-Williams, 1995; Orr et al., 1995). Jecker et al. (1995, p. 12) indicate that serious ethical conflict occurs when one or both parties view "the other's values as not only different, but wrong or extremely offensive, and therefore are unable to accommodate them." They advocate a case-by-case approach, using a fair procedure agreed on by both sides to fashion a "negotiated settlement." The procedure used should assume initially a "nonjudgmental stance" and should be conducted publicly. Besides these recommendations, the literature offers clinicians little guidance in deciding whether they have reached an impasse and if they have, what they should do next.

Often clarity regarding the type and strength of the provider objection and the source and strength of the patient's or family's wish is sufficient to suggest responses that satisfy the health-related moral commitments and practices of both the patient (or family) and the provider. For example, when providers' cross-cultural health care ethics prioritize preservation of provider-patient relationships, they tend to respond with efforts to persuade, educate, build trust, compromise, accede to the patient's wishes, or transfer care to a provider whom the patient or family trusts more fully (see Chapters 4, 6, 8, and 12). When either protection of the patient's physical health interests or respect for professional integrity are prioritized, the range of responses includes instead overriding the patient's or family's wish, refusing to agree, and involving state authorities or seeking a court order to impose a refused intervention (see Chapters 5 and 7).

A discussion of the attitudes and communication skills that support culturally responsive health care follows. Three case stories then illustrate the application of these skills in cross-cultural ethics.

## VII. Develop attitudes culturally responsive to the groups you serve

The attitudes practitioners convey, both verbally and nonverbally, affect their ability to deliver culturally responsive health care. Patients and their families are more trusting and more willing to communicate openly when they feel respected. While cultural concepts of respectful behavior differ, practitioners can demonstrate respect by appearing open, nonjudgmental, and curious about patients' understandings of their illnesses and their preferred healing methods. Displaying patience and empathy are especially valuable with patients who are immigrants or refugees struggling with immense loss, adapting to a new culture, and navigating the complexity of life in the United States (see Chapters 3, 4, 6, 7, 8, and 10–13).

Providers are more likely to be successful when they adopt an attitude of cultural humility (Tervalon & Murray-Garcia, 1998). Western concepts of health, disease, and treatment and concepts of the ideal practitioner-patient relationship have changed over time and will continue to change. Cultural humility helps practitioners remember that the biomedical view is one cultural perspective, and that other perspectives also have validity.

Acknowledging instances in which Hmong beliefs have been demonstrated to be correct and U.S. health care beliefs mistaken can bolster providers' humility. In the 1980s, for example, Hmong parents wanted newborns to sleep on their backs and nurses repeatedly turned babies onto their stomachs; but in the 1990s, the U.S. health care establishment decided that it is better for babies to sleep on their backs to avert sudden infant death syndrome (SIDS). In the 1980s, Hmong patients asked for tetracycline to improve their peptic ulcer symptoms and doctors refused; then in the 1990s, physicians discovered bacteria-inducing peptic ulcers that responded to multiple antibiotics, including tetracycline. In the 1980s, Hmong women wanted to squat to deliver their babies, and some U.S. providers refused to let them, but now others recognize that squatting is an excellent practice to open the pelvic outlet. Also, Hmong patients begged for medical rather than surgical treatment for ectopic pregnancies, appendicitis, and pregnancy terminations, and now there are various options to the once surgical imperatives.

Cultural humility also calls on providers to attend to the unequal power that exists between themselves and their patients, especially those from different cultures (Tervalon & Murray-Garcia, 1998). Unequal power causes problems between patients and providers. It is important that providers adopt an attitude of openness to power sharing (Brody, 1992; Marshall et al., 1998; Orr et al., 1995). Health care professionals occupy positions of respected knowledge, with concurrent social authority. They often come from middle- and upper-class backgrounds, and their current positions allow them to stay at that level or move up the socioeconomic class ladder. Generally, practitioners are so focused on the written word they cannot imagine a world without literacy. And, health care providers are licensed by the state, with government agencies supporting their expertise and authority.

In contrast, Hmong refugees in the United States generally have limited social authority. Many—especially middle-aged adults and elders—are non-English speakers with limited formal education and little income. Moreover, their views of health, disease, and treatment are not sanctioned by the state. When some Hmong people describe conflicts with health care professionals, they object to the "top-down" communication style they often are subject to: nurses tell without listening, people assume without asking, and doctors explain while coercing. In short, some Hmong people feel as though they are being treated as less than human. Their most frustrating experiences have been with court-ordered treatments for children. Over the telephone, in a matter of minutes, physicians can obtain court orders, without judges ever talking with the parents and considering their perspective. Resentful, angry, and depressed, some Hmong families turn away from these dehumanizing experiences and look for other venues for fulfillment, care, and cure (see Chapters 5 and 7).

Health care professionals need to examine their motivations and actions and look out for potential abuses of power. To this end, they can reflect on their personal and professional biases and prejudices and monitor their actions and emotional reactions to patients. Health provider support groups, Balint groups,* ethics committees, and community resources are some available avenues for help.

The structure and policies of health care institutions play a key role in supporting patients' abilities to use their power in clinical settings (Huff & Kline, 1999b; U.S. DHHS, 2000c). For example, hiring medically trained interpreters and bilingual-bicultural workers, developing patient education videotapes and other materials about health and the health care system in the languages of the communities served, and developing culturally responsive risk management practices that can reduce the power differences between patients and providers are important organizational components of culturally responsive health care. (See below, "Recommendations for Health Care Administrators and Educators.")

---

*Balint groups were started in England by Michael Balint, a psychoanalyst, and general practitioners who felt that the most important healing tool physicians have is themselves. They recommended that physicians, in an effort to promote healing by improving the doctor-patient relationship, present their personal feelings and reactions about individual patients to other physicians in discussion groups.

## VIII.  Learn communication skills culturally responsive to the groups you serve

For health care providers to apply their awareness of themselves and their knowledge of others' health beliefs, practices, and values to interactions in health care encounters requires learning and applying culturally responsive communication skills (Gudykunst & Mody, 2002). People usually interpret verbal communication and nonverbal gestures according to their own cultural context. Nonverbal and verbal communication can easily be misinterpreted, leading to misunderstandings that undermine the trust necessary for successful cross-cultural relationships.

The following descriptions of common nonverbal and verbal forms of communication are general guides that apply to many relationships. The reader is cautioned, however, that communication styles within both the Hmong culture and the health care practitioners' culture continue to change, and so these generalities do not apply in all cases. For example, many Hmong are acquiring new communication styles as they participate more in U.S. society and have relationships with U.S. peers. Clinicians must observe the nonverbal and verbal communication patterns of patients and family members, and take their cues from them.

### Nonverbal communication

Nonverbal expressions and gestures are replete with multiple meanings, even opposite meanings, to persons of different cultures. Generally, practitioners need to be alert to such nonverbal forms of communication as eye movements, body positions, smiles, reactions to touch, and discomfort with sensitive topics. When mistakes occur, practitioners should apologize to the patient, plead ignorance, and express a willingness to learn as rapprochement, saying, "Excuse me, I don't understand, but I want to learn," or "Please accept my apology and explain to me about . . ." Later, they can discuss the incident with knowledgeable people, such as bilingual-bicultural workers, and incorporate the information into future interactions.

GREETINGS    Greeting people with a smile and a nod is sufficient for most Hmong people. However, greeting with a handshake is acceptable, and handshakes have become the preferred greeting between Hmong men.

HEAD MOVEMENTS    Nodding a head conveys yes, but it may mean, "Yes, I understand," or "Yes, go on," rather than "Yes, I agree with you and I will do as you say." Hmong people often nod their heads to express respect and politeness or to encourage the speaker to continue speaking so they can ultimately understand the confusing foreign words. It is important not to assume that patients who nod are agreeing with the particular explanation, directive, or recommendation.

SMILING AND LAUGHING    Smiling and laughing can mean enjoyment, but they can also express embarrassment, shyness, or fear, particularly at moments of conflict. Hmong people who smile and laugh during a conflict may be expressing their discomfort not their enjoyment, while providers may interpret the laughter as ridicule.

HAND GESTURES     Hand gesturing for someone to "come here" with the palm and fingers up can be insulting, since this is a common Asian gesture used to call animals. Instead, Hmong people hold their palms down and move their fingers back and forth pointing at the ground.

EYE CONTACT     Making direct eye contact is usually considered respectful in U.S. culture, but in Hmong culture it may be experienced as rude, like staring. To show respect for elders or people of the opposite gender, Hmong people customarily look down at the floor to communicate that they are listening intently and processing what is being said and make eye contact for brief periods to express sincere interest. Particularly when talking with someone about personal private matters of the body and illness, health care workers should look away periodically to show respect and help patients be comfortable.

FACIAL EXPRESSIONS     Making facial expressions is acceptable in U.S. culture, but Hmong may consider these expressions disrespectful. Hmong facial expressions tend to appear neutral, calm, and collected; as one Hmong woman said, "Hmong eyebrows, mouths, and noses do not go all over the place like Americans." Health care providers must be careful not to misinterpret Hmong patients' facial expressions as a flat affect and overdiagnose depression or misinterpret pleasant neutral smiles and underdiagnose depression.

TONE OF VOICE     Speaking loudly, displaying anger, or wearing a displeased facial expression are considered disrespectful and dehumanizing to the Hmong. When people in positions of authority (such as health care providers) communicate in this manner, they sow seeds of disrespect and distrust. Conversely, a soft gentle voice is experienced as respectful and can engender trust. Health care providers should take care not to raise their voices.

TOUCHING     Touching certain parts of the body may be considered disrespectful or insulting to the Hmong. For example, touching an adult's head is insulting because the head is the highest point and most sacred part of the body, and rubbing a child's soft fontanel can disrupt the soul that resides there. However, gently stroking a child's head with the palm of the hand forward indicates love and care for the child. Health care providers can examine people's heads after obtaining their permission or prefacing the exam with a short, "May I" or "Excuse me." In addition, examining a head with just one or two fingers can indicate sensitivity to and respect for a person's personal space.

Touching sexual body parts is regulated by strict social rules. Hmong society strongly disapproves of men touching women, especially if the women are married. Women who easily succumb to or freely make themselves available to men are not respected in the community. Even women who easily consent to pelvic or breast examinations by male doctors may be rebuked, ostracized, divorced, or disciplined by their husbands or extended family members, both male and female. Providers should ask patients for permission and for any preferences (such as a same gender provider or chaperone) when examining sexual parts of the body and should consider modifying their usual approach, including conducting discreet examinations under gowns or around clothes.

### Verbal communication

To work effectively in multicultural settings, providers need skills to work with interpreters and need to acquire some language skills. Speaking a few words of the patient's language communicates respect and a desire to reach out, which can assist the development of a trusting therapeutic relationship. It is important for health care providers to be aware of cultural differences in communication styles and topics of conversation so that they can adjust their approaches to meet patients' cultural expectations (see Huff & Kline, 1999a). No culture is homogenous, however, and individuals may have different reactions to common communication styles and topics.

WORKING WITH INTERPRETERS    Providing patients with trained healthcare interpreters is crucial to establishing culturally responsive provider-patient relationships. The way procedures, therapies, medicines, or diagnoses are explained to patients can influence patients' responses. Likewise, the manner in which patients' thoughts and questions are explained to providers can influence providers' reactions and responses to patients' perspectives and desires (see Chapter 4; Marshall et al., 1998; Woloshin, Bickell, Schwartz, Gany, & Welsh, 1995).

Learning to work with interpreters is as essential as learning how to use a stethoscope or take a blood pressure. The ideal arrangement is to work with interpreters proficient in the health-related concepts of both cultures and trained to provide first-person singular translation. Consider the steps outlined in Table 16.4 when working with health care interpreters (see also Andrulis, Goodman, & Pryor, 2002; Boston City Hospital, 1987, 1990; California Healthcare Interpreters Association, 2002; Center for Cross-Cultural Health, 1997; Cross Cultural Health Care Program, 1998; Downing, 1992; Jackson, 1998; Kaufert & O'Neil, 1990; Kaufert & Putsch, 1997; Like, 2000; Putsch, 1985; Youdelman & Perkins, 2002).

The reality is that trained health care interpreters are not available in all clinical settings at all times. At the very least, institutions should have contracts with telephone communication services that provide trained medical interpreters. Providers should refrain from using the patient's family members as interpreters. Family members may not interpret information that may be important to health care providers because they may be embarrassed by "old-country" behaviors or beliefs, or because they have their own interpretations and agendas that interfere with their ability to translate accurately. Working with a child or adolescent interpreter is problematic because it inverts the normal social and power relationship between adults and children and because adults may not express all physical or emotional problems to children. Also, many children and adolescents do not know the acceptable terms for body parts, illness symptoms, disease terms, or cultural nuances and idioms. Nonetheless, in emergencies providers may have to choose between working without any interpretation and working with nonqualified interpreters, including family members.

GREETINGS    If a verbal greeting is added to a smile or a handshake, Hmong people often comment upon the situation with phrases such as: "Oh, you have come? *[Koj tuaj los?]*" or "Have you eaten yet? *[Koj puas tau noj mov?]*" and "Where are you going? *[Koj mus qhov twg?].*" The traditional greeting "Are you eating well and are you well? *[Koj puas noj qab nyob zoo?]*" has been shortened to the now ubiquitous *"Nyob zoo."*

INTRODUCTIONS    Practitioners should begin with introductions and determine the patient's primary language and whether a trained interpreter should be involved. Trust and respect are further supported by engaging in personal conversation with the patient and family prior to any conversation about the person's health issues. If an interpreter is involved, explain early on how communication will proceed.

Hmong patients frequently ask Hmong professionals about their kinship and geographic origin in Laos. Hmong providers need to spend time establishing kinship relationships and historical connections with Hmong patients before discussing medical issues. It is especially important for Hmong providers to respond and address patients by the social title that properly describes their social relationship.

STYLES OF ADDRESS    Establishing how the patient would like to be addressed is a good way to demonstrate respect and begin a trusting relationship. The Hmong have an extensive list of social titles based on age, generation, and relationship be-

## Table 16.4. Working with an Interpreter

- Match people of same age and same gender as much as possible.
- Meet with the interpreter beforehand to establish ground rules and afterward to wrap-up, clarify, and learn from one another.
- Ensure that the interpreter uses first-person singular, verbatim translation.
- Greet the patient in his or her own language.
- Introduce everyone present.
- Allow the interpreter and the patient to exchange cultural greetings.
- Arrange seats in a triad and address the patient, not the interpreter.
- Explain to everyone how the communication will flow.
- Explain expectations toward confidentiality.
- Express one idea at a time, and pause for interpretation.
- Speak slowly, clearly, and in a calm voice.
- Use common terms and simple language structure.
- Define terms, draw pictures, and show physical evidence.
- Encourage the interpreter to tell you what he or she does not understand.
- Check understandings by periodically asking the patient to repeat what has been said.
- Ask the same questions in different ways to clarify inconsistent or unconnected responses.
- Do not expect the interpreter to resolve differences or conflicts.

tween the two people involved (see Heimbach, 1979, and Lee, 1986, for a complete explanation of White Hmong social relationships). The Hmong rely so much on these social titles that, for example, if you wanted to look for Pa Xiong in the community, you would have to know that she is the mother of Pao Chua Vang, wife of Yia Yee Vang, daughter of Tsu Leng Xiong, and daughter-in-law of Tong Xe Vang. While it is acceptable to call people by the name on their chart, to show respect, health care providers can call older men Txiv Ntxawm (Uncle, or father's younger brother), older women Niam Tais (Auntie, or grandmother on the mother's side), and any woman by her relationship with her husband (Niam Txuj Yis) or her children (Neeb Niam). (For assistance with pronunciation, see Heimbach, 1979; McKibben, 1994; Saturn River Front Academy, 2000; Hmong Lessons, n.d.)

REASONS FOR THE VISIT    It is important for practitioners to inquire about the reasons for the visit in a manner that expresses interest and displays a respectful attitude. By asking for and listening to patients' and family members' stories about their illness experiences, providers can display genuine desires to hear the patient's or family's perspectives, connect with them and their suffering, obtain valuable information, and improve therapeutic relationships.

Initially talking about the Hmong patient's reasons for the health care visit may be considered rude. Beginning by asking about an aspect of the patient's personal life— particularly family members—can facilitate social connections. Providers need to be prepared to briefly answer personal questions that patients may ask them in return.

In soliciting information from Hmong patients about reasons for the visit, providers may have to change the way they ordinarily frame questions. For example, the translation of the seemingly neutral question, "Why have you come here today?" can sound rude and accusatory, akin to "Why have you come here when I do not feel like seeing you?" Patients may react, "Why! I came here because I am sick. If I am not sick why would I come to you!" Better questions to ask are: "How can I help you today?" or "What illness are you here for today?" as they convey a sincere willingness to help. Also, addressing the patient's reason for the visit (e.g., a headache) before addressing other health problems (e.g., kidney insufficiency or high blood pressure) tends to express respect and develop patient trust.

SENSITIVE TOPICS    Asking direct questions about sensitive issues can cause Hmong patients to lose face. Indirect questions are more effective. For example, the practitioners might ask a question in the context of a story: "I know a Hmong Christian family who was concerned about soul loss and conducted a soul-calling ceremony. Is this true for you?" or "I know some people think we draw too much blood. Is this a concern for you?" Similarly, using respectful euphemisms for sexual terms can facilitate communication. Use of appropriate Hmong terms by trained medical interpreters and others demonstrates respect for the patient and family.

RISKS AND BENEFITS    Communicating with Hmong patients and families about risks and benefits should be phrased in the affirmative as much as possible. Rather than saying, "If you don't do this, you will die," it is preferable to say, "I am recommending this because I think it will help you get well the fastest way with the least difficulty." Expressing that there is a risk of death if a procedure or approach is not followed can be expressed by "I think this is the best option for you at this time. If you choose not to [or, If we wait too long], I will feel very sorry for you because I don't know whether I can help you later."

BAD NEWS    Speaking about dire future consequences can make it appear that the practitioners are inviting those things to happen, particularly if they are upset or angry. Practitioners can express their perspective and advice in ways that convey meaning without using the shocking words such as "will die" (see Chapters 5, 7, 13, and 15). Cultural phrases such as "when you are 120 years old" or "when your time comes" can be used to allude to death. To express grave situations, analogies can be used, such as, "Despite all that we are doing, it seems the sky is only getting darker and darker, not brighter" or "It seems the sun is only setting more and more."

COMPLIMENTS    Praising a baby's beauty can be upsetting to animist families. Parents do not want to attract the attention of evil spirits to their beautiful baby, since evil spirits are known to scare babies or take them to the spirit world. So, when praising a baby, Hmong will say the opposite. For example, people say, "Yeah, talking about you, you ugly seed," which everyone knows means, "Yeah, talking about you, you cute little one." When a baby is born, people express their congratulations with "Glad, your baby has come to be with us" or "I am very happy for you," rather than "Your baby is so cute!"

## IX.  Develop skills in applying culturally responsive knowledge, skills, and attitudes to particular clinical encounters

To provide culturally responsive care to a specific patient, practitioners can use the information they know about the cultural group to guide their efforts to learn about the patient's and family's particular experiences and beliefs about the ailment and reactions to recommended assessments and treatments. They can ask questions based on their knowledge of the patient's health care beliefs and values, being careful not to assume what the individual patient and family think, need, want, or fear. One useful approach is a modified version of the LEARN model: Listen, Explain, Acknowledge, Recommend, and Negotiate (Berlin & Fowkes, 1983).*

---

*Levin, Like, and Gottlieb (2000) offer another mnemonic for working in multicultural settings, ETHNIC: Explanation, Treatment, Healers, Negotiate, Intervention, and Collaboration. In addition, Stuart and Lieberman (1993) present a mnemonic for assisting physicians to address psycho-socio-cultural issues in patient care, BATHE: Background, Affect, Trouble, Handling, and Empathy.

## Listen to the patient's or family's responses to questions about their perspectives

Practitioners should attempt to elicit the patient's or family's perspectives of the disease (the bodily discomforts), the illness (their experience of bodily discomforts), and their explanatory models (ideas about cause, timing, and mode of onset of symptoms, patho-physiological processes, severity of illness, and appropriate treatments [Kleinman, 1980]), as well as their moral commitments and practices (e.g., risk-benefit assessments and decision-making practices). The following questions may be useful for eliciting Hmong patients' perspectives. (These questions, while influenced by Kleinman's eight questions [Kleinman, Eisenberg, & Good, 1978], have been expanded and tailored for relationships with Hmong patients.)

*"What do you [or other people] think is wrong?"*    To questions such as, "What do you [or others] call this problem?" Hmong patients and family members may respond, "I don't know. You're the doctor. You tell me." Practitioners can respond by saying that they will render an opinion but they value the patients' ideas and want to understand the patients' fears, concerns, and desires. Practitioners who project an open and interested attitude of, "Teach me about yourself, this illness, and how it affects you," rather than an authoritative attitude of, "I am the one who will tell you," encourage trusting relationships.

*"What do you [or other people] think has caused the problem?"*    For the Hmong, practitioners can inquire about natural and supernatural etiologies (see Chapter 1). It is important to ask about people's religious affiliations, since their understandings of their physical or mental problems can be different if they are Christian or Hmong animist or if they combine both religious orientations. Once religious affiliation is established, practitioners can follow with more specific questions, such as, "Do you think the weather, spirits, or soul loss might have caused these symptoms?" Sometimes asking what others think provides valuable information. A patient may be uncertain about the cause but can explain what his or her relatives think.

*"How has this problem affected your life?"*    For Hmong, social-role obligations are important and assuming the sick role is related to an inability to perform such duties. Practitioners can ask, "Are you able to work, watch children, or cook rice as usual?"

*"What are you [or other people] afraid of?"*    For the Hmong, fears can be about traditional or new diseases. Providers can ask, "Are you concerned this is *mob laug* or *ua qoob*? Are you worried about diabetes *(ntshav qab zib)* or hypertension *(ntshav siab)*?" (See Chapters 5 and 8.) Fears can be about impaired functions in this life (impaired ability to work or make love) or the next life (bad karma or bodily mutilations that can be carried into the next reincarnations).

*"What healing methods have you tried?"*    Providers can ask Hmong people, "Have you tried herbal medicines, magic healing, or shamanic rituals? Have you sought the

assistance of a minister or a prayer group at church?" Also, inquiring about the responses to these methods can be informative.

*"What do you [or other people] think will help?"*    People often have ideas about what they want for assistance, whether from their doctor or from others, that can be elicited by such questions as, "How can I help?" or "Are there Hmong treatments you would like to try before agreeing to my suggestions?"

*"Who usually makes [or, helps you make] decisions about your health care?"*    Cultures vary on what information is told to whom for what types of decision-making processes. Questions to ask Hmong people include, "When this information comes back, whom do you want me to talk to?" or "Would you like a conference so we can discuss this with others?" or "Whom do you want to invite?" Asking is necessary, especially as culture is changing. Some people want the extended family to make the decisions for them while others want to make decisions separate from their family members (see Chapters 3, 6, 7, 9, 11, and 15).

*"What concerns do you have about seeking U.S. health care services for this problem?"*    The community's concerns about diagnostic and therapeutic approaches abound. Asking directly can yield answers and understanding. "What are you concerned about if we do the operation [or, specifically, the endoscopy; the biopsy]?" But sometimes asking indirectly can be helpful. "Have you heard other people's concerns about these services?"

### Explain the biomedical conceptualization of the problem

Once clinicians understand the history and the patient's or family's perspective and conduct a physical exam, they need to explain their views of the patient's condition, build on the patient's and family's ideas, and address the patient's and family's fears and concerns.

Hmong families in Laos were used to having all of the information they needed to make decisions for the sick. In the United States, doctors and nurses have new ideas for them to consider, and families usually want to understand the information: What does the blood test indicate? What is wrong with the urine? What do the X rays look like? What does the sick liver look like? Practitioners should provide concrete information, including explanations, pictures, copies of lab tests, and X rays, and show slides of pathological specimens (see Chapter 13). This information empowers the patient and family to make decisions from their own perspective.

### Acknowledge similarities and differences
### between the provider's and the patient's perspective

Practitioners should acknowledge where the patient's or family's perspective is similar and where different from theirs. It is important to emphasize commonalities (e.g., "We both want your child's fever to come down") and clarify differences (e.g., "I believe this is not a life-threatening condition"). When practitioners fail to listen to the patient's beliefs and fears initially, they cannot perform this step and their focus remains on themselves.

### Recommend a course of action

Practitioners need to explain the options and recommend a course of action that incorporates the patient's perspective where possible to "enhance the acceptability of the treatment plan" (Berlin & Fowkes, 1983). As practitioners recommend diagnostic tests, they must ask permission ("I would like to draw blood from your arm in order to . . . ; is that OK with you?") and explain their rationale for their recommendations in terms that reflect as much as possible the patient's understanding of the problem and desired outcome. The goal is to try to frame the recommendation, taking into consideration the patients' orientation or explanatory models, so patients can understand the recommendation (see Chapter 12).

### Negotiate options

Providers may feel that many of the recommendations in this book would be difficult to implement, since they may challenge providers' personal or professional values. Addressing women by their relationships to their husbands, for example, might run counter to providers' individualist bent or feminist commitments. Calling a baby "an ugly seed" may go against providers' inclinations to praise lovely infants. Changing communication styles—hand gestures, eye contact, or approach to asking questions—may challenge providers' identity. In general, however, these examples of patient or family wishes that challenge merely the personal or cultural preferences of practitioners should be accommodated.

Negotiation is necessary when patients and practitioners reach different decisions about what is best for the patient and for accomplishing the patient's goals. To start, it is necessary to find out how patients feel about the recommended course of action and then to discuss important differences, concerns, and possible alternatives. Kleinman, Eisenberg, and Good (1978, p. 257) assert that "this process of negotiation may well be the single most important step in engaging the patient's trust, preventing major discrepancies in the evaluation of therapeutic outcome, promoting compliance, and reducing patient dissatisfaction."

Negotiation with Hmong patients might lead practitioners to consider pursuing various options for diagnostic tests. For example, they can ask: "If you do not want me to draw two tubes of blood, how about one tube?" or "If not from your arm, how about from your finger?" or "If not today, how about at the next visit?" Providers may alter their customary behaviors and do exams under clothes, ask permission to examine the patient's head, reduce the number of routine pelvic exams, and obtain family input before deciding how or whether to tell dire news to the patient. And finally, they can consider pursuing alternative therapeutic options, for example, "If we don't operate now, how about taking medicine first and if that doesn't work, then consider the operation?"

When patients create the plans together with clinicians, they are more likely to adhere to the specifics. And if they do not follow the plan, then clinicians can pursue the challenges or obstacles at subsequent visits, by asking such questions as: "What happened that you did not take the medicine as you had thought you would?" or "What happened that you were not able to keep the appointment for the CT Scan that you had wanted?" (see Chapters 3–7).

Before deciding how to act in cases of patient reluctance or disagreement with recommended plans, practitioners should try to comprehend the patient's assessments, values, beliefs, needs, and fears. Eliciting this information may require interviewing patients and family members with a different interpreter or referring them to community agencies, cross-cultural psychologists, clinical social workers, or experienced colleagues.

Input from other providers, cultural consult teams, ethics committees with cultural expertise, and community liaisons can also assist with these assessments. Why, for example, is the patient leaving the hospital against medical advice? Does the clinician's disagreement with the patient or family stem from cross-cultural differences concerning trust, respect, roles, disclosure, best interests and risks/benefits, or decision making? Is there any reason to question the decision-making capacity of the patient or family? How likely is the patient or family to compromise or accede to the health care professional's recommendations?

It is also important that health care practitioners reexamine their own assessments, values, and beliefs that influence their reaction to the situation. Does the practitioner feel that the patient's or family's wishes challenge his or her personal preferences, moral beliefs, conscience, or professional integrity? With increased insight into the beliefs and moral commitments of the patient and themselves, practitioners are in a better position to re-evaluate the differences. What can they modify about their own reaction and evaluation of the situation? (See O'Connor, 1995; Orr et al., 1995.) Can they now accede to the patient's wishes? Or do they still disagree? Is their disagreement primarily personal or professional? Because cross-cultural conflicts can be emotionally challenging, practitioners should attend to their reactions to these situations so they do not carry the emotional scars from one difficult situation into another (see Chapter 5).

### Evaluate cross-cultural ethical conflicts and appropriate responses

The points to consider when evaluating and addressing serious cross-cultural ethical conflicts are discussed above. Table 16.5 offers a worksheet to assist with this activity and illustrations of its use with three case stories.

The contrasting patterns of the shaded areas in the completed parts of the table illustrate that cross-cultural ethical challenges to professional integrity vary in strength and do not always outweigh the source and strength of the patient's or family's wishes. In the vaginal bleeding case (Chapter 4), Mrs. Yang's refusal of a biopsy and a hysterectomy did not pose a significant challenge to the providers' professional integrity that outweighed the strength of her treatment wishes. The patient's perspective, in this case, should prevail.

### Table 16.5. Compare Patient or Family Wish and Challenge to Professional Integrity

*Template*

| Strength of Patient's or Family's Wish | | | Strength of Challenge to Professional Integrity | | |
|---|---|---|---|---|---|
| *Type of Wish* | *Patient's/ Family's Decision-making Capacity* | *Source and Strength of Wish* | *Type of Challenge to Professional Integrity* | *Strength of Empirical Support* | *Strength of Professional Agreement* |
| Refusal | Meets biomedical criteria | Strong | Weak | Weak | Weak |
| Request for a standard intervention | Meets criteria of patient's cultural group | Moderate | Moderate | Moderate | Moderate |
| Request for a prohibited or non-validated and risky intervention | Adult of impaired capacity / Child | Weak | Strong | Strong | Strong |

*Patient should prevail* ↑ ↓ *Practitioner should prevail*

*Vaginal bleeding case: Patient refuses surgery*

| Strength of Patient's or Family's Wish | | | Strength of Challenge to Professional Integrity | | |
|---|---|---|---|---|---|
| *Type of Wish* | *Patient's/ Family's Decision-making Capacity* | *Source and Strength of Wish* | *Type of Challenge to Professional Integrity* | *Strength of Empirical Support* | *Strength of Professional Agreement* |
| Refusal | Meets biomedical criteria | Strong | Weak | Weak | Weak |
| Request for a standard intervention | Meets criteria of patient's cultural group | Moderate | Moderate | Moderate | Moderate |
| Request for a prohibited or non-validated and risky intervention | Adult of impaired capacity / Child | Weak | Strong | Strong | Strong |

*Patient should prevail* ↑ ↓ *Practitioner should prevail*

## Hospice case: Family requests surgery

| Strength of Patient's or Family's Wish | | | Strength of Challenge to Professional Integrity | | |
|---|---|---|---|---|---|
| Type of Wish | Patient's/ Family's Decision-making Capacity | Source and Strength of Wish | Type of Challenge to Professional Integrity | Strength of Empirical Support | Strength of Professional Agreement |
| Refusal | Meets biomedical criteria | Strong | Weak | Weak | Weak |
| Request for a standard intervention | Meets criteria of patient's cultural group | Moderate | Moderate | Moderate | Moderate |
| Request for a prohibited or non-validated and risky intervention | Adult of impaired capacity / Child | Weak | Strong | Strong | Strong |

Patient should prevail ↑

Practitioner should prevail ↓

## Heart defect case: Parents refuse surgery for child

| Strength of Patient's or Family's Wish | | | Strength of Challenge to Professional Integrity | | |
|---|---|---|---|---|---|
| Type of Wish | Patient's/ Family's Decision-making Capacity | Source and Strength of Wish | Type of Challenge to Professional Integrity | Strength of Empirical Support | Strength of Professional Agreement |
| Refusal | Meets biomedical criteria | Strong | Weak | Weak | Weak |
| Request for a standard intervention | Meets criteria of patient's cultural group | Moderate | Moderate | Moderate | Moderate |
| Request for a prohibited or non-validated and risky intervention | Adult of impaired capacity / Child | Weak | Strong | Strong | Strong |

Patient should prevail ↑

Practitioner should prevail ↓

In the hospice case (Chapter 13), the strength of the family's request for a curative operation for an adult terminally ill with gallbladder cancer is not morally weighty, because the wish is a request for a nonvalidated and risky surgical intervention and is based on powerful emotions and incomplete information about the efficacy of surgery. At the same time, the challenge the treatment wish poses to professional integrity is moderately strong and outweighs the strength of the family wishes. Therefore, in this case, the provider's perspective should prevail.

In the heart defect case (Chapter 7), the source and strength of the parents' refusal to permit further cardiac procedures and an operation to repair a potentially life-threatening hole in their daughter's heart is significant. The challenge to professional integrity is also significant. If the case is an example of a tie between a strong treatment wish and a strong challenge to professional integrity, then the criteria we recommend for good cross-cultural health care relationships suggests that the family's wishes should prevail. However, if the provider's objection not only is significant but also outweighs the strength of the family's treatment wishes, the provider may justifiably seek a court order to override the family's wishes and provide the refused interventions.

The physician who comments on this case study in Chapter 7 concludes that the parents' treatment wishes were idiosyncratic and not clearly rooted in deeply held cultural and spiritual beliefs. On this view, the challenge to the physician's professional integrity outweighs the family's wishes, and a court order is justified to compel treatment of the seriously ill child over the parents' objections.

# Recommendations for Health Care Administrators and Educators

Health care delivery is influenced by formal institutional policies and procedures, as well as the informal structures and functions of clinics, hospitals, public health organizations, educational institutions, insurance companies, and managed care organizations. It is important that providers ask and be aware of the value commitments of the institutions with which and for which they work. For example, what is the institution's commitment to delivering culturally responsive health care and decreasing ethnic and racial health disparities? In what ways does the institution support clinicians in providing culturally responsive health care?

The day-to-day structure and function of health care institutions can greatly influence the delivery of culturally responsive care (U.S. DHHS, 2000c). For example, health care institutions that are structured to rely on patients' possessing good written and spoken English-language skills may find that they provide lower quality and more expensive health care for nonliterate and minimally literate people because of miscommunication and misunderstanding about their diagnoses, prognoses, medicine instructions, location of services, and responsibilities for payment (Rudd, Moeykens, & Colton, 1999; Smedley et al., 2002). Even highly literate people can have difficulty understanding complex health information, but people with poor literacy skills are more adversely affected. The limited supply of trained interpreters and limited reimbursement by third-party payers means that people who do not speak English or have limited English proficiency (LEP) are denied an essential key to accessing culturally responsive health care (Youdelman & Perkins, 2002).*

Similarly, the focus on rigid schedules and specific appointments causes difficulties for patients who do not read or who do not have calendars, telephones, or independent means of reliable transportation and do not conceptualize time as linear and dividable into rigid prescribed units.

Health care institutions are implementing policies, procedures, and structural changes to improve the delivery of culturally responsive health care to people with limited English-language skills. In fact, institutions that receive federal financial assistance are required by Title VI of the 1964 Civil Rights Act to provide equal access to health care services by all people, regardless of race, sexual orientation, religion, or national origin—which includes people with LEP. The Office for Civil Rights in the U.S. Department of Health and Human Services issued a Policy Guidance titled "Title VI Prohibition Against National Origin Discrimination as It Affects Persons with Limited-English Proficiency" and the Office of Minority Health developed the CLAS standards (U.S. DHHS, 2000c, 2001c, 2001d).

These documents explain the basic legal requirements of Title VI and what recipients of federal dollars, such as hospitals, nursing homes, and managed care organizations, can do to comply with the civil rights law. The Office for Civil Rights cites

---

* LEP is defined as not being able to "speak, read, write, or understand the English language at a level that permits [people] to interact effectively with health care providers and social service agencies" (quoted in U.S. DHHS, 2002b, p. 32).

examples of practices that may violate Title VI, such as subjecting LEP persons to unreasonable delays in the delivery of services. Such delays can occur because an interpreter is not available or an institution fails to inform LEP persons of the right to receive free interpreter services or a clinic requires people to provide their own interpreters.

The suggestions listed below can help health care institutions—those that deliver clinical services and those that train health care professionals—improve their service and comply with federal law. They are consistent with the CLAS Standards (U.S. DHHS, 2001d) and with the recommendations to collect accurate health services data and adopt quality measurements (National Quality Forum, 2002). (For further information about the following suggestions, see Kaiser Family Foundation, 2003; Nerenz et al., 2002; Perot & Youdelman, 2001; U.S. DHHS, 2001a, 2002a, 2002b; Youdelman & Perkins, 2002.)

## Develop policies and practices

- Create institutional mission and value statements that include promotion of culturally responsive health care and equitable access to health care services.
- Require an annual review of departmental diversity plans.
- Create continuing education goals on culturally responsive health care for all staff.
- Collect self-identified data about patients' ethnicity and primary language in order to track health care outcomes and discriminatory care that occurs in the institution. Partner with state and national institutions that are tracking this type of information.
- Monitor and report on the quality of care for all patients, with special attention to racial and ethnic groups.
- Allow traditional healers to practice healing rituals within the institution, if patients and families desire it.
- Clarify the administration's support for exceptions to standards of practice in the interests of delivering culturally responsive health care.
- Expand visiting hours and number of visitors to accommodate a family's need to be with their sick family members.
- Allow family members to be present in procedure rooms when the observation of procedures could decrease fear and concern, with supervision as needed.

## Provide services that support culturally responsive health care

- Hire bilingual-bicultural persons for positions throughout the institution (e.g., support personnel, providers, and administrators).
- Provide bilingual receptionists, triage nurses, and answering services in order to attend to patients' immediate needs.
- Hire trained medical interpreters who can provide face-to-face interpretation.
- Subscribe to a telephone interpreter service that is available twenty-four hours a day, seven days a week to augment interpreter personnel.

- Post signs in the languages of the communities served.
- Routinely identify and document patients' primary language and need or desire for interpreter services in charts and computerized records.
- Allow walk-in appointments at clinics (not just emergency departments) for people whose needs and concepts of time do not fit institutionalized appointment schedules.
- Expand patient advocacy departments to include cultural consult teams.
- Provide space for large numbers of visiting family members.
- Provide transportation for people to access a full range of health care services.
- Provide child-care activities on site.
- Add a cultural perspective to clinical ethics committees and consult teams.
- Make the institution esthetically pleasing to the cultural groups served and offer traditional food.
- Monitor the effects of programs on patient satisfaction and health care outcomes.

## Provide staff education

- Require training in culturally responsive care for all personnel, including bilingual-bicultural staff.
- Provide non-bilingual staff with pictures and phrase sheets for communication with LEP patients.
- Require proficiency in communicating with interpreters for all employees with patient and family contact.
- Require training in culturally responsive communication skills for all practitioners.
- Educate practitioners in pertinent epidemiological and clinical information about cultural groups served.
- Provide staff with community resource lists.
- Assess skills in culturally responsive care in employee evaluations.
- Evaluate the effects of culturally responsive education on patient care, patient satisfaction, staff satisfaction, and health care outcomes.
- Monitor the effects of programs on patient satisfaction and health care outcomes.

## Provide patient education

- Educate patients and families about the health care system.
- Inform patients about available interpreter services, patients' rights, and the patient advocacy department.
- Provide non-English-speaking patients and families with educational videotapes in their own language.
- Develop consent forms in easy-to-understand English and in people's first language, and create videotapes or audiotapes for nonliterate people.
- Evaluate effects of education on patient care and health care outcomes.

### Engage in community outreach and education

- Conduct community needs assessment in partnership with community members and organizations.
- Create community outreach programs that connect patients and health care workers.
- Partner with community organizations to provide community health education based on the community's concerns and beliefs.
- Link with community organizations to educate staff and support institutional efforts.
- Include community representatives on institutional committees, for example, boards of directors, ethics committees, and institutional review boards (IRBs).

In addition to hospitals and clinics, professional education programs—medical schools, nursing schools, and technical schools—can recruit, enroll, and support a diverse student body, staff, and teachers (Cohen, Gabriel, & Terrell, 2002; IOM, 2001b). Increasingly, such institutions are providing classes and continuing nursing and medical education in various aspects of cultural diversity and multicultural communication skills, including working with interpreters. (See Gilbert, 2003.) Indeed, many nursing schools, medical schools, and residency programs are embracing cultural competence and are championing educational efforts, but more needs to be done. (See Berger, 2001; Carillo, Green, & Betancourt, 1999; Culhane-Pera, Like, Lebensohn-Chivalro, & Loewe, 2000; Huff & Kline, 1999b; Leininger, 1995b; Like, Steinger, & Rubel, 1996; Leuning, Swiggum, Wieger, & McCullough-Zander, 2002.)

Resistance to these recommendations has many sources. Administrators may have concerns that there is insufficient time, money, or human resources to implement them. Providing services that are not culturally responsive, however, can also be costly. Poor relationships between practitioners and patients can result in wasted time, energy, and dollars as unnecessary tests and referrals are ordered, as more visits are required to understand the patients' condition, as patients delay seeking services until they are in crises, and as lawsuits are filed for medical malpractice or violation of civil rights. Long-range business considerations often support increasing institutions' cultural responsiveness: appealing to minority consumers; competing for private purchasers' business; responding to public purchasers' demands; and improving cost-effectiveness (Brach & Fraser, 2002).

Responding to a variety of clinical, ethical, and business commitments, many health care institutions—including managed care organizations, hospitals, and community clinics—are implementing policies and activities to improve their ability to provide culturally responsive care. (For example, see Chong, 2002; Kaiser Family Foundation, 2003; U.S. DHHS, 2001a, 2002a, 2002b.) Efforts to measure cultural competence and evaluate the influence of programs and activities on patient care are ongoing (U.S. DHHS, 2001b). Together, individual health care providers, administrators, educators, and communities can make tremendous differences, but policy makers are essential partners in comprehensive efforts to deliver culturally responsive health services.

# Recommendations for Public Policy Makers

Social, political, and economic issues influence the major determinants of health in this country. People in the upper socioeconomic class have the best health, the lowest rates of disease, and the best health care, while people in the lower socioeconomic class have the worst health, the highest burden of all diseases, and the worst health care. People of non-European-American heritage have higher morbidity and mortality rates and lower usage rates of health care facilities and procedures than European-Americans. These disparities of health and health care services are unjust. Redressing these disparities requires the development and implementation of supportive policies by government and nongovernment agencies. (For example, see Andrulis, 1999; Brach & Fraser, 2000; Huff & Kline, 1999b; Lavizzo-Mourey & Mackenzie, 1996; Lecca, Quervalu, Nunes, & Gonzales, 1998; New Jersey Legislature, 2003; U.S. DHHS, 2002a, 2002b.)

The U.S. Department of Health and Human Services has taken several steps to improve the quality of health care for people from all racial and ethnic backgrounds. Its efforts include the Initiative to Eliminate Racial and Ethnic Health Disparities (U.S. DHHS, 2000b); Healthy People 2010, a program that puts the goal of eliminating health disparities on the national agenda (U.S. DHHS, 2000a); and the National Standards on Culturally and Linguistically Appropriate Services (CLAS) (U.S. DHHS, 2000c, 2001d). More recently, the Centers for Medicare and Medicaid Services began requiring that Medicare+Choice organizations address either clinical health care disparities or culturally and linguistically appropriate services for their Quality Assessment Performance Improvement project (U.S. DHHS, 2002b; Agency for Healthcare Research and Quality, 2003). For examples of partnerships between governmental and nongovernmental organizations to implement policies to reduce health disparities, see U.S. DHHS, 2002a. At the state level, policy efforts are under way to require mandatory cultural competency training for medical licensure (New Jersey Legislature, 2003). For other, more detailed resources on the responsibilities of organizations and policy makers to support culturally responsive health care see, for example, Andrulis, Goodman, & Pryor, 2002; Brach & Fraser, 2000; Huff & Kline, 1999b; Lavizzo-Mourey & Mackenzie, 1996; and Lecca, Quervalu, Nunes, & Gonzales, 1998.

Policy makers can work toward improving culturally responsive health care by advocating for such policies as:

- Third-party payers (insurance companies, managed care organizations, Medicaid/Medicare funds, etc.) that reimburse for health care interpreters
- Third-party payers that reimburse transportation costs
- Support for the training of qualified health care interpreters and the development of national uniform standards of practice
- Medicaid and Medicare contracts that require health care organizations to provide clear guidelines for culturally responsive care
- Policies that require training in patient-centered communication skills for continued state licensure for physicians, nurses, and other clinicians

- Accreditation requirements that hospitals and professional training programs provide training in the delivery of culturally responsive health care
- Programs to recruit and support members of diverse cultural groups in professional schools and positions of leadership
- Enforcement of federal laws that require institutions to be responsive to constituencies' needs for interpreter services

To redress the root causes of health disparities in this country policy makers should embrace a wide understanding of the social and economic factors that influence health. They need to advocate for political and economic policies that help communities be healthier, with decent housing, living-wage jobs, convenient affordable transportation systems, and clean, safe environments. Refugees and immigrants need help to adjust to their new society, with language classes, job skills training, child care, and financial assistance. Policies and programs are needed to help stem addictions to tobacco, alcohol, gambling, and illicit drugs. In short, advocating for culturally responsive health care can have broad implications for the health of all people and may benefit from close coordination between local, state, regional, and national policy makers.

## Conclusion

Those interested in promoting health and improving health care for patients from all cultural backgrounds must act to reduce personal, institutional, political, and economic barriers to delivering culturally responsive health care. Work is needed at the individual, institutional, and public policy levels.

The solutions are multiple. Be aware of the cultural basis for differences in health status and health-related beliefs, practices, and values. Understand the cultural perspectives of the cultural groups served. Learn to communicate effectively across cultural and linguistic differences. Learn to negotiate and to work effectively through serious cross-cultural ethical conflicts. Attend to the policies, procedures, and values of health care institutions where practitioners, patients, and families interact. Advocate for organizational and system changes that support culturally responsive care. Engage in partnerships with community organizations. Together these activities empower patients to seek—and health care professionals to deliver—culturally responsive health care.

# References

Agency for Healthcare Research and Quality. (2003). *Oral, linguistic, and culturally competent services: Guides for managed care plans.* Retrieved April 4, 2003, from *www.ahrq.gov/about/cods/cultcomp.htm*

Andrulis, D. P. (1999). Cultural competence assessment of practices, clinics, and health care facilities. In E. J. Kramer, S. L. Ivey, & Y. Ying (Eds.), *Immigrant women's health: Problems and solutions.* San Francisco: Jossey-Bass, 330–335.

Andrulis, D., Goodman, N., & Pryor, C. (2002, May 6). *What a difference an interpreter can make: Health experiences of uninsured with limited English proficiency.* Boston: The Access Project. Available from *www.healthlaw.org/immigrant.shtml*

Appelbaum, P. S., Lidz, C. W., & Meisel, A. (1987). *Informed consent: Legal theory and clinical practice.* New York: Oxford University Press.

Beauchamp, T. L., & Childress, J. F. (1994). *Principles of biomedical ethics* (4th ed.). New York: Oxford University Press.

Benjamin, M. (1990). *Splitting the difference: Compromise and integrity in ethics and politics.* Lawrence: University Press of Kansas.

Benjamin, M. (1995). Conscience. In W. T. Reich (Ed.), *Encyclopedia of bioethics* (Rev. ed.). New York: Simon and Schuster Macmillan, I, 469–473.

Bennett, M. J. (1986). A developmental approach to training for intercultural sensitivity. *International Journal of Intercultural Relations, 10,* 179–196.

Bennett, M. J. (1993). Towards ethnorelativism: A development model of intercultural sensitivity. In R. M. Paige (Ed.), *Education for the intercultural experience.* Yarmouth, ME: Intercultural Press, 21–71.

Berger, J. T. (1998). Cultural discrimination in mechanisms for health decisions: A view from New York. *Journal of Clinical Ethics, 9*(2), 127–131.

Berger, J. T. (2001). Multicultural considerations and the American College of Physicians ethics manual. *Journal of Clinical Ethics, 12*(4), 375–381.

Berlin, E. A., & Fowkes, W. S. (1983). A teaching framework for cross-cultural health care. *Western Journal of Medicine, 139,* 934–938.

Betancourt, J. R., Green, A. R., & Carillo, J. E. (2002). *Cultural competence in health care: Emerging frameworks and practical approaches.* Field report. Retrieved January 31, 2003, from *www.cmwf.org/programs/minority/betancourt_culturalcompetence_576.pdf*

Blackhall, L. G., Frank, G., Murphy, S., & Michel, V. (2001). Bioethics in a different tongue: The case of truth-telling. *Journal of Urban Health, 78,* 59–71.

Blackhall, L. G., Frank, G., Murphy, S. T., Michel, V., Palmer, J. M., & Azen, S. P. (1999). Ethnicity and attitudes towards life sustaining technology. *Social Science and Medicine, 48,* 1779–1789.

Blackhall, L. J., Murphy, S., Frank, G., Michel, V., & Azen, S. (1995). Ethnicity and attitudes toward patient autonomy. *Journal of the American Medical Association, 274*(10), 820–825.

Blacksher, E. (1998). Desperately seeking difference. *Cambridge Quarterly of Healthcare Ethics, 7,* 11–16.

Boston City Hospital, Department of Interpreter Services, & Boston Area Health Education Center. (1987). *The bilingual medical interview I: The geriatric interview.* Boston: Boston Area Health Education Center.

Boston City Hospital, Department of Interpreter Services, & Boston Area Health Education Center. (1990). *The bilingual medical interview II: The geriatric interview.* Boston: Boston Area Health Education Center.

Brach, C., & Fraser, I. (2000). Can cultural competency reduce racial and ethnic health disparities? A review and conceptual model. *Medical Care Research and Review, 57* ( Supplement 1), 181–217.

Brach, C., & Fraser, I. (2002). Reducing disparities through culturally competent health care: An analysis of the business case. *Quality Management in Health Care, 10*(4), 15–28.

Brock, D. W., & Wartman, S. A. (1990). When competent patients make irrational choices. *New England Journal of Medicine, 322*(22), 1595–1599.

Brody, H. (1992). *The healer's power.* New Haven, CT: Yale University Press.

California Healthcare Interpreters Association. (2002). California standards for healthcare interpreters: Ethical principles, protocols, and guidance on roles and intervention. Retrieved February 9, 2003, from *www.calendow.org/pub/publications/ca_standards_healthcare_interpreters.pdf*

Campinha-Bacote, J. (1999). A model and instrument for addressing cultural competence in health care. *Journal of Nursing Education, 38*(5), 203–207.

Campinha-Bacote, J. (2003). Many faces: Addressing diversity in health care. *Online Journal of Issues in Nursing, 8*(1) Manuscript 2. Retrieved February 9, 2003, from *http://nursingworld.org/ojin/topic20/tpc20_2.htm*

Campinha-Bacote, J., & Munoz, C. (2001). A guiding framework for delivering culturally competent services in case management. *The Case Manager, 12*(2), 48–52.

Caralis, P. (1993). The influence of ethnicity and race on attitudes toward advance directives, life-prolonging treatments, and euthanasia. *Journal of Clinical Ethics, 4*(2), 155–165.

Carillo, J. E., Green, A. R., & Betancourt, J. R. (1999). Cross-cultural primary care: A patient-based approach. *Annals of Internal Medicine, 130*(10), 829–834.

Carrese, J. A., & Rhodes, L. A. (1995). Western bioethics on the Navajo reservation. *Journal of the American Medical Association, 274,* 826–829.

Center for Cross-Cultural Health. (1997). *Caring across cultures: The provider's guide to cross-cultural health care.* Minneapolis, MN: Center for Cross-Cultural Health.

Chong, M. (2002). A model for the nation's health care industry: Kaiser Permanente's Institute for Culturally Competent Care. *Permanente Journal, 6*(3), 47–50.

Clouser, K. D., Hufford, D. J., & O'Connor, B. B. (1996). Medical ethics and patient belief systems. *Alternative Therapies, 2*(1), 92–93.

Cohen, J. J., Gabriel, B. A., & Terrell, C. (2002). The case for diversity in the health care workforce. *Health Affairs, 21*(5), 90–102.

Collins, K. S., Hughes, D. L., Doty, M. M., Ives, B. L., Edwards, J. N., & Tenney, K. (2002, March). *Diverse communities, common concerns: Assessing health care quality for minority Americans.* Findings from the Commonwealth Fund 2001 health care quality survey. Available from *www.cmwf.org/publist/publist2.asp?CategoryID=11*

Crawley, L., Marshall, P., & Koenig, B. (2001). Respecting cultural differences at the end of life. In T. E. Quill and L. Snyder (Eds.), *Physician's guide to end-of-life care.* Philadelphia: American College of Physicians–American Society of Internal Medicine.

Crawley, L., Marshall, P. A., Lo, B., & Koenig, B. A. (2002). Strategies for culturally effective end-of-life care. *Annals of Internal Medicine, 136,* 673–679.

Cross, T. L., Bazron, B. J., Dennis, K. W., & Isaacs, M. R. (1989). *Towards a culturally competent system of care: A monograph on effective services for minority children who are severely emotionally disturbed.* Washington, DC: Child and Adolescent Service System Program (CASSP) Technical Assistance Center, Georgetown University Child Development Center.

Cross-Cultural Health Care Program. (1998). Communicating effectively through an interpreter. Seattle, WA: PacMed Clinics.

Culhane-Pera, K. A., Like, R., Lebensohn-Chivalro, P., & Loewe, R. (2000). Multicultural curricula in family practice residencies. *Family Medicine, 32*(3), 167–173.

Culhane-Pera, K. A., & Vawter, D. E. (1998). A study of health care professionals' perspectives about a cross-cultural ethical conflict involving a Hmong patient and her family. *Journal of Clinical Ethics, 9*(2), 179–190.

Downing, B. T. (1992). *Guidelines for working with interpreters with reference to patient-doctor interviews.* Unpublished manuscript, University of Minnesota, Minneapolis.

Dula, A., & Goering, S. (Eds.). (1994). *It just isn't fair: The ethics of health care for African Americans.* Westport, CT: Praeger.

Epstein, R. (1999). Mindful practice. *Journal of American Medical Association, 282*(9), 833–839.

Fadiman, A. (1997). *The spirit catches you and you fall down: A Hmong child, her American doctors, and the collision of two cultures.* New York: Farrar, Straus, and Giroux.

Fetters, M. D. (1998). The family in medical decision making: Japanese perspectives. *Journal of Clinical Ethics, 9*(2), 132–146.

Flack, H. E., & Pellegrino, E. D. (Eds.). (1992). *African-American perspectives on biomedical ethics.* Washington, DC: Georgetown University Press.

Galanti, G. A. (1997). *Caring for patients from different cultures: Case studies from American hospitals* (2nd ed.). Philadelphia: University of Pennsylvania Press.

Gardenswartz, L., & Rowe, A. (1999). *Managing diversity in health care manual: Proven tools and activities for leaders and trainers.* San Francisco: Jossey-Bass.

Gervais, K. G. (1998). Changing society, changing medicine, changing bioethics. In R. DeVries & J. Subedi (Eds.), *Bioethics and society: Constructing the ethical enterprise.* Upper Saddle River, NJ: Prentice Hall, 216–232.

Gilbert, M. J. (Ed.). (2003). Principles and recommended standards for cultural competence education of health care professionals. The California Endowment, Woodland Hills, CA. Available from *www.caldendow.org/pub/frm_htm*

Goldman, R. E., Monroe, A. D., & Dube, C. E. (1996). Cultural self awareness: A component of culturally responsive patient care. *Annals of Behavioral Science and Medical Education, 3,* 37–46.

Gostin, L. (1995). Informed consent, cultural sensitivity, and respect for persons. *Journal of the American Medical Association, 274*(10), 844–845.

Grisso, T., & Appelbaum, P. S. (1995). Comparison of standards for assessing patients' capacities to make treatment decisions. *American Journal of Psychiatry, 152,* 1033–1037.

Grisso, T., & Appelbaum, P. S. (1998). *Assessing competence to consent to treatment: A guide for physicians and other health professionals.* New York: Oxford University Press.

Gudykunst, W. B., & Mody, B. (2002). *Handbook of international and intercultural communication.* (2nd ed.). Thousand Oaks, CA: Sage Publications.

Heimbach, E. E. (1979). *White Hmong-English dictionary.* Ithaca, NY: Southeast Asia Program Publications, Cornell University.

Helman, C. G. (2000). *Health and illness: An introduction for health professionals* (4th ed.). Woburn, MA: Butterworth-Heineman.

Hern, H. E., Koenig, B. A., Moore, L. J., & Marshall, P. A. (1998). The difference that culture can make in end-of-life decisionmaking. *Cambridge Quarterly of Health Care Ethics, 7,* 27–40.

Hmong Lessons. (n.d.). Retrieved January 27, 2003, from *http://members.aol.com/nyablaj/hmong.html*

Huff, R. M., & Kline, M. V. (1999a). The cultural assessment framework. In R. M. Huff & M. V.

Kline (Eds.), *Promoting health in multicultural populations: A handbook for practitioners.* Thousand Oaks, CA: Sage.

Huff, R. M., & Kline, M. V. (1999b). *Promoting health in multicultural populations: A handbook for practitioners.* Thousand Oaks, CA.: Sage.

Hyun, I. (2002). Waiver of informed consent, cultural sensitivity, and the problems of unjust families and traditions. *Hastings Center Report, 32*(5), 14–22.

Institute of Medicine, Committee on Quality of Health Care in America. (2001a). *Crossing the quality chasm: A new health system for the 21st century* [Electronic version]. Washington, DC: National Academy Press. Retrieved October 17, 2001, from *www.nap.edu/catalog/10027.html*

Institute of Medicine. (2001b). *The right thing to do; the smart thing to do: Enhancing diversity in the health professions.* Washington, DC: National Academy Press.

Jackson, C. (1998). Medical interpretation: An essential clinical service for non-English-speaking immigrants. In S. Loue (Ed.), *Handbook of immigrant health.* New York: Plenum Press.

Jecker, N. S., Carrese, J. A., & Pearlman, R. A. (1995). Caring for patients in cross-cultural settings. *Hastings Center Report, 25,* 6–14.

Kagawa-Singer, M., & Blackhall, L. J. (2001). Negotiating cross-cultural issues at the end of life: "You got to go where he lives." *Journal of the American Medical Association, 286*(23), 2993–3001.

Kaiser Family Foundation. (1999a). *Key facts: Race, ethnicity and medical care.* Retrieved February 7, 2003 from *www.kff.org/content/1999/1523/KEY%20FACTS%20BOOK.pdf*

Kaiser Family Foundation. (1999b). *A synthesis of the literature: Racial and ethnic differences in access to medical care.* Retrieved February 7, 2003, from *www.kff.org/content/1999/1526/SYNTHESIS%20OF%20LITERATURE.pdf*

Kaiser Family Foundation. (2003). *Compendium of cultural competence initiatives in health care.* Retrieved February 9, 2003, from *www.kff.org/content/2003/6067*

Kaufert, J. M., & O'Neil, J. D. (1990). Biomedical rituals and informed consent: Native Canadians and the negotiation of clinical trust. In G. Weisz (Ed.), *Social science perspectives on medical ethics.* Boston: Kluwer, 41–63.

Kaufert, J. M., & Putsch, R. W. (1997). Communication through interpreters in healthcare: Ethical dilemmas arising from differences in class, culture, language, and power. *Journal of Clinical Ethics, 8*(1), 71–87.

Kirton, E. S. (1985). *The locked medicine cabinet: Hmong health care in America.* Unpublished doctoral dissertation, University of Santa Barbara, Santa Barbara, CA.

Kleinman, A. (1980). *Patients and healers in the context of culture: An exploration of the borderland between anthropology, medicine, and psychiatry.* Berkeley: University of California Press.

Kleinman, A. (1988). *Illness narratives: Suffering, healing, and the human condition.* New York: Basic Books.

Kleinman, A. (1995). Anthropology of bioethics. In W. Reich (Ed.), *Encyclopedia of bioethics.* New York: Macmillan, 1667–1674.

Kleinman, A., Das, V., & Lock, M. (1997). *Social suffering.* Berkeley: University of California Press.

Kleinman, A., Eisenberg, L., & Good, B. (1978). Culture, illness, and care: Clinical lessons from anthropologic and cross-cultural research. *Annals of Internal Medicine, 88,* 251–258.

Klessig, J. (1992). The effect of values and culture on life-support decisions. *Western Journal of Medicine, 157,* 316–322.

Koenig, B. A., & Gates-Williams, J. (1995). Understanding cultural difference in caring for dying patients. *Western Journal of Medicine, 163*(3), 244–249.

Kune-Karrer, B. M., & Taylor, E. H. (1995). Toward multiculturality: Implications for the pediatrician. *Pediatric Clinics of North America, 42*(1), 21–30.

Kunstadter, P. (1980). Medical ethics in cross-cultural and multi-cultural perspectives. *Social Science and Medicine, 14B (4),* 289–296.

Lane, S., & Rubinstein, R. (1996). Judging the other: Responding to traditional female genital surgeries. *Hastings Center Report 26*(3): 31–40.

Lavizzo-Mourey, R., & Mackenzie, E. R. (1996). Cultural competence: Essential measurements of quality for managed care organizations. *Annals of Internal Medicine, 124*(10), 919–920.

Lecca, P., Quervalu, I., Nunes, J. V., & Gonzales, H. F. (1998). *Cultural competency in health, social, and human services: Directions for the twenty-first century.* New York: Garland.

Lee, G. Y. (1986). White Hmong kinship terminology and structure. In B. Johns & D. Strecker (Eds.), *Hmong world I.* New Haven, CT: Yale Southeast Asia Studies.

Leininger, M. (1988). Leininger's Theory of Nursing: Cultural care diversity and universality. *Nursing Science Quarterly, 1*(4), 152–160.

Leininger, M. (1995a). Culture care assessment to guide nursing practices. In M. Leininger (Ed.), *Transcultural nursing: Concepts, theories, research & practices* (2nd ed.). New York: McGraw-Hill, 115–148.

Leininger, M. (Ed.). (1995b). *Transcultural nursing: Concepts, theories, research, and practices.* New York: McGraw-Hill.

Leuning, C. J., Swiggum, P. D., Wieger, H. M., & McCullough-Zander, K. (2002). Proposed Standards for Transcultural Nursing. Transcultural Nursing Society. *Journal of Transcultural Nursing 13*(1), 40–46.

Levin, S. J., Like, R. C., & Gottlieb, J. E. (2000). ETHNIC: A framework for culturally competent clinical practice. *Patient Care, 34*(9), 188–189.

Lieban, R. W. (1990). Medical anthropology and the comparative study of medical ethics. In G. Weisz (Ed.), *Social science perspectives on medical ethics.* Boston: Kluwer, 221–239.

Like, R. C. (2000). For working with medical interpreters. In Appendix: Useful clinical interviewing mnemonics. *Patient Care, 34*(9), 188.

Like, R. C., Steiner, R. P., & Rubel, A. J. (1996). Recommended core curriculum guidelines in culturally sensitive and competent health care. *Family Medicine, 27,* 291–297.

Lo, B. (1995). *Resolving ethical dilemmas: A guide for clinicians.* Baltimore: Williams & Wilkins.

Lock, M. (2002). *Twice dead: Organ transplants and the reinvention of death.* Berkeley: University of California Press.

Loustaunau, M. O., & Sobo, E. J. (1997). *The cultural context of health, illness, and medicine.* Westport, CT: Bergin & Garvey.

Macklin, R. (1999). *Against relativism: Cultural diversity and the search for ethical universals in medicine.* New York: Oxford University Press.

Marshall, P. A. (1992). Anthropology and bioethics. *Medical Anthropology Quarterly, 6*(1), 49–73.

Marshall, P. A., & Koenig, B. A. (1996). Bioethics in anthropology: Perspectives on culture, medicine, and morality. In C. F. Sargent & T. M. Johnson (Eds.), *Medical anthropology: Contemporary theory and method.* Westport, CT: Praeger, 349–373.

Marshall, P. A., Koenig, B. A., Grifhorst, P., & Van Ewijk, M. (1998). Ethical issues in immigrant health care and clinical research. In S. Loue (Ed.), *Handbook of immigrant health.* New York: Plenum Press, 203–226.

McKibben, B. (1994). *English-White Hmong dictionary Phua Txhais Lux Askiv-Hmoob Dawb.* Provo, UT: Author.

Meleis, A. F., & Jonsen, A. R. (1983). Ethical crises and cultural differences. *Western Journal of Medicine, 138*(6), 889–893.

Muller, J. H., & Desmond, B. (1992). Ethical dilemmas in a cross-cultural context: A Chinese example. *Western Journal of Medicine, 157*(3), 323–327.

National Quality Forum. (2002). *Improving healthcare quality for minority patients.* Available from *www.qualityforum.org/news/qfacrnew2.htm*

Nerenz. D. R., Gunter, M. J., Garcia, M., Green-Weir, R. R., Widsom, K., & Joseph C. (2002, July). *Developing a health plan report card on quality of care for minority populations.* The Commonwealth Fund. Available from *www.cmwf.org/publist/publist2.asp? CategoryID=11*

New Jersey Legislature. (2003). Proposed bills in Senate (S411) and Assembly (A2297). Retrieved February 7, 2003, from *www.njleg.state.nj.us/bills/BillsByNumber.asp*

Nie, J-B. (2000). The plurality of Chinese and American medical moralities: Toward an interpretive cross-cultural bioethics. *Kennedy Institute of Ethics Journal, 10*(3), 239–260.

Novack, D. H., Suchman, A. L., Clark, W., Epstein, R. M., Najberg, E., & Kaplan, C. (1997). Calibrating the physician: Personal awareness and effective patient care. *Journal of American Medical Association, 278*(6), 502–509.

O'Connor, B. B. (1995). *Healing traditions: Alternative medicine and the health professions.* Philadelphia: University of Pennsylvania Press.

O'Connor, B. B. (1998). Healing practices. In S. Loue (Ed.), *Handbook of immigrant health.* New York: Plenum Press, 145–162.

Orona, C. J., Koenig, B. A., & Davis, A. J. (1994). Cultural aspects of nondisclosure. *Cambridge Quarterly of Healthcare Ethics, 3,* 338–346.

Orr, R. D., Marshall, P. A., & Osborn, J. (1995). Cross-cultural considerations in clinical ethics consultations. *Archives of Family Medicine, 4,* 159–164.

Pellegrino, E. D. (1992). Intersections of Western biomedical ethics and world culture. In E. Pellegrino, P. Mazzarella, & P. Corsi (Eds.), *Transcultural dimensions in medical ethics.* Frederick, MD: University Publishing Group, 13–19.

Perkins, H. S., Supik, J. D., & Hazuda, H. P. (1993). Autopsy decisions: The possibility of conflicting cultural attitudes. *Journal of Clinical Ethics, 4*(2), 145–154.

Perkins, H. S., Supik, J. D., & Hazuda, H. P. (1998). Cultural differences among health professionals: A case illustration. *Journal of Clinical Ethics, 9*(2), 108–117.

Perot, R. T., & Youdelman, M. (2001, September). *Racial, ethnic, and primary language data collection in the health care system: An assessment of federal policies and practices.* The Commonwealth Fund. Available from *www.cmwf.org/publist/publist2.asp? CategoryID=11*

Putsch, R. W. (1985). Cross-cultural communication: The special case of interpreters in health care. *Journal of the American Medical Association, 254*(23), 3344–3351.

Rudd R. E., Moeykens, B. A., & Colton T. C. (1999). Health and literacy: A review of medical and public health literature. In J. Comings, B. Garners, & C. Smith (Eds.), *Annual review of adult learning and literacy.* New York: Jossey-Bass. Retrieved February 7, 2003, from *www.hsph.harvard.edu/healthliteracy/litreview_final.pdf*

Saturn River Front Academy. (2000). *Hmong pronunciation guide.* St. Paul Public Schools. Available from *http://ww2.saturn.stpaul.k12.mn.us/hmong/pronunciation.html*

Smedley, B. D., Stith, A. Y., & Nelson, A. R. (Eds.) (2002). *Unequal treatment: Confronting racial and ethnic disparities in health care.* Washington, DC: National Academies Press.

Spector, R. E. (2000). *Cultural care: Guides to heritage assessment and health traditions.* Upper Saddle River, NJ: Prentice Hall Health.

Stuart, M. R., & Lieberman, J. A. (1993). *The fifteen minute hour: Applied psychotherapy for the primary care physician.* (2nd ed.). New York: Praeger.

Tervalon, M., & Murray-Garcia, J. (1998). Cultural humility versus cultural competence: A critical distinction in defining physician training outcomes in multicultural education. *Journal of Health Care for the Poor Underserved, 9*(2), 117–125.

U.S. Department of Health and Human Services. (2000a). *Healthy people 2010: Understanding and improving health.* (2nd ed.). Washington, DC: U.S. Government Printing Office. Available from *www.healthypeople.gov/document/tableofcontents.htm*

U.S. Department of Health and Human Services. (2000b). *Initiative to eliminate racial and ethnic disparities of health.* Available from *www.raceandhealth.hhs.gov/*

U.S. Department of Health and Human Services. Office of Minority Health. (2000c). *National standards on culturally and linguistically appropriate services (CLAS) in health care. Federal Register, 65*(247), 80865–79. Available from *www.omhrc.gov/clas*

U.S. Department of Health and Human Services. Health Resources and Services Administration. (2001a). *Cultural competence works: Using cultural competence to improve the quality of health care for diverse populations and add value to managed care arrangements.* Available from *www.ask.hrsa.gov/detail.cfm?id=HRS00249*

U.S. Department of Health and Human Services. Office of Minority Health. (2001b). *Health Resources and Services Administration study on measuring cultural competence in health care delivery settings: A review of the literature.* Retrieved March 17, 2003, from *www.hrsa.gov/OMH/cultural/cultural.htm*

U.S. Department of Health and Human Services. Office for Civil Rights. (2001c). *Policy guidance: Title VI prohibition against national origin discrimination as it affects persons with limited-English proficiency.* Retrieved March 18, 2003, from *www.hhs.gov/ocr/lep/guide.html*

U.S. Department of Health and Human Services. Office of Minority Health. (2001d). *National standards on culturally and linguistically appropriate services (CLAS) in health care: Final report.* Retrieved February 2, 2003, from *www.omhrc.gov/omh/programs/2pgprograms/finalreport.pdf*

U.S. Department of Health and Human Services. (2002a). *Healthy people 2010: Memorandum of understanding (MOU) goals.* Retrieved February 7, 2003, from *www.healthypeople.gov/Implementation/mous*

U.S. Department of Health and Human Services. Centers for Medicare and Medicaid. (2002b). *Medicare managed care manual.* Chapter 5, *Quality assessment: Appendices.* Retrieved February 2, 2003, from *http://cms.hhs.gov/manuals/116_mmc/mc86c05exhibits.asp#s2003*

van Ryn, M., & Burke, J. (2000). The effect of patient race and socio-economic status on physicians' perceptions of patients. *Social Science and Medicine, 50,* 813–828.

Vawter. D. E. (1996). The Houston citywide policy on medical futility [letter]. *New England Journal of Medicine, 276*(19), 1549–1550.

Vawter, D. E., & Babbitt, B. (1997). Hospice care for terminally ill Hmong patients: A good cultural fit? *Minnesota Medicine, 80*(11), 42–44.

Veatch, R. M. (1989). *Cross cultural perspectives in medical ethics: Readings.* Boston: Jones and Bartlett.

Veatch, R. M. (2000). *Cross-cultural perspectives in medical ethics* (2nd ed.). Boston: Jones and Bartlett.

Woloshin, S., Bickell, N. A., Schwartz, L. M., Gany, F., & Welch, H. G. (1995). Language barriers in medicine in the United States. *Journal of the American Medical Association, 273*(9), 724–728.

Yeo, G. (1995). Ethical considerations in Asian and Pacific Island elders. *Clinics in Geriatric Medicine, 11*(1), 139–154.

Youdelman, M., & Perkins, J. (2002, May). *Providing language interpretation services in health care settings: Examples from the field.* The Commonwealth Fund. Retrieved February 2, 2003, from *www.cmwf.org/publist/publist2.asp?CategoryID=11*

## Further Resources

### Web Sites

California Endowment home page. *www.CALENDOW.ORG* [April 4, 2003].

Center for Cross-cultural Health home page. *www.crosshealth.com* [March 18, 2003].

Commonwealth Foundation home page. *www.commonwealthfoundation.com/* [April 4, 2003].

Diversity Rx home page. *www.diversityrx.org* [October 17, 2002].

Ethnomed. *Ethnic medicine information from Harborview Medical Center* home page. *www.ethnomed.org* [March 18, 2003].

Management Sciences for Health. *The providers guide to quality & culture*. Available from *http://erc.msh.org/* [October 17, 2002].

National Center for Cultural Competence home page. Georgetown University Child Development Center. (1999–2002). *www.georgetown.edu/research/gucdc/nccc/* [April 30, 2002].

State University of New York Institute of Technology. (2001). *CulturedMed*. Available from *www.sunyit.edu/library/html/culturemed/* [June 13, 2002].

University of Medicine and Dentistry of New Jersey. Robert Wood Johnson Medical School Center for Healthy Families and Cultural Diversity home page. *www2.umdnj.edu/fmedweb/chfcd/INDEX.HTM* [April 29, 2001].

### Motion Pictures

American Academy of Family Physicians. (2000). *Quality care for diverse populations*. Leawood, KS.

Greene, J. & Newell, K. (2001). *Community voices: Exploring cross-cultural care through cancer*. Fanlight Productions distributor. Available from *www.fanlight.com*

Koskoff, H. (2002). *The culture of emotions*. Fanlight Productions distributor. Available from *www.fanlight.com*

# Editors and Contributors

## Editors

Kathleen A. Culhane-Pera, M.D., M.A., is a family physician at Ramsey Family and Community Medicine Residency and West Side Community Health Center. She holds a master's degree in anthropology. Dr. Kathie, as she is known in the Hmong community, has worked with the Hmong since 1983 and has conducted ethnographic research with Hmong in Northern Thailand. She lives in St. Paul with her husband, Tim, and two children, Sam and Megan.

Dorothy E. Vawter, Ph.D., Associate Director, Minnesota Center for Health Care Ethics, directs the Minnesota Center's collaborative work on cross-cultural health care ethics. She has published on cross-cultural health care in *The Journal of Clinical Ethics* and *Minnesota Medicine* and co-chaired three conferences for clinicians on traditional Hmong health beliefs and practices. She completed her doctoral studies at Georgetown University and the Kennedy Institute of Ethics.

Phua Xiong, M.D., graduated from the University of Minnesota Medical School in 1996 and is a family practice physician at the St. Paul Family Medical Center in St. Paul. Dr. Xiong, who is dedicated to providing culturally responsive care, teaches others about the Hmong and Hmong health care, and acts as cultural broker, advocate, and liaison for both Hmong and Americans.

Barbara Babbitt, B.S.N., R.N., M.A., spent many years working in both medical and psychiatric nursing. In 1995 she began working with the Minnesota Center for Health Care Ethics in the areas of cultural diversity and health care decisionmaking. Out of this work grew a commitment to improve health care delivery to Minnesota's growing immigrant and refugee populations. In partnership with other healthcare professionals she continues to research, plan, and implement changes in the way health care is delivered to culturally diverse individuals and families.

Mary M. Solberg, Ph.D., M.S.W., is a member of the religion faculty at Gustavus Adolphus College. She was Project Editor for the *Encyclopedia of Bioethics* and a co-editor of *Ethical Challenges in Managed Care: A Casebook*. Dr. Solberg is the author of *Compelling Knowledge: A Feminist Proposal for an Epistemology of the Cross*. Living in Europe and Latin America, working with refugees, and forming part of a cross-cultural family have all deeply affected her work as an ethicist and theologian.

## Contributors

Elizabeth C. Walker Anderson, B.A., was born in Taiwan and grew up in Southeast Asia. She spent eight years in Thailand interviewing refugees seeking resettlement in the United States. For two years she was a Political Asylum Officer for the INS. More recently, she was the Director of International Services at Regions Hospital in St. Paul. Ms. Walker helped found the Center for Cross-Cultural Health and is completing a law degree.

Bruce Bliatout, Ph.D., M.P.H., M.S.Hyg., Dr. Ac., a Hmong-American, is the Director of the TB Prevention and Treatment Center, Multnomah County Health Department, Oregon. He has served for 17 years on the Governor's Medical Assistants Advisory Board of the State of Oregon and for 20 years on the Board of Directors of the Hmong-American Association of Oregon. Dr. Bliatout is the author of *Hmong sudden unexpected nocturnal death: A cultural study* and numerous articles on cultural health.

Helen B. Bruce, R.G.N., S.C.M., M.T.D., C.N.M. is a native of Scotland and has been a midwife for more than 30 years. As a new immigrant she found great privilege working with a group of midwives in St. Paul, Minnesota, where her particular responsibility was to the Southeast Asian immigrant populations, many of whom were Hmong.

Donald Brunnquell, Ph.D., is the Director of the Office of Ethics for Children's Hospitals and Clinics in Minnesota, where his work involves consultation, education and policy development. He received his doctorate in child clinical psychology from the University of Minnesota in 1981 and is a Licensed Psychologist in Minnesota. As the 1991 recipient of a Bush Foundation Leadership Fellows grant, he completed a master's degree in philosophy with a concentration in ethics. Dr. Brunnquell is an Instructor for the Institute of Child Development and Clinical Assistant Professor in Clinical Psychology at the University of Minnesota, where he teaches ethics in applied psychology.

Karen G. Gervais, Ph.D., is the Director of the Minnesota Center for Health Care Ethics. She received her B.A. from Oberlin College and her Ph.D. in philosophy from the University of Minnesota. In 1987 she published *Redefining Death* (Yale University Press). She was a coeditor of *Ethical Challenges in Managed Care: A Casebook* (Georgetown University Press, 1999).

Mymee Her, Ph.D., was born in Laos and emigrated to the United States at age nine, where she struggled growing up in both Hmong and American cultures. She is married, has three children, and lives in Fresno, California. Dr. Her holds a Ph.D. in clinical psychology and has eight years of experience working with members of Hmong and other cultures.

Chue Pao Heu is Mymee Her's father. At an early age, he learned to be a community leader so he could advocate for his family. With siblings to support, Mr. Heu became a nurse and provided medical services to the Hmong in the mountains of Laos. In 1976 he brought his family to the United States and lives in Fresno, California.

Peter Kunstadter, Ph.D., is a medical anthropologist and director of the Asian Health Program at the University of California San Francisco-Fresno Medical Education Program. Since 1985 he has conducted field research on culture, health services, epidemiology and demography with Hmong in Thailand and since 1987 with Hmong refugees in California.

Dr. Kunstadter has also worked with other highland minority groups in Thailand and among Native Americans.

Stephen Kurachek, M.D., is a board-certified pediatrician (pediatric pulmonary medicine and pediatric critical care medicine from Boston Children's Hospital). He has directed pediatric intensive care units and currently sees patients at a multi-ethnic pediatric intensive care unit in Minneapolis. Dr. Kurachek has a pediatric pulmonary practice in the inner city and also participates in an inner-city chest clinic.

Pacyinz Lyfoung received a J.D. from the University of Minnesota Law School and formerly worked as a legal aid housing staff attorney. She is the co-founding executive director of Asian Women United of Minnesota, the first Pan Asian battered women's program, now one of only eight existing Pan Asian women's shelters in the nation. She is currently working as a policy staff for the Minnesota Housing Finance Agency and continues to be active with several Asian women's groups on a volunteer basis.

Mayly Lyfoung Lochungvu, a Hmong woman, emigrated from Laos to France in 1975 and lived there for 16 years. She moved to St. Paul in 1991. Ms. Lochungvu holds a B.S. in computer science and since 1995 has worked as a Natural Family Planning Practitioner at the Twin Cities Natural Family Planning Center. Since 1998 she has worked as a multilingual, multicultural interpreter at HealthEast St. Joseph's Hospital, where she bridges the gap between healthcare providers and patients of diverse cultural backgrounds.

Deborah K. Mielke, M.D. is a family practice physician at the Model Cities Health Center in St. Paul, Minnesota, where, with the expert support of Hmong staff and interpreters, she has cared for Hmong patients over the past 15 years. In teaching family practice residents at Regions Hospital, Dr. Mielke promotes the idea of compassionate, intercultural medicine.

Christopher L. Moertel, M.D., is medical director of hematology and oncology at Children's Hospitals and Clinics–St. Paul. He has worked closely with the Hmong community in St. Paul since 1990, concentrating on iron deficiency anemia in Hmong children.

Mai Neng Moua is the editor of *Bamboo Among the Oakes (2002)* and *Paj Ntaub Voice*, the Hmoob (Hmong) arts journal of writing and visual artwork by Hmong writers and artists in the United States. Ms. Moua has a B.A. from St. Olaf College in Northfield, Minnesota and is currently working on a M.A. from the Hubert H. Humphrey Institute of Public Affairs at the University of Minnesota.

Vang Leng Mouanoutoua, Ph.D., is a senior psychologist with Fresno County Mental Health Services. He teaches cultural competence principles and cultural diversity at California State University-Fresno. He has also conducted workshops on Southeast Asian cultures, domestic violence, Hmong youth suicide, acculturation problems, and Southeast Asian mental health issues.

Elanah Dalyah Naftali, Dr.P.H., R.D., is cross-trained in nutrition, child development, epidemiology, and program evaluation. Her research interest in cross-cultural public health interventions led to her involvement in an iron-deficiency anemia prevention project in the Hmong community of St. Paul. She has since expanded her love for cross-cultural work to the domain of religious studies and is currently a chaplain at a large trauma care center in Philadelphia.

Kevin A. Peterson, M.D., M.P.H., is an assistant professor in the Department of Family Practice and Community Health at the University of Minnesota Medical School in Minneapolis. He practices at a postgraduate residency training site in St. Paul with a large Hmong population.

Gregory A. Plotnikoff, M.D., M.T.S., Medical Director of the Center for Spirituality and Healing, is an Associate Professor of both Clinical Medicine and Pediatrics at the University of Minnesota. Dr. Plotnikoff serves patients of all ages at the Community-University Health Care Center, an inner-city primary care clinic. He is a 2002 Bush Foundation Leadership Fellow and has been recognized as "One of the 100 Most Influential People in Healthcare" by *Minnesota Physician* magazine.

Marline A. Spring, Ph.D., is an applied anthropologist at the University of Minnesota, Minneapolis. She has worked with Hmong and other Southeast Asian refugees and immigrants for two decades, and more recently with those from East Africa. Dr. Spring has developed ethnographic, research-based health education for immigrants and presently coordinates research on violence among Somali and Oromo immigrants. Her other research interests include ethnopharmacology, chronic illnesses, and reproductive, mental, and dental health.

Carol A. Tauer, Ph.D., is professor emerita of philosophy at the College of St. Catherine in St. Paul. She holds a Ph.D. in philosophy from Georgetown University with a specialization in bioethics. She has served on ethics panels for the National Institutes of Health and has been a member of the Committee on Ethics of the American College of Obstetricians and Gynecologists since 1997.

Mao Heu Thao is a Hmong Health Coordinator at the Saint Paul-Ramsey County Department of Public Health in Minnesota. For the last twelve years, she has provided health education for the Hmong community through media campaigns and health fairs. Ms. Thao holds a B.A. in health education and administration.

Va (Valerie) Thao is a licensed practical nurse who has worked as a Health Education Program Assistant at the Saint Paul–Ramsey County Department of Public Health in Minnesota for the last ten years. As a student, Ms. Thao worked with Dr. Culhane-Pera, researching Hmong parents' concepts of childhood illnesses and their reactions to medical evaluations and treatments.

Cher Vang is an Enforcement Officer for the Minnesota Department of Human Rights. Previously, he was a Parent Representative and Community Liaison at Children's Hospitals and Clinics, St. Paul. Before moving to Minnesota, Vang counselled minority students at Merced College and Hmong and Lao clients at the Stanislaus County Mental Health in Modesto, California. Vang holds a B.A. in Social Work from Augsburg College, Minneapolis, and an M.A. in Public Administration from Golden Gate University, San Francisco.

May Lee Vang, A.A., graduated from two two-year programs in registered nursing and midwifery in Laos. She was a diabetes educator for six years at the West Side Community Health Center in St. Paul and completed a team management course in diabetes mellitus in 1995 at the International Diabetes Center. Since 1996, Ms. Vang has been an Outreach Coordinator at the Phalen Village Clinic in St. Paul. She has conducted many health education activities in the Hmong community.

Thomas Vang, M.S., is a Human Services Counselor for the Wilder Foundation's Social Adjustment Program for Southeast Asians in St. Paul. He received a M.S. degree in Guidance and Counseling from the University of Wisconsin, Stout.

Patricia F. Walker, M.D., DTM&H, is a graduate of Mayo Medical School and the Mayo Graduate School of Medicine. She is board-certified in Internal Medicine. While a Bush Medical Fellow, 1995 to 1998, Dr. Walker earned a Certificate in Health Care Management and two degrees in Tropical Medicine and Hygiene. She is currently the Director of the Center for International Health at Regions Hospital, St. Paul.

Joseph Westermeyer, M.D., practiced general medicine and surgery in Laos from 1965 to 1967. In 1969 he earned an M.A in anthropology; in 1970 he completed psychiatric training and received an M.P.H. and a Ph.D. Dr. Westermeyer returned to Laos annually from 1971 to 1975, conducting psychiatric research and consulting for the Ministry of Health. From 1976 to 1989, he directed an International Clinic at the University of Minnesota, where over 2,000 refugees received psychiatric care.

Chue Monica Xiong, R.N., was born in Laos and emigrated to Thailand with her family in 1976. She became interested in nursing while observing her older brother care for the sick at a refugee hospital. In 1980 she and her family emigrated to Duluth, Minnesota. She received her R.N. in 1992 and worked with the Southeast Asian Prenatal Project at Ramsey Hospital, St. Paul, Minnesota, on the nurse midwifery team.

Yer Moua Xiong, M.P.H., spent a year in a refugee camp in Thailand before emigrating to the United States with her family in 1979. She is currently a student at the University of Minnesota Medical School and plans a career in primary care with an emphasis in cross-cultural health.

Nkaj Zeb Yaj is a Hmong shaman and a Yang community and family leader. In his nineteen years in the United States, he has helped to bridge the gap between traditional Hmong healing and Western biomedicine by teaching Hmong and U.S. health care professionals about working effectively with Hmong patients and by providing traditional treatment to Hmong, both in the hospital and in the community.

Deu Yang, L.P.N., is a Personal Care Attendant Case Manager Nurse at U-Care in Minneapolis, MN. For many years, she was a prenatal health educator at Model Cities Health Center, providing clinical perinatal services and prenatal classes, community prenatal outreach, and hospital assistance. She continues to be active in community health education with the Hmong Health Care Professionals Coalition. She is married, has six children and two grandchildren.

# Index